A TEXT BOOK OF

HERBAL DRUG TECHNOLOGY

As Per PCI Regulations

Third Year B. Pharm.
Semester - VI

Dr. V. M. Shinde
M. Pharm., M.Sc., Ph.D.
Assistant Professor of Pharmacognosy,
Bharati Vidyapeeth University,
Poona College of Pharmacy, Pune 411 038.

Mrs. K. S. Bodas - Yadav
M. Pharm.,
Assistant Professor in Pharmacognosy,
Sinhgad College of Pharmacy,
Vadgoan (Bk.), Pune 411 041.

NIRALI PRAKASHAN
ADVANCEMENT OF KNOWLEDGE

N4060

HERBAL DRUG TECHNOLOGY **ISBN 978-93-89686-37-1**

First Edition : **November 2019**

Published By :

NIRALI PRAKASHAN

Abhyudaya Pragati, 1312, Shivaji Nagar,
Off J.M. Road, Pune – 411005
Tel - (020) 25512336/37/39, Fax - (020) 25511379
Email : niralipune@pragationline.com

➢ DISTRIBUTION CENTRES

PUNE

Nirali Prakashan (For orders within Pune) : 119, Budhwar Peth, Jogeshwari Mandir Lane, Pune 411002, Maharashtra
Tel : (020) 2445 2044, 66022708, Fax : (020) 2445 1538; Mobile : 9657703145
Email : niralilocal@pragationline.com

Nirali Prakashan (For orders outside Pune) : S. No. 28/27, Dhayari, Near Asian College Pune 411041
Tel : (020) 24690204 Fax : (020) 24690316; Mobile : 9657703143
Email : bookorder@pragationline.com

MUMBAI

Nirali Prakashan : 385, S.V.P. Road, Rasdhara Co-op. Hsg. Society Ltd.,
Girgaum, Mumbai 400004, Maharashtra; Mobile : 9320129587
Tel : (022) 2385 6339 / 2386 9976, Fax : (022) 2386 9976
Email : niralimumbai@pragationline.com

➢ DISTRIBUTION BRANCHES

JALGAON

Nirali Prakashan : 34, V. V. Golani Market, Navi Peth, Jalgaon 425001, Maharashtra,
Tel : (0257) 222 0395, Mob : 94234 91860; Email: niralijalgaon@pragationline.com

KOLHAPUR

Nirali Prakashan : New Mahadvar Road, Kedar Plaza, 1st Floor Opp. IDBI Bank, Kolhapur 416 012
Maharashtra. Mob : 9850046155; Email : niralikolhapur@pragationline.com

NAGPUR

Nirali Prakashan : Above Maratha Mandir, Shop No. 3, First Floor,
Rani Jhanshi Square, Sitabuldi, Nagpur 440012, Maharashtra
Tel : (0712) 254 7129; Email : niralinagpur@pragationline.com

DELHI

Nirali Prakashan : 4593/15, Basement, Agarwal Lane, Ansari Road, Daryaganj
Near Times of India Building, New Delhi 110002 Mob : 08505972553
Email : niralidelhi@pragationline.com

BENGALURU

Nirali Prakashan : Maitri Ground Floor, Jaya Apartments, No. 99, 6th Cross, 6th Main,
Malleswaram, Bengaluru 560003, Karnataka; Mob : 9449043034
Email: niralibangalore@pragationline.com

Other Branches : Hyderabad, Chennai

niralipune@pragationline.com | www.pragationline.com

Also find us on www.facebook.com/niralibooks

PREFACE

We are delighted to present the book entitled 'Herbal Drug Technology' specially written for T. Y. B. Pharm Semester VI students as per the syllabus prescribed by Pharmacy Council of India, New Delhi.The book is divided into five units comprising thirteen chapters which contains basic information regarding each topic mentioned in the syllabus.

Last two decades have witnessed lot of changes in subject pharmacognosy. Today, herbal drugs are widely accepted in framework of modern medicine. On this background, there is no surprise for inclusion of 'Herbal Drug Technology' in Pharmacy Council of India's new syllabus. As popularity of herbal drugs is on rise, there are certain issues which need attention. This book will address these issues.

Unit I includes the use of herbs as medicine, good agricultural practices, biodynamic agricultural and Indian systems of medicines. Unit II is related with neutraceuticals, herbal drug and herb food interactions. Unit III covers herbal cosmetics, excipients and formulations of herbal origin. Unit IV focuses on evaluation of herbal drugs, patenting and regulatory issues which are important from regulatory point. Last Unit V covers current situation of herbal drug industry in India. It also includes good manufacturing practices for Indian system of medicines. As herbal drugs are becoming popular worldwide, this book will be very crucial in explaining different basics concepts to students and users.

Authors have written this book by keeping undergraduate student in mind. The key features of this book include use of simple language, self-explanatory tables along with comprehensive text and diagrams to make learning effortless.

Authors owe a special debt of gratitude Hon. Prof. Shivajirao Kadam, Prof. K. R. Mahadik, Prof. A. P. Pawar and other staff members of Bharti Vidyapeeth Deemed University, Poona College of Pharmacy, Pune and Sinhgad Technical Education Society for providing good infrastructure and facilities to carry out our work.

We express our deep gratitude and love to our family members. Without their support and encouragement this would not have been possible.

Last but not the least, we express my sincere gratitude to Publisher Shri. Dineshbhai Furia, Shri. Jigneshbhai Furia, Nirali Prakashan, Pune for providing opportunity. We also express our sincere thanks to entire team of Nirali Prakashan, Pune for their excellent cooperation in bringing out this book.

The valuable comments and fruitful suggestions are welcomed for further improvement of the book. We hope this book will be helpful to students and teachers of pharmacy.

November, 2019

Dr. V. M. Shinde
Mrs. K.S. Bodas-Yadav

SYLLABUS

UNIT-I

Herbs as Raw Materials

Definition of herb, herbal medicine, herbal medicinal product, herbal drug preparation Source of Herbs Selection, identification and authentication of herbal materials Processing of herbal raw material.

Biodynamic Agriculture

Good agricultural practices in cultivation of medicinal plants including Organic farming.

Pest and Pest management in medicinal plants: Biopesticides/Bioinsecticides.

Indian Systems of Medicine

a) Basic principles involved in Ayurveda, Siddha, Unani and Homeopathy

b) Preparation and standardization of Ayurvedic formulations viz Aristas and Asawas, Ghutika,Churna, Lehya and Bhasma.

UNIT-II

Nutraceuticals

General aspects, Market, growth, scope and types of products available in the market. Health benefits and role of Nutraceuticals in ailments like Diabetes, CVS diseases, Cancer, Irritable bowel syndrome and various Gastro intestinal diseases.

Study of following herbs as health food: Alfa alfa, Chicory, Ginger, Fenugreek, Garlic, Honey, Amla, Ginseng, Ashwagandha, Spirulina

Herbal-Drug and Herb-Food Interactions

General introduction to interaction and classification. Study of following drugs and their possible side effects and interactions: Hypercium, kava-kava, Ginkobiloba, Ginseng, Garlic, Pepper & Ephedra.

UNIT-III

Herbal Cosmetics

Sources and description of raw materials of herbal origin used via, fixed oils, waxes, gums colours, perfumes, protective agents, bleaching agents, antioxidants in products such as skin care, hair care and oral hygiene products.

Herbal Excipients

Herbal Excipients – Significance of substances of natural origin as excipients – colorants, sweeteners, binders, diluents, viscosity builders, disintegrants, flavors & perfumes.

Herbal Formulations:

Conventional herbal formulations like syrups, mixtures and tablets and Novel dosage forms like phytosomes

UNIT-IV

Evaluation of Drugs WHO & ICH guidelines for the assessment of herbal drugs Stability testing of herbal drugs.

Patenting and Regulatory Requirements of Natural Products:

a) Definition of the terms: Patent, IPR, Farmers right, Breeder's right, Bioprospecting and Biopiracy

b) Patenting aspects of Traditional Knowledge and Natural Products. Case study of Curcuma & Neem.

Regulatory Issues - Regulations in India (ASU DTAB, ASU DCC), Regulation of manufacture of ASU drugs - Schedule Z of Drugs & Cosmetics Act for ASU drugs.

UNIT-V

General Introduction to Herbal Industry

Herbal drugs industry: Present scope and future prospects.

A brief account of plant based industries and institutions involved in work on medicinal and aromatic plants in India.

Schedule T – Good Manufacturing Practice of Indian systems of medicine

Components of GMP (Schedule – T) and its objectives.

Infrastructural requirements, working space, storage area, machinery and equipments, standard operating procedures, health and hygiene, documentation and records.

CONTENTS

❖❖❖

UNIT-I

Chapter...1

HERBS AS RAW MATERIALS

Objectives

- To understand the concept of herb, herbal medicine, herbal medicinal product and herbal drug preparation.
- To know different sources of herbs.
- To study selection, identification and authentification of herbs.
- To understand processing of herbal raw material.

1.1 DEFINITION OF HERB

Herb can be defined as, "any plant which has leaves, stem, flowers, roots and seeds; used for different purposes like flavoring, food, medicine or perfume". Botanically, herb is any seed-bearing plant which does not have a woody stem and dies down to the ground after flowering or completion of life cycle. Means herbs are seasonal plants. According to Oxford dictionary, "herb is any plant with leaves, seeds or flowers used for flavouring, food, medicine or perfume". Plants used as spice, aromatic and food are also considered as herb in day to day life. Botanically, Tulsi (*Ocimum sanctum*) can be considered as herb while Neem (*Azadirachata indica*) is tree not herb. Other examples of herbs can be Onion, Ginger, Asparagus, Turmeric, Bramhi etc.

Now-a-days, as herbal wave is spreading worldwide, use of herbal medicines is increasing. One needs to understand, there are many terms associated with herbal medicine. Herbal drugs/ Phytomedicine/ Herbal Medicinal Products (HMP) or herbal remedies are drugs obtained from plants.

Following are few examples of herbal drugs:

- Senna (*Cassia angustifolia* and other species) leaves and pods are used for constipation.
- Ginseng (*Panax* species) is used as tonic to improve immunity and strength.
- Ginkgo (*Ginkgo biloba*) is used for improving brain function and memory.
- Ashwagandha (*Withania somnifera*) is used for memory and learning.
- Hypericum (*Hypericum perforatum*) is used for treatment of depression.

On the other hand, isolated compounds from above herbs are not considered as herbal drugs and regulated as modern licensed medicines. We all know that, Digitalis is herbal medicine. But when one isolate digoxin or other glycosides from plant and prescribe in pure form, they are isolated drugs, thye are no more herbal medicines. In this case, it becomes new chemical entity (NCE) as per modern system of medicine.

Following isolated compounds are not considered as herbal drugs:

- Quinine from Cinchona (*Cinchona* species) is used for malaria.
- Taxol form Taxus (*Taxus brevifolia*) is used to treat cancer.
- Morphine from Opium (*Papaver somniferum*) is used as painkiller.
- Digoxin from Digitalis leaves (*Digitalis purpuria*) is used for congestive heart failure.

Natural product is wide term which includes drugs obtained from plants, animals as well as minerals. There is lot of confusion between herbal drugs and Ayurvedic drugs. All herbal drugs can not be considered as Ayurvedic medicines. Every country or regulating authority has prescribed certain rules to avoid confusion related to herbal drugs. In India, according to Drug and Cosmetic Act, 1940, there are 54 authoritative books which are called as classical books. If drug or formula is mentioned in these books, then and then only it is considered as Ayurvedic medicine. For example, *Arogya Kalpadruma, Ashtang Hridaya, Bhava Prakash,* Ayurvedic formulary of India, Ayurvedic pharmacopoeia of India etc. These and other books are considered as authoritative books of Ayurveda. Same thing applies to Siddha and Unani system also. According to Drug and Cosmetic act, these are commonly called as 'ASU drugs' (Ayurvedic Siddha Unani). For example, Ashwagandha, Bramhi considered as Ayurvedic drugs because they are mentioned in old classic Ayurvedic texts while Digitalis, Ginkgo, Taxus are not Ayurvedic drugs. India has documented all traditional knowledge in digital form in TKDL (Traditional Knowledge Digital Library). The drugs which are not documented in this TKDL are not considered as Traditional drugs.

1.2 HERBAL MEDICINE

Herbal drugs which are derived from plants are called as herbal medicinal products (HMP).

In European Union (EU), the agency called as European Medicines Agency (EMA) controls the evaluation and supervision of medicinal products. Before 2004, EMA was also known as European Medicines Evaluation Agency (EMEA). EMA has formed Committee on Herbal Medicinal Products (HMPC) to give several guidelines about herbal drugs use, safety and other issues. The Directive 2001/83/EC has provided definitions for HMPs, herbal substances and herbal preparations.

Herbal Medicinal Product exclusively contain active herbal ingredient, one or more herbal substance, one or more herbal preparation, one or more herbal substances in combination with one or more herbal preparations.

HMPs may also contain vitamins and minerals, provided that the action of the vitamins or minerals is ancillary to that of the herbal active ingredients. Chemical moieties can be obtained by extraction and purification from plant material. Such isolated or purified and chemically defined constituents or mixtures are not considered as HMPs. HMPs are different from isolated chemicals. Because of this specific separate guidelines have been established, which cover particular aspects related to HMPs. Herbal substances and herbal preparations are complex mixtures of natural constituents which altogether form the "active substance". This includes those constituents that may arise from natural transformations.

Herbal medicinal products are medicinal products that exclusively contain as active substances (one or more) herbal substances and/or (one or more) herbal preparations. Herbal substances and herbal preparations contain (complex) mixtures of primary (e.g. sugar, cellulose) and secondary (e.g. terpenes, glycosides) constituents. Because these mixtures of herbal constituents originate from the environment, they are considered as natural products. Therefore, use of herbal substances and preparations in small amounts in medicinal products is considered as safe to the environment. The HMPC acknowledges there may be exceptional cases where further justification to the absence of an environmental risk and assess this risk.

Some important Definitions according to Article 1 of Directive 2001/83/EC: Questions & Answers on the EU framework for (traditional) herbal medicinal products, including those from a 'non-European' tradition Page 2/20.

Extracts: These are preparations of liquid (liquid extracts and tinctures), semi-solid (soft extracts and oleoresins) or solid (dry extracts) consistency, obtained from herbal drugs (or animal matter) which is usually in a dry state.

Genuine (Native) herbal preparation: This refers to the preparation without excipients, even if for technological reasons the genuine herbal preparation is not available. However, for soft and liquid herbal preparations the genuine herbal preparation may contain variable amounts of (extraction) solvent.

Herbal medicinal products: These are medicinal products which exclusively contains one or more herbal substances as active ingredients or one or more herbal preparations, or one or more such herbal substances in combination with one or more such herbal preparations.

Herbal substances: These are the substances mainly whole, fragmented or cut plants, plant parts, algae, fungi, lichen in an unprocessed, usually dried form but sometimes fresh. Herbal substances also contain certain exudates which are not subjected to any specific treatment. Herbal substances are precisely defined by the plant part used and the botanical source including genus, species, variety and author.

Herbal drug preparations: Preparations obtained by subjecting herbal substances to treatments such as extraction, distillation, expression, fractionation, purification, concentration or fermentation are called herbal drug preparations. Examples of herbal drug preparation are powdered herbal substances, tinctures, extracts, essential oils, expressed juices and processed exudates.

1.3 SOURCES OF HERBS

India is one of 17 mega biodiversity countries in the world which contribute about 7% of world total biodiversity. India has 15 agro-climatic zones ranging from Himalayan to marine and desert to rain forest ecosystems. India has vast number of medicinal plants. According to database of NMPB (National Medicinal Plant Board), out of 17000-18000 flowering plants species in India, more than 7000 are medicinal.

Herbs can be obtained through different sources. Herbs can be collected from wild sources or from cultivated source such as field or green house. Cultivation of herb is becoming common practice all over world because it gives consistent good quality raw material. Cultivated herbs are generally free from contamination. Propagation of herbs can be carried out by sexual or asexual method.

Table 1.1: Various Sources of Drugs

Sr. No.	Source	Significance	Example
1.	Plant	Most important source of drugs, widely available, large structural diversity, sustainable, renewable, cost effective source.	Digitalis, Cinchona, Ephedra, Opium, Senna, Aloe, Rhubarb, Rauwolfia, Belladonna.
2.	Animal	Provides many important drugs, enzymes from ancient time.	Honey, Bees wax, Spermaceti, Wool, Wool fat, Cod liver oil, Shark liver oil, Musk, Lakh, Cantharidine, Cochineal, Lard, Suet, Catgut, Gelatin, Vaccines, Sera, Blood.
3.	Marine	Huge source of many potential drugs, marine algae, plants, animals, fungi are not yet exploited or searched.	Agar, Algae, Toxins, Antibiotics.
4.	Mineral	Naturally occurring minerals, salts, oxides are used as medicine from ancient time. They are stable and effective on various diseases.	Zink oxide, Calamine, Shilajit, Sulphur, Bhasma.
5.	Micro-organism	Now-a-days lot of new drugs are discovered from micro-organisms.	Antibiotics, antimicrobials, enzymes, vitamins.
6.	Modern approaches	Plant tissue culture, biotechnological approaches.	Insulin, hormones, secondary metabolites, antibiotics produced by fermentation.

Table 1.2: Important Drugs Isolated from Natural Products

Name of drug	Plant name	Common use
Atropine	Belladonna (*Atropa belladonna*)	Anticholinergic
Cocaine	Cocoa (*Theobroma cocoa*)	Local anaesthetic
Codeine	Opium (*Papaver somniferum*)	Analgesic, antitussive
Digoxin	Digitalis species	Cardiotonic
Emetine	Ipecacunha species	Antiamebic agent
Ephedrine	Ephedra species	Bronchodilator
Morphine	Opium (*Papaver somniferum*)	Analgesic
Papaverine	Opium (*Papaver somniferum*)	Smooth muscle relaxant
Physostigmine	*Physostigma venenosum*	Ophthalmic cholinergic
Pilocarpine	Jaborandi (*Pilocarpus microphyllus*)	Ophthalmic cholinergic
Quinidine	Cinchona species	Cardiac depressant
Quinine	Cinchona species	Antimalerial
Reserpine	Sarpagandha (*Rauwolfia serpantina*)	Antihypertensive
Sennoside A and B	Senna (*Cassia augustifolia* and other species of senna)	Laxative
Tubocurarine	Curare (*Chondrodendron tomentosum* and other species)	Skeletal muscle relaxant
Vinblastine, Vincristine	Periwinkle (*Vinca rosea* and other species of vinca)	Anticancer

Table 1.3: Drugs Isolated from Plant Parts

Sr. No.	Part of plant	Example
1.	Roots	Shatavari, Rauwolfia, Ipecacuanha, Aconite, Jalap, Ginseng, Ashwagandha.
2.	Woods	Quassia, Sandalwood, Sassafras, Red sanders
3.	Barks	Cinchona, Kurchi, Cinnamon, Quillaia, Frangula (*Rhamnus frangula*), Oak (*Quercus petrea*).

Contd...

4.	Rhizomes	Ginger, Valerian, Podophyllum, Turmeric, Vacha, Motha (Nutgrass), Devils claw (*Harpagohytum procumbens*), Kava kava (*Piper mythysticum*), Rhubarb (*Rheum palmatum*), Sarsaparilla (*Smilax ragelii*), Echinacea (*Echinacea angustifolia*).
5.	Flowers	Clove, Pyrethrum, Artemisia, Saffron, Dhataki.
6.	Fruits	Colocynth, Fennel, Bael, Karela, Amla, Hirada, Black pepper, Gokharu.
7.	Leaves	Senna, Digitalis, Vasaka, Eucalyptus, Balm (*Melissa officinalis*), Nightshade (*Atropa belladonna*), Ginkgo (*Ginkgo biloba*), Green Tea (*Camellia sinensis*), Peppermint (*Mentha piperita*), Bearberry (*Arctostaphylos uva-ursi*).
8.	Seeds	Nux-vomica, Strophanthus, Isabgol, Castor, Mucuna, Mustard
9.	Entire drugs	Ephedra, Ergot, Cantharides, Belladonna, Kalmegh, Neem, Brahmi, Warmwood (*Artemisia annua*).
10.	Dried latices	Opium, Gutta-percha, Papain.
11.	Resins	Balsam of Tolu, Myrrh, Asafoetida, Benzoin, Guggul.
12.	Dried Juices	Aloes, Kino, Red gum.
13.	Gums	Acacia, Tragacanth, Ghatti gum, Guar gum.
14.	Dried extracts	Gelatin, Catechu, Agar, Curare, Aloe.

Table 1.4: Important Unorganized Drugs

Drug	Description	Example
Gums	Pathological product, produced by plant as response to injury. Gums are plant hydrocolloids and may be anionic or non-ionic polysaccharides. On hydrolysis (acidic hydrolysis or prolonged boiling with water), gum yield sugar and uronic acids which form salts with calcium and magnesium. Soluble or partly soluble in water, insoluble in alcohol and in most of the organic solvents.	Gum Acacia, Tragacanth, Gum Karaya, Gum Ghatti, Guar Gum
Mucilages	Physiological product similar to gums, produced by plant as normal metabolism. Mucilage is produced inside the cells of the plant. Mucilages are esters of sulphuric acid, wherein ester group is a polysaccharide complex. Mucilages form slimy masses with water, but do not dissolve.	Isabgol, Squill, Agar, Chondrus

Contd...

Extracts	Solid or semisolid mass obtained by extraction of drug either by water or other solvent.	Agar, Sodium alginate, Catechu, Gelatin,
Resins, oleo resins, oleo gum resins	They are solids, liquids and semi-viscous materials, clear, translucent yellow or brown materials insoluble in water and soluble in most of the organic solvents.	Resins: Podophyllum resin, Jalap resin, Colophony, Sandarac, Guaiacum; Oleo resin: Capsicum, Podophyllum, Ginger; Balsam: Tolu, Benzoin, Storax, Peru; Oleo-gum resins: Myrrh, Asafetida
Latices	Product contained in special secretory tissues of certain plants. It is usually a white aqueous suspension, oil globules are suspended. These natural suspensions of milky consistency may contain alkaloids, proteins, sugars, mineral and alkaloidal salt in the true solution, whereas gums, starch and resins in the suspended form.	Rubber, Chicle gum, Opium, Papain, Gutta percha.
Juices	Obtained from fleshy leaves, fruit, stems of the trees (Kino) by cutting or crushing.	Aloe, Kino

For herbs collected from natural places need to take certain precautions. First important step is botanical identification. Correct botanical identification is very important for ensuring good quality assurance of herbal formulations. In case of some herbs, collection from wild sources is not feasible. In such cases, herbs can be propagated in field to ensure best quality raw material and regular supply.

Table 1.5: Comparison between Sexual Seed and Asexual Vegetative Propagation

Sr. No.	Sexual Propagation (Seed propagation)	Asexual Propagation (Vegetative propagation)
1.	In this method, seeds are used for propagation; plants are raised by using seeds.	In this method, vegetative part of the plant such as stem, root, leaf is used to develope new plant.
2.	Comparatively cheaper method of propagation.	Asexual propagation involves high cost.
3.	Plants start bearing seed or fruit late.	Seed or fruit bearing starts early.
4.	Plants are long lived.	Generally, plants may or may not be long lived.

Cond...

5.	Plants are uniform in growth and yield capacity.	Plants are uniform in growth and yield, but growth is not vigorous.
6.	Because of cross-pollination and genetic exchange, there are chances to improve plant variety.	Because of vegetative propagation, there is no chance for improvement in the variety.
7.	Generally, plants are sturdier and bigger.	Plants are not always sturdy and big.
8.	Because of natural variation, harvesting is difficult.	Generally, harvesting is easy.
9.	Seed propagation sometimes take long germination time.	Germination time is not longer.
10.	Example: Orange, Papaya, Castor, Foodgrains.	Example: Grapes, Rose, Sugar cane, Potato.

1.4 SELECTION OF HERBAL MATERIAL

According to World Health Organization data, more than 60% of world population is directly or indirectly using plant based medicines. On this background, it is very important to select right plant material for development of herbal drug. Selection of plant can be done by various approaches like randomized approach, ecological approach, chemo systemic approach, ethanobotanical (traditional knowledge based) approach.

Randomized selection:

In this, plant material is selected randomly from forest for discovery of new medicine. Success rate is low but this approach offers wide variety of diversity and plant material is available readily.

Zoopharmacognosy (Ecological approach):

Zoopharmacognosy is observation of animal behaviour for discovery and development of new drug. Observation of Chimpanzee in African forest lead to discovery of antimalarial properties of *Trichilia rubescens* leaves. This is also called as ecological approach. Ecological observation include like production of certain secondary metabolite by plant for insect repellence. Obviously, these toxic secondary metabolites can be used for treatment of some human ailments. Very few plants can be selected by this approach, yet this is good approach as it saves time and high success rate.

Chemosystemic approach:

Distribution of chemical constituents is common in certain groups of plant. This approach is also called as phylogenetic or chemotaxonomic approach. If plants belonging to certain taxa is therapeutically active, then there is high chance that other plants from same taxa can be active. For example, *Emblica officinalis* (Euphorbiaceae) commonly called as Amala contains ascorbic acid, gallic acid and tannins. So one can expect other genus and species. Species of Euphorbiaceae can also contain similar chemical compound and activity.

This approach is not decisive, but definitely gives some idea related to chemical diversity and possible activity of plant.

Ethanopharmacology:

Ethanopharmacology is branch of science which observes knowledge of people, their traditions and beliefs for discovery and development of drugs. Ethanopharmacology is also related with reverse pharmacology approach. In this approach, drug which is already in use from several years is taken and studied or explored for possible drug development. Ethanobotany involves study of certain plants with respect to ethnic group of people. Ethanobotany helps to classify plants systematically. Ethanopharmacology combines knowledge of people and pharmacological techniques. Ethanomedicine involves study of use of medicines by different ethnic groups including traditional medicines.

This type of selection of plant material increases success rate because plant is already known for activity and saves time and efforts.

1.5 IDENTIFICATION AND AUTHENTICATION OF HERBAL DRUGS

Correct botanical identification of drug is very important for good quality of finished product. Substitution or adulteration with morphologically or chemically similar plant is becoming common in herbal drug industry. Evaluation of drug is of critical importance on this background.

Table 1.6: Evaluation Methods

Sr. No.	Method	Characteristic or Parameters
1.	Taxonomic method	Botanical name, vernacular names, site of collection of plant material, details of collector, habitat, season of collection, altitude and part collected.
2.	Herbarium voucher sample	Voucher sample in a herbarium or a research institute for future references.
3.	Macroscopic method	Shape, size, colour, odour, texture, surface characteristics, fracture characteristics, taste and such organoleptic properties.
4.	Microscopic method	Light microscopy and polarized microscopy, structural, cellular and internal tissue features.
5.	Physicochemical methods	Total ash, water soluble ash, acid insoluble ash and sulphated ash and other parameters.
6.	Chromatographic methods	High Performance Liquid Chromatography (HPLC), Capillary Electrophoresis (CE) and Thin Layer Chromatography (TLC), GC-MS, LC-MS.

Contd...

7.	Spectroscopic methods	Infrared Spectroscopy, Electron Spectroscopy for Chemical Analysis, Inductively Coupled Plasma Mass Spectrometry (ICP-MS), Atomic Absorption Spectrometry (AAS), X-ray Diffraction Analysis (XRD), X-ray Fluorescence Analysis (XRF).
8.	Molecular markers	Primary and secondary metabolites and other macromolecules such as nucleic acids. Restricted Fragment Length Polymorphism (RFLP), PCR-Based techniques; Random amplified polymorphic DNA (RAPD), Amplified fragment length polymorphism (AFLP) and Real time PCR (RT-PCR).
9.	Immunoassays	Enzyme linked Immunosorbent Assay (ELISA), Poly Acrylamide Gel Electrophoresis (PAGE).

Identification of herbal material is combination of art and science. Correct botanical identification is first and one of the most important steps for ensuring good quality finished product. If the starting raw material is not original or good quality; then finished product quality cannot be guaranteed. Identification of herb can be done by different ways. Although there are several methods available, no one method is suitable for all herbs. Most of the time combination of these methods can be employed for correct identification.

Macroscopy:

Macroscopy involves checking external appearance or sensory characters like colour, odour, taste, size, shape, fracture etc. Botanical identification of herb is generally done by trained person like botanist. For correct botanical identification, entire plant along with root and flower is needed. Botanical identification is based on morphology which involves checking various parts of herbs like leaves, flower, root and others. Leaves and flowers are most important parts which help in identification of plant. Herb can be observed for colour, size, shape and arrangement of leaves and flower. Arrangement of leaves on stem and branching is called phylotaxy. Different types of arrangement of leaves like alternate, distichous, opposite, decussate, whorled types of leaves arrangement can be helpful to identify herb correctly. Different types of shapes of leaves like oval, oblong, obovate, round, linear, lanceolate, elliptical, spatulate, cordate, hastate are one of the simplest tool to identify plants. Even margins of leaves can be observed to identify herbs. Margins like entire, serrate, dentate, sinuate, ciliate, spinose help in identification of herb. In some cases, different species of plants can be identified only after flowering.

Microscopy:

Microscopy plays very crucial role in identification of drug those are morphologically similar. Microscope can be employed for checking sections of leaves, root and stem to confirm identity of herb. Microscopy can be also used to check stomata, trichome, calcium oxalate crystals, which may be unique to that herb. Certain leaf constants like stomatal index, palisade ratio, vein islet number are important for correct identification of herb. Indian senna and Alexandrian senna can be differentiated by using microscopic parameters. Indian senna has vain islet number 19.5 to 22.5 while Alexandrian senna has 25 to 29.5. Indian senna have stomatal index 17 to 20 while Alexandrian senna have 11.4 to 13.3. Likewise many other plants can be identified by microscopy. Shape of calcium oxalate is useful to identify plant for example- rosette shaped crystal is present in *Datura stramonium*, needle shaped crystal are presents in *Iris germanica*, raphaides are present in *Urginea maritima*, monoclinic prism shape is present in *Hyoscaymus niger*, sand shaped present in *Atropa belladonna*.

Microscopy is especially useful in case of powdered drugs. Starch grains, size and length of fibers, staining reactions like lignified xylem and phloem can be studied by using microscope.

Phytochemistry:

After macro and microscopy, preliminary phytochemical analysis helps to identify plant. Preliminary phytochemical analysis helps to reveal chemical constituents. Also analytical techniques are used to identify marker compound which is specific to particular herb. UV, MASS, NMR, HPLC, HPTLC are routinely used in industry for identification of herbs.

DNA fingerprinting:

Use of biotechnological tools for correct identification of herbs is the upcoming latest technology. Molecular markers like RAPD, ISSR, RFLP uses DNA fingerprinting for identification of herb at molecular level. Molecular markers are nothing but sequence of DNA which is unique to each plant. First, plant DNA is isolated and then amplified with the help of PCR and then screened for similar and different patterns. Plants also have unique DNA patterns similar to human. Pattern of this DNA can be identified in the form of DNA barcoding or DNA fingerprinting. DNA barcoding identify plant as species or even subspecies level or molecular level, even when small part of plant without flower is available. More recent technology like genomics, proteomics, transcriptomics and metabolomics technique can identify plant at genetic level.

1.6 PROCESSING OF HERBAL RAW MATERIALS

Processing is the entire journey for raw herbal material from field into finished product. Processing involves many steps according to nature of herbs. Each and every herb is different, so different methods of processing are employed for individual herbs. After correct botanical identification of herb, collection can be done. Now-a-days, generally collection is done from cultivated plants. Herb material collected needs some special precaution. If fresh herb is not supposed to be used immediately, it should be dried to prevent deterioration. Again method of drying is selected depending upon nature of herb. After drying, it can be cleaned for certain impurities. Dressing or garbling is done in order to make herb more presentable before sending to market. Storage of herbs also needs special precaution. Before storage, herb material should be packed in suitable material. After this step, herbal material is ready for market. It can undergo extraction procedure as per requirement. Extraction method can be selected according to nature of herb. Extracts are then characterized by means of other chromatographic techniques. Now, after determining content of one or more ingredients, these extracts can be called as standardized extracts. Standardized extract show uniformity in pharmacological action and do not have much variation. These extracts can be converted into suitable herbal formulation or can undergo further isolation procedure.

Collection of Crude Drugs:

Collection of crude drugs is very crucial factor to determine quality. After correct botanical identification, collection can be done. Time, place and method of collection are critical to determine quality of the drug. Chemical constituents in any plant are subjected to change according to time of collection, season, geography, stage of maturity, sex, age of plant. One should collect the plant material when chemical constituents are in maximum concentration. While collecting the drug one has to consider Convention on Biodiversity (CBD) which was effective from 1992, which ensures conservation of biodiversity and prevent over exploitation of biodiversity. According to government laws, some endangered varieties of plant and animal are banned for collection. European Union has prescribed guidelines for Good Agriculture Practice for Medicinal and Aromatic Plants in 1998. These guidelines specify propagation, collection, harvesting, processing, storage, quality assurance of drugs. In India, there are several laws like Plant variety and Farmers right protection act. Apart from this, intellectual property right protection is considered by geographical indication act. Immediately after collection, it is advisable to keep reference sample/ herbarium for further use.

Table 1.7: Time of Collection for Herbal Drugs

Sr. No.	Plant part	Time of collection	Example
1.	Leaves	Before maturity, before flowering	Digitalis, Vinca, Tea, Belladonna, Senna, Tulsi.
2.	Flowers	Before pollination or maturity, preferably in morning before sunrise	Clove bud, Rose, Chamomile, Arnica, Saffron.
3.	Roots	When aerial growth of plant stops, i.e. spring	Withania, Ginseng.
4.	Rhizomes	When aerial growth of plant stops, when rhizome has maximum reserve food material	Ginger, Turmeric, Jalap.
5.	Stem	After maturity	Kalmegh, Ephedra.
6.	Bark	Spring or early summer, after damp weather when it separates readily from wood	Ashoka, Arjuna.

Cond...

7.	Seed	After maturity, washed and freed from pulp	Nux Vomica, Cocoa.
8.	Fruit	Ripe, half ripe or fully mature	Coriander, Dill, Bael.
9.	Resin	Immediately after oozing from plant, in dry weather	Balsam of Peru, Balsum of Tolu.
10.	Gum	After oozing, when it dries or hardens, in dry weather	Acacia, Tragacanth
11.	Latex	After oozing out, after coagulation	Papaya, Opium.
12.	Heartwood	After maturation	Sandal wood.
13.	Pod	After maturation	Senna

Harvesting of Crude Drugs:

Harvesting is an operation which is actual collection of crude drugs from field. Harvesting is an operation which is actual collection of crude drugs from field. Harvesting also involves processing of drugs like removal of seed coat, cover etc. Now-a-days harvesting is carried out by machines as compared to conventional methods.

Table 1.8: Types of Harvesting

Sr. No.	Types of harvesting	Example	Advantages/ Disadvantages
1.	Manual, skilled workers	Flowers, Leaves like tea leaves, vinca, senna leaves, digitalis, belladonna, cinchona.	Selectivity, sorting by hand/ Laborious, time consuming, costly.
2.	Mechanical diggers	Roots, rhizomes, tubers e.g. potato, ginger, sugarcane.	Economic, washing is possible.
3.	Mechanical shakers	Fruits like apple, olive and some flowers.	Free from soil, good quality.
4.	Seed striper, separator	Seeds, barks like cork.	Saves time and labour.
5.	Machine harvester, mowers, thrashers, winnowers	Seeds, grains, some fruits	Saves time and labour.

Dressing/Garbling of Crude Drugs:

Garbling or dressing means preparation of drug for market by removing sand, dirt, extraneous matter, insects, stalks and other impurities. It may involve grading of material based on size, shape and weight. Removal of stalk in case of leaf drug like senna, fennel, sand and clay in case of underground drug is done before packing of drug. This can be done with special size of sieves and shakers. Before going to market, drug should be presentable.

Garbling also involves some special treatment given to different drugs to make drug more acceptable in market:

Table 1.9: Special Treatment Given to Some Drugs

Sr. No.	Drug	Garbling procedure
1.	Ginger	Removal of clay and liming of ginger for improvement in colour.
2.	Bees wax	Exposure to sunlight for bleaching.
3.	Clove	Removal of clove stalks from cloves.
4.	Shark liver oil	Filtration, centrifugation, purification and adjusting vitamin content.
5.	Cinnamon	Scraping polishing of bark to remove wood part.
6.	Powdered drugs	Removal of iron pieces by magnet.

Drying of Crude Drugs:

Drying is simple procedure and consists of removal of moisture. Drying of crude drugs generally followed immediately after collection. As a general rule leaves, herbs, flowers are dried at 20 to 40°C and barks, roots and stem can be dried at 30 to 65°C.

Advantages of Drying:

- Drying increases shelf life and storage of drug.
- It helps in size reduction and powdering of crude drugs.
- Drying is recommended before transport of drug as it reduces weight and saves space before packing.
- Drying retards growth of microorganism and maintains uniform quality of drug.

Table 1.10: Types of Drying

Sr. No.	Type of Drying	Specifications	Example
1.	Drying under sun	Low cost but time consuming and possibility of contamination with dust, generally in practice in tropical countries; fading of colour due to sunlight is possible.	Acacia gum, barks, seeds and few fruits.

Contd...

2.	Drying under shade/ open air drying	Avoid photo degradation of heat/ light sensitive drugs but takes long time for drying.	Senna, Digitalis, Clove, Cardamom, Cinnamon, Colocynth, Chinese Rhubarb, Fennel, Dill, Caraway and other volatile oil containing drugs.
3.	Tray dryer/ hot air oven	Quick method for large scale drying, hot air circulated through drug.	Cinchona bark, Belladonna.
4.	Spray dryer	Suitable for heat sensitive material, liquid or slurry.	Milk, protein, enzyme drugs, Papaya latex, tannins, several extracts are dried by this method.
5	Vacuum dryer/ freeze dryer	Suitable for heat and moisture sensitive drugs	Digitalis leaves, Tannic acid, taxus, biological products.

Application of Drying:

- If herbal drug is sensitive to heat then use of oven drying was found to have less phytochemicals as compared to freeze drying.
- Recent study on effect of drying process on the composition of Black Pepper ethanolic extract by High Performance Liquid Chromatography (HPLC) have shown higher impurities in oven dried samples.
- Herbal drugs are often freeze-dried (lyophilized) for use and a variety of freeze-dried drugs are marketed to the consumers. Freeze-drying prevent loss of certain certain chemicals and preserves the medicinal qualities of plants, and is considered superior to other preservation methods.
- Some botanical samples are freeze dried before their use as food, spices, or in research studies.
- Freeze drying can affect different plants and different constituents in a variety of ways. Freeze drying is preferred method in case of Dill (*Anethum graveolens*) extract compared to hot air drying. Another report indicated that, the thymol contents of the plant increase after freeze drying. Most researches indicate the reduction or degradation of the volatiles after freeze drying.
- Regarding the other components, in most plants, freeze drying preserves their phenolic and antioxidant contents. Recent research suggests that freeze drying is better method in drying of carotenoids. Freeze drying of *Echinacea purpurea* causes more retention of cichoric acid, a moisture sensitive acid, than air drying.
- There are some limitations of freeze-drying. According to some reports, if medicinal compounds like volatiles, phenolics and carotenoids which are not preserved properly may increase the mutation rate in unicellular organisms and may reduce some activities.

Packaging of Crude Drugs:

After garbling, grading of crude drugs can be carried out in most of the cases. Different grade material is then packed according to requirement and further use. Packaging is important for storage and transport of crude drug. Proper packing helps in increasing shelf life of crude drug.

Table 1.11: Types of Packaging Materials

Sr. No.	Packaging material	Plant name and part	Advantages
1.	Gunny bags	Roots, seeds (coffee bean), small branches, barks	Allow rough handling, supply air to keep material live and fresh, cost effective.
2.	Tin or metal containers	Volatile oil, resins, balsams	Prevent oxidation and photo degradation, increases shelf life.
3.	Plastic containers	Whole plant	Drugs sensitive to oxidation, packed in airtight containers.
4.	Polythene bags/ zip lock/ self-sealable	Extracts, powders	Suitable for hygroscopic material, can be opened and packed as required.
5.	Wooden boxes, cardboard	Fruits	Delicate, fragile drugs.

Storage of Crude Drugs:

Storage of crude drugs is very important aspect to maintain quality of drug and increase shelf life. If crude drug is not stored properly, loss can be upto approximately 5 to 10 per cent. Different drugs because of their different physical and chemical nature need separate storage conditions. Most common enemies of crude drug are oxygen, light, moisture (humidity) and temperature. Drug containing fixed oil, cod liver oil, shark liver oil should be stored in container in which air is replaced by inert gas. Proper care should be taken while storing volatile oil containing drugs which is liable to lose aroma with increase in temperature. Generally for oil, amber coloured glass bottles or stainless steel containers are most suitable material for storage.

- Drugs which contain oil can catch fire if stored at high temperature e.g. Pista.
- Tuber and bulb crops are important food vegetables cultivated and consumed in most areas of the world.
- Potatoes (*Solarium tuberosum L.*), yams (*Dioscorea spp.*), sweet potatoes (*Ipomea batatus L.*), and ginger (*Zingiber officinale L.*) form the economically important tuber crops, whereas onions (*Allium cepa L. var. cepa*), shallots (*A.cepa L. var. ascalonicuni*), and garlic (*A. sativum L.*) constitute the major bulb crops. Because of their high water content and the difficulty of storing, processing and transportation, postharvest losses of tuber and bulb crops are potentially very high.

- At the same time seeds and nuts also need special environment for storage. Improper storage in case of opium may decrease morphine content. Drugs like Ergot, Cascara, Sarsaparilla, Indian Hemp, Taxus, Echinacea are very sensitive to storage conditions.
- One has to consider loss due to physical factors in failure of storage like mechanical injuries sustained by the drug handling operations have a major influence on storage quality.
- Apart from the direct losses caused by mechanical damage, roughly handled drugs lose weight more rapidly in storage and are more prone to attack by rot-producing microbial pathogens.
- Sprouting, rooting, transpiration, and respiration are the major physiological factors contributing to both qualitative and quantitative deterioration in tuber and bulb drugs.

Common Precautions in Storage of Crude Drug:

- Crude drugs should be stored in optimum storage conditions which include cool and dry environment.
- Crude drugs should be protected from direct sunlight and excessive temperature variation.
- Properly sealed containers which are impermeable for insects and mites can be employed to increase storage life.
- Regular cleaning with insecticide like pyrethrin, fumigation with ethylene oxide, irradiation of storage drug and place will also increase storage life of crude drug.

Summary of Storage Conditions of Crude Drug:

Table 1.12: Storage Conditions of Crude Drugs

Criteria	Effect	Precaution
Temperature	High temperature increases degradation of drug. Most of drugs like proteins, enzymes, peptides are very sensitive to heat, high temperature also cause loss of volatile oil from crude drug.	Cool temperature, avoid excess temperature, shocks should be avoided.
Light	Increase photodegradation, photolysis, decomposition, bleaching of drug, loss of vitamin.	Avoid direct sunlight, use of amber coloured bottle, opaque non-transparent container.
Oxygen	Responsible for oxidation of drug, rancidity of fixed oil, resinification of volatile oil.	Replace oxygen by inert gas like nitrogen to prevent oxidation.
Moisture	Responsible for increase in weight of crude drug cargo, facilitates hydrolytic degradation of drug, encourage growth of fungus, mold and bacteria.	Proper packing, use of dehydrating agents like silica gel, cobalt chloride, calcium sulphate, calcium chloride or lime can be provided with crude drugs.

Role of Moisture in Storage of Crude Drug:

As general rule, drug should be dried enough to increase shelf life. Naturally dried crude drug may contain up to 12 per cent moisture. Most of the carbohydrates containing drugs, powdered drugs are hygroscopic in nature and liable for attack of moisture. In general, the growth of bacteria and fungi are favoured by warm, humid conditions.

- Hygroscopic drugs like Cocoa, Coffee, various nuts, Grains, Acacia gum, Starch and Squill powder should be protected from moisture.
- Some drugs like Digitalis, Indian hemp, Echinacea, Sarsaparilla, Taxus, Gentian and Ergot are very sensitive for degradation, need special attention.
- Moisture loss due to transpiration, and to a lesser extent to respiration, increases with storage temperature; evaporative losses are generally proportional to the water vapour pressure deficit in the surrounding air.
- Matured tubers with a well-formed skin, and properly cured bulbs with a tight, dry outer scale lose less water in storage due to transpiration than do immature tubers or bulbs having exposed fleshy scales. In addition, sugar formation can occur in potatoes when stored at temperatures below 7°C by conversion of starch.
- In potatoes, bacterial soft rot caused by *Erwinia* spp. may assume very serious proportion under warm tropical storage conditions, leading to substantial loss.
- At lower storage temperatures, rotting of onions is mainly due to *Botrytis allii* whereas at higher temperatures the black mold (*Aspergillus niger*) and bacterial species (*Erwinia caratovora, Pseudomonas* spp., *Xanthomonas* spp.), cause soft rotting are the main microorganisms responsible for spoilage.

Use of Chemicals in Storage of Crude Drugs:

Use of chemicals is no more preferred method for storage now-a-days. But in certain cases, chemicals like methyl bromide can be used for killing pests before storage of crude drugs. But growing list of resistant strains has questioned the effective use of chemicals in the control of postharvest losses of stored products. For environmental and health reasons, the consumer rejection of chemical pesticides is growing. Because of this, use of radiation and other methods are becoming popular.

- Chemicals can be used in case of insect strains include *Tribolium castaneum, T. confusum, Sitophilus oryzae, S. granarius, S. zeamais, O. surinamensis, Rhyzopertha dominica, Dermestes maculatus, Callosobruchus chinensis, Trogoder magranarium, S. cerealelle, Plodia interpunctella, E. cautella,* and *E. kuehniella.*
- Application of certain chemicals like maleic hydrazide, chemical inhibitors of cell division such as Chlorpropham, Propham and Tecnazene (tetrachloro nitrobenzene) are used on potatoes as a postharvest application for control of sprouting. Metabolic loss, sprouting, can cause huge loss in case of potato, onion, yam, garlic.

Use of Radiation in Storage of Crude Drugs:

Use of radiation is also called as 'cold pasteurization'. In 1930, French patent was issued to Otto Wiist (a German) for the use of ionizing radiation to preserve foods. Radiation is used for drugs which can have problem in heat pasteurization.

- Some beetles from the family Bruchidae of insects. Order Coleoptera are most sensitive to radiation, while moths (Lepidoptera) are the most resistant for radiation.

- Storage of apples, peaches, pears, and nectarines has been studied with regard to the control of ripening, of certain physiological disorders, and to reduction of decay caused by fungal pathogens.
- Moth species, *P. interpuntella, C. cautella, E. kuehniella, Ectomyelois ceratonae, Corcyra cephalonica,* and *Amyelois transitella*, are the most common insect pests of dried fruits and nuts. These can be treated with radiation. The beetle species *T. castaneum* and *Carpophilus hemipterus* are also associated with dried fruits and nuts.
- Radiation is more useful in case of international trade of dried fruit and nuts. Dried dates have problem of infestation more than 12 species of insects including the fig moth, *Cadra cautella (E. cautelld)*, saw toothed grain Beetle and *Oryzaephilus surinamensis*. Although drying of drug is considered good to increase shelf life but radiation is proving useful in this case. Similarly, dried apricot, dates, figs and raisins, tobacco, coconut, spices, mushrooms can also irradiated to increase storage life and retain quality.
- At temperatures of 5-15°C, the dormancy of onions, shallots, and garlic is shortened and can result in a more vigorous sprout growth. Irradiation decreases sprouting thereby increasing shelf life.

Different Methods for Storage of Crude Drugs:

Table 1.13

Method	Mechanism involved	Specification	Example
Heating	Killing Micro organism	Quick and reliable method but External appearance, properties of drug may change	Pasteurization (milk), Sterilization (canned foods, drugs)
Radiation (shelf-life extension)	Inhibition	Properties of drug (look, taste, smell) remains same as that of non-irradiated drug. Drug can be contaminated after radiation treatment (if exposed to pest again)	Fish, spices
Radiation (serilization)	Killing Micro organism	Properties of drug (look, taste, smell) remains same as that of non-irradiated. Drug can be contaminated after radiation exposure (if exposed to pest again)	Shelf-stable prepared meals
High pressure pasteurization	Killing of microbes	External appearance, properties of drug may change	Fruit juices, sauces
Low temperature refrigeration	Inhibition	Good for storage	Dairy products

Contd...

Freezing for longer term storage	Inhibition	Good for temperature sensitive drugs, keeps vitamins and taste intact but not suitable for all drug candidates	Fish
Atmosphere modification, vacuum packaging	Inhibition	Most suitable method for packing, increase shelf life	Dates
Modified atmosphere packaging	Inhibition	Can keep seeds, tubers live and fresh	Seeds, nuts, tubers, pork
Controlled atmosphere	Inhibition	Most suitable method for packing	Fruits, vegetables
Acidification fermentation	Inhibition	Limited applications, can not be suitable for all drugs	Dairy products, pickles
Reduced water activity Dried foods	Inhibition	Decrease weight, good for transport and packing	Dehydrated vegetables, leaves, fruits
Increased osmolality, Sugar conserves	Inhibition	Simple method but can change original taste of drug, also increase in calories	Jams, gellies
Cured and salted foods	Inhibition	Low cost, long lasting method but can alter original taste of drug	Fish
Use of preservatives	Inhibition	Control of pest throughout life time of product, Chemicals are not acceptable by consumer as well as regulatory agencies, has certain limitations like pH, taste	Bakery products (propionate in bakery products, benzoate in fruit products, nitrite (cured meats), sulfite (meats, wine), antibiotic (nisin), Compartmentalization
Water-in-oil emulsions	Inhibition	Gives stability to drug but suitable only for liquid drugs	Butter

Recent Advancement in Storage of Drugs:

Use of Modified Atmospheric Packaging (MAP):

- This consists of modification of atmosphere by either lowering the level of oxygen, raising the level of carbon dioxide, or by an altered level of the inert gases. Modified atmosphere have been used to control insects in grains, dried fruits and nuts.

- This can include different techniques, such as vacuum packaging, controlled-atmosphere packaging, and modified atmosphere or gas packaging. Mainly fruits and vegetables can have benefits of a modified atmosphere as a result of natural respiration. Storage and quality of food is increased by inhibiting chemical, enzymatic, and microbial spoilage.
- Different gases can be used in most MAP applications like oxygen (O_2), nitrogen (N_2), and carbon dioxide (CO_2). Nitrogen is most preferred as an inert gas for storage of crude drugs. But in some rare cases oxygen can be used as it will generally stimulate the growth of aerobic bacteria and to prevent the growth of strictly anaerobic bacteria. Use of nitrogen can prevent oxidative rancidity and also inhibit the growth of aerobic microorganisms. CO_2 is both water- and lipid-soluble, and its role is primarily to inhibit the growth and metabolism of microorganisms. Carbon dioxide inhibits the growth rate of aerobic Gram-negative bacteria such as *Pseudomonas* spp.,
- Sometimes combination of one or more technique can be used like fish oil such as Cod (*Gadus morhua*), Haddock (*Melanogrammus aeglefinus*), Halibut (*Hippoglossus hippoglossus*), California (*Paralichthys californicus*), Indian mackerel (*Rastrelliger kanagurta*), Sole (English, gray, lemon, Petrale) use of irradiation with MAP or vacuum packaging is very effective. Issue of rancidity in fatty fish after irradiation can be overcome by excluding O_2 during irradiation and storage.
- Modification of pH is another way to increase storage life. If food/ drug have high water content but a pH below 4.5, it is not necessary to heat severely. Reason is, spores of *Clostridium botulinum* cannot grow out at pH values below 4.5, so there is no need to heat-inactivate them. Combination methods like use of mild heating and refrigerated storage or removal of oxygen and reduced temperature and increased acidity is excellent method for storage.
- Reduction of water, pH and addition of nitrite followed by refrigeration is also used as combination method. Few drugs can be stored by heating and then addition of sodium chloride or nitrite to increase shelf life.
- A combination of irradiation and exposure to nitrogen, accelerate the mortality of flour beetle *Tribolium spp*. In case of cocoa beans and dates, irradiation in combination with heating by infrared radiation or microwaves can be a commercially viable technology.
- For berries fruits, grapes, gamma irradiation can often be combined with other physical treatments (e.g., hot-water dip, controlled atmosphere) or chemical agents to control postharvest diseases. The resulting 'combination treatments' may involve synergistic or additive effects leading to decreased treatment requirement for one or more of the combined agents. This is also useful for control of fungal diseases in fruit like papaya, banana, figs and mangoes.
- Combination of heat, chemical and radiation is necessary to control deteriorating in cherries, citrus fruits, mangoes, cauliflower, asparagus, dill, coriander and broccoli. Root drugs like carrots, beet roots, and turnips may benefit from radiation processing by inhibiting sprouting and the consequent shrinkage and loss of quality.

Commonly Found Organisms in Stored Crude Drugs:

Crude drugs may be obtained from marine or other water sources. Potential human concern are mainly gram-positive organisms like *Bacillus cereus, Clostridium botulinum, Clostridium perfringens, Listeria monocytogenes, Staphylococcus aureus* and gram-negative bacteria *Aeromonas hydrophila, Campylobacter jejuni, Escherichia coli, Salmonella, Shigella, Vibrio, Yersinia enterocolitica.*

Table 1.14: Types of Micro-organims found in Crude Drugs

Organism	Example	Contamination
Mould	*Rhizopus* spp., *Mucor* spp., *Penicillium* spp., *Eurotium* spp., *Thamnidium* spp.	Peanut, Corn, Wheat, Rice, other grains, Cereals, Oils seeds, Acorus.
Bacteria	*Salmonella* spp., *E coli*	Most of crude drug including Acacia, Agar, Starch, Sterculia, Digitalis, Tragacanth, Galatin, underground drugs.
Mite (Arachinida)	*Acarus siro* (flour mite)	Common in cereal, grains.
Moth (Lepidoptera)	*Ephestia kuehniella* (flour moth), *E. Cautella* (fig moth), *E. elutella* (Cocoa moth), *P. interpunctella* (Indian meal moth)	Almond, Ground nut, Cocoa, Ginger, Capsicum, Tobacco.
Beetles	Sap feeding (*Carpophilus* spp.), Merchant grain (*Oryzaephilus* spp.), Furniture (*Stegobium* and *Anobium* spp.), Spider (*Ptinus* spp.), Flour (*Tribolium* spp.)	Dried fruits, Grains, Tobacco, Flour, Ginger, Almond, Nutmeg, Rhubarb and other vegetable drugs.

QUESTIONS

1. What is herb? Give any five examples.
2. What do you mean by herbal medicine?
3. Which are differnt sources of herbal drugs?
4. Which are different criteria for selection of herbal material?
5. Explain different approaches for identification and authentification of herbal drugs.
6. Write in detail processing of herbal raw material.
7. Write a note on collection of herbal drugs.
8. Write note on harvesting of crude drugs.
9. What is garbling of crude drug?
10. Write note on drying of curde drug.
11. Which are different types of drying methods and its application.
12. Which are recent trends in packaging of crude drugs.
13. Write a note on storage of crude drug.
14. Which are different points need to consider for storage of crude drugs.
15. Which are different factors affecting storage of crude drugs.
16. Which are different recent advancement in storage of crude drugs.

❖❖❖

Chapter...2

BIODYNAMIC AGRICULTURE

Objectives

- To understand the concept of good agriculture practices.
- To understand basic principals of organic farming.
- To understand pest and management of pest.
- To understand concept of biopesticides and bioinsecticides.

2.1 INTRODUCTION

Biodynamic agriculture is a type of agriculture technique, where farm is considered as living entity, where sustainable, ecological methods are used for soil fertility, plant growth, and livestock care. It includes various concepts drawn from the ideas of Rudolf Steiner (1861–1925).

Biodynamic agriculture includes use of manure and compost which are prepared ecologically. The word sustainable is derived from the Latin, *sustinere*, meaning to keep in existence, long-term support. Sustainable agriculture is capable of maintaining its productivity and usefulness to human for long period of time.

Biodynamic agriculture is environment friendly, resource-conserving, economical, socially supportive and commercially competitive. These methods do not use any synthetic chemical fertilizers and pesticides. Biodynamic farming involves greater earthworm population and less energy used for production as compared with other farming.

Table 2.1: Different methods of farming

Parameter	Organic farming	Chemical, inorganic or synthetic farming	Biodynamic farming
Cost	Low	High	Low
Method	Need special training	Easy to use	Special treatment
Fertilizers	Naturally occurring manure, green manure	Synthetic granules or liquid	Special preparations like BD-500, BD-501, BD-502 etc.

Cond...

Soil life	High	Low	High
Energy consumed	Medium	High	Low
Sustainable method	Yes	No	Yes
Use of genetically modified plant	May be	Yes	No
Use of green house	May be	Yes	No
Crop rotation	May be	No	Yes
Cosmic forces and planting calendar	No	No	Yes

Biodynamic agriculture involves:

- Use of natural methods like soil building.
- Use of natural composting, manures.
- Crop rotations to increase yield and soil health.
- Use of field sprays (referred to as BD-500 and BD-501) or additives for manure composting.
- Maintenance of biological rhyme of farm.
- Prohibition of any synthetic fertilizers and pesticides.
- Management of pest by natural ways.
- Involves certification of product to ensure quality.

Concept of Biodynamic Agriculture:

The concept of biodynamic agriculture was first proposed by German philosopher Rudolf Steiner in 1924. He was founder of the movement called as 'anthroposophy'. This movement involves a holistic and spiritual interpretation of agricultural systems with special central role of human. To check the idea of biodynamic agriculture, a group of more than 800 farmers was formed in Europe and America named as 'Agricultural Experimental Circle of Anthroposophical Farmers and Gardeners of the General Anthroposophical Society'. With aim of restoring, maintaining and enhancing ecological harmony movement was started worldwide. The term *bio* indicates farm as living entity while term *dynamics* indicates energy. Theme of this practice mainly includes crop diversification, the avoidance of chemical soil treatments and off-farm inputs generally, and decentralized production and distribution with more harmony with nature.

Based on Rudolf Steiner's idea, organization was formed in 1928 named as 'Demeter International'. This is now one of the largest certification organizations for biodynamic agriculture and organic certifiers. 'Demeter' is name of Greek goddess of grain and fertility. Demeter Biodynamic Certification is used in more than 50 countries to verify that biodynamic products meet international standards in production and processing for ecological label for organic foods. This certification ensures preservation of biodiversity, ecosystem and live-stock integration.

Biodynamic agriculture prohibits use of genetically modified plants and organisms. Farm is considered as holistic organism and thus products certified are of high quality.

Biodynamic farming has increased polyphenol content and radical scavenging activity as compared to conventional farming in Chicory (*Cichorium intybus*) and some other plants.

Effect of Cosmic Forces:

Biodynamic farming involves consideration of effect of light and cosmic forces from sun, earth, moon and other stars on plant growth. Position of moon, ascending or descending is taken into consideration. Soil preparation, sowing, harvesting is to be done with rhythm of nature. Constellations (Group of stars) are also considered before starting most agriculture activity.

Cow Pat Pit (CPP)

This is one of the techniques of biodynamic agriculture which involves compost with cow manure mixed with crushed egg shell and basalt powder. In this, 12 inch pit cow dung is fermented for 3 to 4 months along with biodynamic preparation BD 502- BD 507. This fermentation allows growth of several bacteria and fungi and enriches soil fertility.

Biodynamic Field Spray:

BD 500: It is also known as 'Cow horn manure'. The Biodynamic agriculture involves preparation of BD-500 which is a fermented cow manure derivative used to improve the soil fertility. This also helps in the formation of a strong root system. Cow horns are filled with fresh lactating cow dung. These horns are buried during descending moon. These horns are allowed to ferment and taken out during winter and kept at dark place in earthen pots. For preparing the spray solution for one ha, 62.5 g of this material is dissolved in 40 L of warm (40°C) water with continuous stirring for 1 hour (alternately in clockwise and anti-clock wise directions). Use of BD 500, improve the overall soil quality and organic matter, microbial biomass and diversity. The difference between organic and BD farming lies essentially in the use of defined sprayed compounds such as 500 and 501. These products are permitted in organic farming by an EC Regulation (834/2007). Preparation BD-500 has enzymatic-specific activities and are rich in microbial cells like genus Bacillus exhibits an auxin-like activity. This acts as the 'prime starter of biodynamic'.

BD 501: It is also known as 'Cow horn silica' and is made from quartz crystals ground to alum powder consistency, packed into a cow horn. This cow horn is then buried during spring equinox and taken out during autumn equinox. The material stored in glass bottle then exposed to the sun by the windowsill was used to prepare the BD 501 spray solution by dissolving 2.5 g in 40 L of water, which was prepared for spray in a similar way as that of BD 500.

Table 2.2: Different Preparations Used in Biodynamic Agriculture

Preparation	Content	Common name	Role
BD 500	Fermented cow dung	Cow horn manure	Development of humus, microorganism, earthworms
BD 501	Ground quartz crystals	Cow horn silica	Aid photosynthesis
BD 502	*Achillea millefolium*	Yarrow blossom	Flowering, fruiting, disease resistance
BD 503	*Matricaria recutita*	Chamomile	Helps to retain nitrogen, calcium, sulphur
BD 504	*Urtica dioica*	Stinging nettle	Enrich soil, chlorophyll formation
BD 505	*Quercus robur*	Oak bark	Restore water balance, fungal diseases
BD 506	*Taraxacum officinale*	Dandelion flower	Flowering, fruiting, soil activity
BD 507	*Valeriana officinalis*	Valerian flower	Activate bacteria. Protection from frost
BD 508	*Equisetum*	Horse tail	Protection from fungus

However some recent studies also report there is no significant difference in conventional, organic and biodynamic farming with respect to flavonoid content, hydroxyl cinnamic acid and anthocyanin patterns were not affected by the type of cultivation. In fact conventionally grown salad yield was found to be more. Comparison of conventional as well as biodynamic viticulture activity was studied in Spain for wine. It was observed that in biodynamic farming there is 80% reduction in diesel use as manual workers are used in production.

Applications:

With use of two biodynamic preparations (BD 500 and BD 501) in Chilli by adopting a biodynamic calendar resulted better fruit quality of Chilli.

Biodynamic preparation and organic manure have increased yield in case of Cumin (*Cuminum cyminum L.*). There was significant increase in number of umbels (seeds), plant height and other parameters.

2.2 ORGANIC FARMING

Organic farming is defined as, "production of crop, animal, and other products without application of harmful chemicals like synthetic chemical fertilizers and pesticides, genetically modified or transgenic species, or antibiotics and growth-enhancing steroids."

Organic farming is also called as ecological farming. Biodynamic farming, which we have already studied, uses specific fermented herbal preparations as compost additives and field sprays in addition to organic farming. Organic farming consists of several principles and practices, which are given by the standards of International Federation of Organic Agriculture Movements (IFOAM) as the principle of health, ecology, fairness and care.

Organic farming does not involve any chemicals right from seed production and even after post harvesting, handling and storage. Product obtained is free from chemical fertilizers, herbicides and pesticides.

Aim behind Organic Farming:

- Production of food of high quality in sufficient quantity.
- Minimization of all forms of pollution.
- Processing of products using renewable resources.
- Production of biodegradable organic products.
- Consideration of the wider social and ecological impact of the organic production.
- Maintenance of long term fertility of soils.
- Maintain the genetic diversity of the plant and wildlife habitats.
- Promotion of the healthy use and proper care of water, water resources, all life therein.
- Use of local renewable resources in production systems.
- To encourage and enhance biological cycles within the farming system, involving micro-organisms, soil flora and fauna.
- Development of a valuable and sustainable aquatic ecosystem.

Effects of Organic Farming:

- Organic fertilizers have been known to improve the biodiversity.
- Organic farming helps to improve soil quality and microbial biomass.
- Organic fertilizers have lower nutrient content and release of nutrient is slow. So they are more effective for long term use.
- Bio-fertilizers contain microbial inoculants of living cells of micro-organism like bacteria, algae, fungi alone or combination which increase crop productivity.
- Nitrogen fixing bacteria like Azotobacter, *Azospirillum* species are nitrogen-fixing organisms, capable of forming an associative relationship with the roots of several crops.
- Organic farming can act on plant growth directly through the production of phytohormones or indirectly through nitrogen fixation or production of bio-control agents against soil-borne phytopathogens for better yield.

Applications

- In one study, vermin composted with coir pith and coir pith composted with microorganisms were used as a growth medium for growth of the medicinal plant *Andrographis paniculata*. The results are helpful for the reclamation of soils from industrial sites in a small scale nursery.

- *Asparagus racemosus* grown through organic farming using organic manures - cow dung, compost and vermin compost without using mineral or chemical fertilizer showed high antioxidant activity and increase in the total phenol and total flavonoid content was highest in the plants from vermin compost treated soil.
- Organically grown *Thymus vulgaris* was found to contain highest value of thymol.
- Treatment of *Ocimum basillicum* roots with rhizobacteria results in increased growth and volatile oil.
- Organic farming of geranium results in increase in fresh weight and oil percentage.
- Organic farming of marjoram (*Majorana hortensis L.*) along with treatment of bio-fertilizers shown almost two fold fresh weight as compared to control.
- Use of poultry manure has significantly increased the herbage, essential oil content and dry matter yield in *Java citronella*.
- Morphological characteristics and essential oil content of German chamomile was found improved with use of the vermin compost. Organic farming helped to improve plant height, early flowering; flowers dry weight, anthodia height and diameter also.
- Vegetative growth and essential oil accumulation was improved in Dragon head (*Dracocephalum moldavica L.*) by using compost.

Integrated pest management (IPM) can be defined as, "the method of cultivation of plant by consideration of all the factors that can provide to the plant efficient use of environmental resources for higher quality and quantity". Biofertilizers are micro-organisms which bring about nutrient enrichments of soil by enhancing the availability of nutrient to crops. A culture medium made of vermiculite, peatmoss, and pearlite is quite suitable for the application of biofertilizers, which gives better plant growth. Cyanobacteria and micorrhizal fungi fix nitrogen in air for plants and increase yield. *Bacillus polymaxa, Pseudomonas striata, Thiobaqcillus, Penicillium* and *Aspergillus* are some examples. Microphos are biofertilizers and release phosphates from bound and insoluble form.

2.3 GOOD AGRICULTURAL PRACTICES IN CULTIVATION OF MEDICINAL PLANTS

In India, about 22% of the production of medicinal plants sourced through cultivation. On this background, there is tremendous scope for improvement in cultivation of medicinal plants. Domestic demand of medicinal plants has been estimated 1,95,000 MT for the year of 2014-15. Total consumption of herbal raw drug in the country for the year 2014-15 has been estimated 5,12,000 MT. Trade of medicinal plants is an important affair involving 1178 species used in trade, of which, 242 species traded in excess of 100 MT / year. The export of medicinal plants during 2014-15 was about 3211 Crore and demand of medicinal plants estimated about 1, 34,500 MT.

Table 2.3: Good Agricultural Practices in Cultivation of Medicinal Plants

Sr. No.	Wild plants	Cultivated species
1.	Wild resources are open for access resource and do not need much investment.	Cultivation needs heavy initial investment.
2.	It is natural resource and free from pesticides.	It can keep genotypes being standardized or improved.
3.	Wild resource is supposed to be more efficacious.	Cultivated plants are not sturdy and may have less effect.
4.	Production volume and cost is not stable.	Production volume and price can be stable for longer periods.
5.	This can be threat to rare, endangered species.	It relieves harvesting pressure on rare and threatened species.
6.	Supply is seasonal and not continuous.	It guarantees continuing supply of raw medicinal materials.
7.	Natural gene pool is maintained.	Reintroduced plants can cause genetic pollution of wild resource.
8.	Wide genetic diversity is observed.	Genetic diversity is narrow.
9.	Risk of adulteration or contamination with different species is involved.	Risk of contamination or mixing is not involved.

Need for Good Agricultural Practices (GAP):

Use of medicinal plants is continuously increasing worldwide. Last few decades, with more number of people using herbal medicines, there is rise in concerns about safety. On this background, quality assurance and quality control of herbal medicines still need attention. Poor quality of herbal medicine is most of the time because of poor quality of starting material. In order to ensure quality, safety and efficacy of herbal medicine, World Health Organization (WHO) had identified importance of agricultural and collection practices. WHO guidelines provide detail description of Good Agricultural and Collection Practices (GACP) for herbal medicines. These are guidelines, which are supposed to be followed. Laws made by country or regulating authority are mandatory and should not be violated. Guidelines are there to help common grower or cultivator to increase quality of medicinal plant.

- Most of the farmers, producers, handlers and labours who collect raw material are not aware with concept of quality.
- Good agricultural practices (GAP) can be a first step to produce good quality herbal medicines. If starting material is of high quality then subsequent problem of poor quality can be less.

- Good agricultural practices can increase safety and efficacy of herbal medicine. Material collected from wild source can be contaminated by other species.
- Good agricultural practices are sustainable practice, saving forest, natural resources also ensuring regular supply of raw material. Protection of endangered species, environment, over harvesting, problems with intellectual property rights can be effectively managed by GAP.
- GAP can provide regular, affordable and sustainable supply of raw material.

2.3.1 Good Agricultural Practices for Medicinal Plants

Selection of Plant Material:

- Plant material should be selected as per specifications in national pharmacopoeia or by specific authority.
- In case of new plant material, identity of the material selected for cultivation should be confirmed and documented.

Botanical Identity:

- Correct botanical identity of medicinal plant including scientific name, genus, species, sub-species, order, family, local name, chemo type, phenotype should be documented.
- Origin or source of seed, plants, name of the cultivar, supplier and specific geographic region should be recorded.
- In case of doubt in identification, voucher specimen should be submitted to national or local herbarium for identification. Example: In India, there are several institutes like Botanical Survey of India, which can identify medicinal plant.
- After botanical identification, if possible, genetic fingerprinting can be done to compare data with authentic sample.

Seed or Other Material:

- Seed or other material used for propagation should be free from any contamination and diseases. Material should be resistant to environmental stress.
- Seeds or other material should be checked for genetically modifications. It should meet country's laws about use of genetically modified plant material. It should be properly labelled and documented.
- Sub-standard, inferior quality, adulterated, mixed varieties or strains should be avoided.

2.3.2 Good Cultivation Practices

Good cultivation requires certain precautions:

- As far as possible, traditional method of cultivation should be followed. In case of new plant material, where traditional method is not available, new method for cultivation can be developed through research.
- **Environmental effect:** Effect of cultivation on land and environment should be considered. Good plant husbandry principles like environmental stability of plant, growth requirements, crop rotation and soil condition should be studied.

- **Climate:** Climatic conditions like length of the day, sunlight, rainfall, water supply, temperature, day and night variation and many more climatic factors should be studied. Influence of soil, rainfall, temperature, sunlight and other environmental factors should be considered before selection of site or place of cultivation.
- **Soil:** Soil and soil fertility, nutrient content of soil, soil type, pH, water retention, should be considered before selecting plant material. Conservation of soil and prevention of soil erosion should be considered while doing cultivation. Land history for previous land use, previous cultivations, should be checked.
- Cultivation can affect ecological balance in particular area. Genetic diversity in surrounding area should be taken into consideration.
- While introducing new variety, ecological effect of cultivation should be studied.
- Impact of cultivation on social and economic life of local people should be considered. In case of large scale cultivation, local people should be benefitted by giving job or wages.
- **Use of fertilizers:** Need of suitable type of fertilizer and its quantity need to be considered. All type of human excreta should not be used in any form as fertilizer. Animal manure should be completely decomposed before using. Fertilizers used should be approved by respective countries. Use of fertilizers should be as less as possible. Care should be taken that, fertilizers should not leach in environment. Use of green manures such as alfalfa should be done for sustainability.
- Irrigation system should be chosen according to plant need. Excessive or under watering of plant should be avoided. Water used should comply with regional quality standards.
- Maintenance of plants should be carried out as and when required. Cutting, pruning, topping should be done when needed to guide plant growth.
- Chemical use should be as less as possible and to be done when there is no other alternative. Integrated pest management should be followed. Only approved pesticides should be used in minimum effective concentration. Use of pesticide should be done by qualified staff. Use of all pesticide and herbicide should be documented. For pesticide residue and use, 'International Plant Protection Convention and Codex Alimentarius' should be consulted. Final product should comply with pesticide and herbicide residue according to regulatory authorities.
- **Harvest:** Medicinal plant should be harvested only during best optimal season to produce best possible product quality. National pharmacopoeia, published standards or other reference books should be considered before deciding time of harvesting. Best time of the season and day for harvest should be determined by quality and quantity of biological active constituents. Care should be taken to ensure no foreign matter, plant, parts are mixing with medicinal plants while harvesting. Harvest plant material should be protected from rail, excessive moisture, humidity. Harvesting material should undergo drying as early as possible to avoid growth of microorganisms. Equipment used for

harvesting should be clean and maintain properly. Harvesting equipment need to be stored in proper place protected from dust, rodents, pests, insects and any other possible source of contamination. After harvesting, medicinal plant material should be kept on clean muslin cloth and contact with soil should be avoided. Underground material should be cleaned to remove adhering soil. Material should be transferred to clean and dry containers and then to central processing facility. Containers should be protected from rodents, birds, pets, insects and other harmful animals. Any damaged material during transport or harvesting should be discarded. Post harvesting inspection need to carry out to eradicate low quality material.

- **Personnel:** In order to ensure best quality of medicinal plant cultivation, plant grower or producer should have adequate knowledge of medicinal plants. All people including field workers or labours involved in propagation, cultivation, harvesting and post harvesting processing should maintain personal hygiene. Such personnel should have received required training regarding hygiene requirement. All personnel involved should wear protective clothing, gloves, goggles, mask, gown, cap or other special equipments required. Protection of environment and conservation of medicinal plant species should be given consideration.

2.3.3 Good Collection Practices

Generally, collection refers to collecting plant material from wild source such as forest. Collection of medicinal plant is associated with number of environmental and social issues. Good collection practices should ensure long term care of wild plant populations and their habitats. There are several examples of damage to endangered species and environment because of improper collection practices. On this background, WHO has provided comprehensive guidelines on Good Collection Practices for medicinal plants to deal with issues related to sustainability and conserving natural resources.

Permission:

- Collection of any plant from wild resources should be done with prior permission from Government authorities.
- While doing this, list of endangered or red list of plants should be considered.
- Convention on International Trade in Endangered Species of Wild Fauna and Flora (CITES) permits for export and import should be followed when required.

Planning:

- Before initiation of collection, proper study of geographical distribution and population of medicinal plant is needed.
- Distance of collection site from processing unit, national collection and transport permit should be obtained.
- All relevant information regarding target plant like taxonomy, genotype, phenotype, biology should be collected.

- Data related to environmental conditions, topology of local forest, geology, soil, climate, other vegetation at the collection site should be studied. Photo copies of target medicinal plants should be given to workers to identify the plant material. Other identification clues or illustration needed to identify plant material, similar morphological species and other related or unrelated species should be studied.
- Arrangement for quick and safe transport facility for people, equipment and plant material should be arranged properly. Expert team with experience of good collecting techniques, transport, cleaning, drying, storage should be ready. Training of all personnel involved in collection should be carried out. Responsibilities of all tasks should be given to respective persons. Social and economic impact of collection on local communities should be checked. Sustainability of environment should be considered before collection.

Selection of Plant Material:

- For source of medicinal plant material, national pharmacopoeia or official reference books should be referred with respect to country where collection is to be carried out.
- Plant variety should match with pharmacopoeia or official book. If plant variety to be collected is new, then it should be identified and documented as per country requirement.
- Herbarium sample should be deposited to regional or national herbaria for identification purpose. Date, time, place and other relevant information regarding collection including name of botanist should be documented.

Collection of Plant Material:

- Good collection practice should ensure long term sustainability of wild plants and environment. Density of plant material, demographic data of plant, part of plant to be collected and other information need to be studied. Rare or endangered plant material should not be collected.
- Medicinal plants should be collected during suitable time and season to ensure maximum biologically active constituents.
- Ecologically sustainable plant part should be collected. For example, instead of main root, lateral roots should be collected to allow further growth of plant. Bark from entire tree should not be collected. Instead, only longitudinal one side bark should be collected to allow growth of tree.
- Collection of medicinal plants from high level contaminated or polluted area should not be carried out.
- While collecting, care should be taken to remove unwanted plant parts or decomposed plant material.
- Collected plant part after collection should be placed in proper container.

- After collection, medicinal plant should be subjected to processing like removal of soil, grading, cutting and quality check.
- Cross-contamination should be avoided all the time. Different plants collected from same place should be kept separately.
- Equipment needed for collection should be maintained properly.

Personnel:

- Local expert should have sufficient knowledge and training. Local expert should work as link between collector and non-local, local people.
- Field worker should have proper training for identification as well as local and scientific name of plant material.
- All people including field workers or labours involved in collection should maintain personal hygiene.
- All personnel involved should wear protective clothing, gloves, goggles, mask, gown, cap or other special required. Protection of environment and conservation of medicinal plant species should be given consideration.

2.3.4 Good Agricultural Practices in Post Harvesting Processing

After harvesting, visual inspection of collected plant material should be carried out for foreign matter, damage. Sorting should be carried out depending upon appearance of drug.

Primary Processing:

- Plant material should be protected from rain, water, moisture or other conditions which can be harmful to plant material. Collected plant material should be immediately unloaded at processing facility. Medicinal plant material may need to be used as fresh, so should be stored in refrigerator. Suitable jars, box or pouch can be used.
- Plant material should be preserved without preserving agents. In case, preserving agents are used it should be documented. All plant material should be inspected during primary processing. Sol, sand, stone or other vegetable matter should be removed.
- Sorting of plant material should be carried out by suitable means like winnowing, sieving or by other suitable means.
- Mechanical devices used for processing should be clean and regularly maintained.
- Processed plant material should be protected from contamination.

Drying:

- Moisture content of medicinal plant should be kept as low as possible or given by pharmacopoeias. Depending upon medicinal plant, suitable method of drying can be chosen. Medicinal plants can be dried in shade or sun or tray dryers according to method suitable for individual drug.
- The drying conditions should be recorded properly for further reference.

- Shade drying should be preferred when crude drug is heat labile, in case of leaves or flowers or volatile oil containing drugs. Plant material should be moved or air circulation should be maintained to avoid mold infestation.
- While sun drying, drug should not be placed on ground. Suitable cloth or material can be used for spreading of drug. Care should be taken to avoid contamination of drug while drying. Dust, animals, rodents, pests should be kept away from drug material while drying.
- For indoor drying various parameters like drying temperature, duration, humidity, moisture content, agitation, plant part used, nature of chemical constituents should be kept in mind.
- Use of direct flame or heat should be avoided. Care should be taken to keep drying temperature below 60°C when necessary.

Processing:

- Processing of collected plant material is very important to improve shelf life, quality of finished product. Processing of plant material may involve various activities like sorting, peeling of skin, boiling, steaming, lime treatment, distillation, removal of stalk, roasting, fermentation, soaking, pickling, chopping, grading, shaping, bundling, drying, garbing or dressing. Proper processed herbal material have less microbial load.
- Antimicrobial treatment used like irradiation should be done with proper care, declared and documented. Only properly trained staff should carry such activity. This operation should be done as per standard operating procedure as per country specifications or regulatory body requirement.
- Location of the processing facility should be free from dust, smoke, pollution and other contaminants. Adequate drainage and connectivity by road is desired. Provision for cleaning of facility should be made.
- Processing building should have good construction. Different operations like drying, milling, roasting should be done in separate building area. Building material should not become contamination source.

Building Premises:

- Building should have adequate space, storage, hygiene, temperature control, humidity control, cleaning facility, ample light. Building should prevent entry of rodent, pollutant, pets, animals, smoke etc.
- Handling area floors, walls, ceilings should be designed, constructed, finished to prevent contamination. Floors should be water proof, non-absorbent, washable, non-toxic, non-slippery. Building should be free from cracks and handling area should be easy to clean and disinfect.
- Windows and other openings should not cause dust entry. Doors, stairs, lifts, fittings, overhead structures should not cause problem for processing. Food preparation, eating, changing facility, animal keeping facility should be separate.

- There should be ample of potable as well as non-potable clean water with suitable pressure.
- There should be effluent and waste disposal system, which is all time maintained. Effluent pipes should be large enough.
- Adequate changing room and toilets facility should be provided.
- Design of changing room and toilet should ensure good hygienic condition.
- Hand washing, hand cleaning, hand drying, elbow operated taps, hot and cold water, towel dispensers, waste bins should be provided at proper places.
- Building should have proper ventilation to avoid excess heat, steam building. Air flow should be unidirectional, that is from clean area to dirty area.
- Natural as well as artificial light system should be provided. Light should be of natural white light without any colour. Light fixtures should not contaminate plant material.
- Waste material should be stored properly and should not mix with plant material, potable water, building premises.

Packaging:

- Processed medicinal plant material should be stored properly in suitable container to avoid contamination as soon as possible.
- Plant material should be packed in clean, dry box, sacks, bag or other container depending upon suitability. Material should comply with regional or national authorities. Packing material should not be polluting and interfere with drug. Fragile plant material should be packed in rigid box.
- Packaging material if reused should be disinfected and dried before use. All packaging material should be stored in proper place protected from pest, rodents, animals and other contamination sources.
- Neat label on packaging material should be placed. Label should contain all relevant information like batch number, date of collection, processing date, relevant certification or other information if any.
- Origin of all batches, dates, weight, analysis or quality reports should be maintained in separate record. All records should be kept for minimum three years or according to requirement specified in national law.

Storage of Plant Materials:

- Generally fresh plant material should be preserved between 2 to 8°C; while frozen material should be kept at -20°C.
- Bulk transport of plant material should be done in proper vehicle.
- Storage area should be fumigated by trained person. All documents related to fumigation such as date of fumigation, chemical used should be documented. Only authorized chemicals should be used for fumigation.

- Organic plant material should be stored and transported separately.
- Temperature and humidity record should be maintained while storing medicinal plant material.

Equipment for Processing:

- All equipments used for processing should be made of the material which is not causing any contamination. Equipments surfaces should be clean, non-absorbent and capable of cleaning or disinfection whenever required. Use of corrosive material should be avoided.
- Design of equipment should prevent contamination or hygienic hazards. Equipment should be able to inspect visually with ease. Installation of equipment should permit easy acess and cleaning.
- Container used should be of good quality, leak proof, easy to clean and close.
- Refrigerated equipments should have temperature recording devices.

Quality Assurance:

- Quality assurance measures should be taken through regular audit carried by expert professional as per regulatory bodies' requirement.

Documentation:

All processes involved in good agriculture practices should be documented. Standard operating process should be documented and followed throughout operation. All documents should carry date, and signature of competent person.

Examples of documented format are given by different authorities:

- Seed and propagation of medicinal plant, herbarium, batch number.
- Site of cultivation or collection.
- Crop history including rotation.
- Use of fertilizers, growth regulators, pesticides, herbicide or other chemicals.
- Harvesting.
- Processing.
- Transport.
- Storage.
- Fumigation.
- Quality audit or inspections.

Photo or video documentation of cultivation, collection can be done. Agreement done between collector and purchaser should be documented.

Personnel:

- All personnel involved should have adequate botanical and agricultural or collection training. All personnel should have training in use of agrochemicals, appropriate harvesting techniques, avoidance of deterioration of harvested medicinal plant materials, post-harvest handling and primary processing stages.

- Personnel should be instructed on all relevant issues regarding sustainability, environmental protection, the conservation of plant species, soil management to conserve fields for cultivation and for soil erosion control and prevention of environmental damage.

Health and hygiene:

- Medicinal plant materials should be handled according to national and/or regional regulations on safety, materials handling, sanitation and hygiene. All personnel should be protected from contact with toxic or potentially allergenic herbs by means of adequate protective clothing, including gloves, eye wear or apron.

Health status:

- Personnel suffering from a disease or illness should not be allowed for working. Medical examination of personnel should be carried out if necessary.

Illness and injuries:

- Personnel with open wounds, inflammations, communicable diseases or skin diseases should not allowed to work till recovery. Persons suffering from known airborne or food-borne diseases like dysentery and diarrhoea should not be allowed to work.
- Health conditions that should be reported to the management while considering possible exclusion from handling of medicinal plant materials include: jaundice, diarrhoea, vomiting, fever, sore throat with fever, visibly infections and discharges from body.

Personal Cleanliness:

- All personnel should follow high degree of cleanliness, clean clothing, gloves, including head covering and footwear.
- All personnel should follow washing of their hands with soap when necessary to prevent any contaminated material to ensure safe operations.
- Smoking, eating, spitting, coughing should not be permitted in medicinal plant processing areas at any cost. Personnel should not use items such as jewellery, watches or other items that can cause possible threat for contamination.
- Visitors to processing and handling areas should wear appropriate protective clothing and adhere to all of the rules personal hygiene provisions mentioned above.

Other Issues Related to GAP:

- Ethical codes or norms of the community or country in which the activities take place should be followed. The provisions of the Convention on Biological Diversity must be followed for sustainability.

- In case of collection or cultivation of indigenous plant material, proper benefits should be given to community or country as per IPR laws.
- In case of endangered or threatened species, one should maintain all documentation according to Convention on International Trade in Endangered Species of Wild Fauna and Flora (CITES).

2.4 PEST AND PEST MANAGEMENT IN MEDICINAL PLANTS

Pests are unwanted creatures from animal or plant origin that affect yield of drug. Insects, weeds, rodents, mollusc, nematode, mites, ticks and fungi are most common type pests. Even unwanted, other plant species are also considered as pest. Pesticides are chemicals used to kill different types of pest. Pesticides can be classified according to type of organism on which they are effective like insecticide, herbicide, rodenticide, molluscicide, nematocide, acaricide and fungicide.

Cockroaches, rats, rodents and other different types of pest are harmful to mankind as they can cause various diseases or serious epidemics like the bubonic plague. Not only human beings but plants are also suffering from these pests. About 10 to 20 % of total food and crop production is destroyed by pest. On this background, use of pesticide becomes inevitable. Pesticides can be synthetic chemicals or natural compounds. After green revolution, use of synthetic pesticide has become a norm and increased continuously. After a decade or two, people are becoming aware about dangers of synthetic pesticides. There are few examples explaining harmful effect of pesticides on human and environment. World health organization's International agency for Research on Cancer has declared many pesticides as probable carcinogen.

Some examples of harmful effects of chemical pesticides:

- Use and adverse effects of 'Agent Orange' or dioxin is still controversial part of Vietnam War.
- More than 1000 people killed and hundreds were born defectives in Kasargod, Kerala because of indiscriminate use of endosulfan.
- Some pesticides like monocrotophos or highly toxic organophosphates which are discontinued in USA but still used in India.
- Pesticides like organochlorides: 1, 3 dichloropropene and other cause kidney damage, cancer, and ground water contamination.
- World's most widely used weed killer glyphosate popular brand name 'Roundup' is also in debate because of recent cases filed against company Monsanto.
- Some pesticides like neonicotinoides are harmful to main pollinators like bees and butterflies and creating problem for ecology.

Not only these, there are many incidents occurred worldwide because of use of pesticides. Over the time, the pest and diseases of plant as well as animals have developed resistance, as a result of which existing pesticides do not give expected results. Because of the problems associated with chemical pesticides, need for naturally occurring pesticides is always increasing.

Table 2.4: Some Common Synthetic Pesticides and Mechanism of Action

Sr. No.	Type	Example	Mechanism of Action
1.	Organochlorides	DDT, Chlordane, Aldrin, Heptachlor	Nervous system stimulation, convulsion, alter membrane permeability.
2.	Organophosphate	Bromophos, Chlorpyrifos, Parathion, Malathion,	Paralysis, bronchoconstriction, muscular weakness, CNS and respiratory depression.
3.	Pyrethrin class	Pyrethrin I, II, Fenvalerate, Permethrin	Seizures, nervous system hyperactivity, loss of co-ordination.
4.	Chlorophenoxy	2,4-D, 2,4,5-T	Muscle weakness, hypotonia.
5.	Bipyridyl	Paraquat, Diquat	Respiratory distress.
6.	Rodenticide	Warfarin, Strychnine	Prevent blood clotting.
7.	Carbamate	Carbaryl	CNS and respiratory depression.

Desired Properties of Pesticide:

- Effective.
- Environmentally safe.
- Must have potent effect on wide spectrum of pest.
- Low mammalian toxicity.
- Lack of neurotoxic activity.
- Low persistence in environment.
- Biodegradability.

Role of Plant Secondary Metabolites:

Use of secondary metabolites from plants is becoming popular because of several reasons. Secondary metabolites are chemicals produced by plant in less quantity and have special role. These secondary metabolites have limited role apart from growth and development of plant. There are several theories behind production of secondary metabolites by plants. More studies on physiology, biochemistry and ecology of secondary metabolites will result in plants with better protection against microbes and herbivores.

- Metabolic waste or as by-product or as excretory pathway.
- UV-Protection and nitrogen storage.

- Attraction of pollinating insects, seed dispersal, roots bacteria.
- Defence from herbivores: insect, mollusc, vertebrates.
- Growth inhibition, repellent, protection from other microbes like virus, bacteria, fungi through exhibiting toxicity, or as deterrent, anti-feedant or growth inhibition, protection from other plants while germination and growth of seedling.

Table 2.5: Some Common Secondary Metabolites and their Mechanism Behind Activity

Sr. No.	Secondary Metabolites	Mechanism Behind Pesticide Activity
1.	Saponin	Membrane disruption, change of protein conformation, inhibition of membrane protein
2.	Pyrrolizidine Alkaloides	Covalent modification, point mutation
3.	Camptothecin	Inhibition of DNA topoisomerase I
4.	Actinomycin D	Inhibition of transcription
5.	Berberin, Emetin, Quinine, Anthraquinine	Intercalation
6.	Nicotine	Modulation of neurocalation
7.	Aconitine	Modulation of ion channel
8.	Cyclopamine	Modulation of ion channel
9.	Phorbol esters	Modulation of regulatory protein
10.	HCN cyanogen	Inhibition of enzyme
11.	Isothiocyanates, sesquiterpenes, lactones	Covalent bonding, change of conformation
12.	Ligands, quinines, anthraquinones, isoquinolines	Non-covalent bonding and change of conformation

Table 2.6: Basic Difference between Plant, Animal and Fungi Cell

	Plant cell	Animal cell	Fungi cell
Hypae	Absent	Absent	Present
Cell wall	Cellulose	Chitin in exoskeleton cellulose	Chitin
Sterol	Sitosterol	Cholesterol	Ergosterol
Storage compounds	Starch in lipid sucrose	Glycogen, lipid trehalose in some	Glycogen, lipid trehalose

Contd...

Microtubules sensitivity	Colchicine	Colchicine	Sensitive to Benzimidazoles and griseofulvin
Nuclei	Diploid	Diploid	Haploid
Centriole	Present	Present	Absent
Lysine	Synthesized by Diaminopimelic acid Pathway	Not synthesized	Synthesized by α-aminodipic acid pathway

This difference between plant, animal and fungi cell is used as base for development of new pesticides. Development of new pesticide is carried out by using these targets which are different in plant, animal and fungi cells. In coming years, biotechnological intervention can give more targets. This target can be checked by using High Throughput Screeing (HTS) to search interaction of new molecules that inhibit these. Pesticide can work by different ways. Some pesticides can inhibit growth of pest while some kill pest after contact or inhalation. Some pesticides have unique mechanism. Antifeedants are compounds after application to plant, pest is not able to eat that plant and die from starvation.

Indian Government have passed 'The Insecticides Act 1968' to regulate the import, manufacture, sale, transport, distribution and use of insecticides with a view to prevent risks to human beings or animals. According to this law, the term 'insecticide' is any substance in the schedule or such other substances or preparations intended for the purposes of preventing, destroying, repelling or mitigating any insects, rodents, fungi, weeds and other forms of plant and animal life not useful to human beings.

Natural Pesticides:

Table 2.7: Types of Natural Pesticides

Sr. No.	Name of plant	Biological source	Active constituents	Uses
1.	Pyrethrum (Insect-flower)	Dried flowers of *Chrysanthemum cinerarifolium* (Compositae)	Pyrethrins I, II, Cinerin I, II	Domestic insect repellent, insecticide and contact-poison
2.	Neem (Margosa)	Aerial parts of *Azadiracta indica* (Maliaceae)	Azadirechtin, Nimbin, Nimbidin	Insecticide, antifeedant, nematicide, antimicrobial, antifungal

Contd...

3.	Derris (Tuba-root)	Rolts and rhizomes *Derris-elliptica* (Leguminosae)	Rotenone (tubatoxin), Tephrosin	Contact poison, insecticide, killing of hoppers, beetles, cater pillers and aphides
4.	Sabadilla (Caustic barley)	Ripe seeds of *Schoenoeauion offioinale* (Liliacae)	Sabadine, Cevadine	Domestic insecticides, killing of bugs, flies
5.	Tobacco	Dried leaves of *Nicotiana tobacum* (Solanaccae)	Nicotin, Nornicotin, Anabasine	Very potent insecticide
6.	Ryania (Ryanicide)	Roots and stems *Rysnia speriost* (Flacourtriceae)	Ryanodine	Insecticide

2.5 BIOPESTICIDES/BIOINSECTICIDES

Biopesticides are nothing but pesticides of biological origin, including microbial pesticides, entomopathogenic, nematodes, baculoviruses, plant derived pesticides or insect pheromones.

After successful implementation of 'Green Revolution; India became self-sufficient in food production. But while the production of food grains increased fourfold, soil and environment health have been affected adversely. According to one survey, application of 250 times more chemical fertilizers and 400 times higher applications of pesticides also happened in some cases. As harmful effects of chemical fertilizers and pesticides are evident, there is growing need for research and development for biological alternatives such as biopesticides and biofertilizers. Indian Government, Ministry of Agriculture has taken initiative under Dr. M.S. Swaminthan from 2004. In 2006, use of biopesticides was only about 12 to 15 %. Detailed framework has been prepared for the application of biotechnology in agriculture for security of food, health, environment and national as well as international trade. Large-scale field testing of released transgenic variety and seeds is under consideration as per agronomic requirements.

Table 2.8: Some Successful Applications of Biopesticides

Sr. No.	Control of Pest	Biopesticides Used
1.	Diamondback moths	*Bacillus thuringiensis*
2.	Mango hoppers, mealy bugs, coffee pod borers	*Beauveria*
3.	*Helicoverpa* on cotton, pigeon-pea on tomato	*Bacillus thuringiensis*

Contd...

4.	White fly on cotton	*Neem*
5.	Sugarcane borers	*Trichogramma*
6.	Rots and wilts in various crops	*Trichoderma*-based products

Tabel 2.9: Some Common Available Biopesticides in India

Sr. No.	Name of biopesticide	Average production (approx.)
1.	Neem 300 PPM	Over 1,000,000 L
2.	Neem 1500 PPM	Over 250,000 L
3.	*Bacillus thuringiensis*	Over 50,000 kg
4.	Nuclear Polyhedrosis Virus	Over 500,000 L.E
5.	*Beauveria*	--
6.	Pheromone traps	Over 500,000
7.	Lures	Over 2 million
8.	*Trichogramma*	1 million
9.	*Chrysoperla* and other biocontrol insects	--

Basic Points Behind use of Biopesticides:

- **Predator organisms:** In this approach, enemies of pest such as parasitoids, predators and insect pathogens are used to kill them.
- **Biochemicals:** These are behaviour-modifying chemicals such as pheromone analogues, antifeedant, repellents, attractants, direct toxicants, and insect growth regulators.
- **Pheromones:** In this approach, monitoring pests through field surveys and surveillance is carried out. This helps to set pheromone traps and lures to tackle the buildup of pests/diseases.

Advantages of Biopesticides:

- Biopesticides are less harmful to crop plant and human.
- They are highly specific in action.
- Biopesticides are very effective in small quantities also.
- Biopesticides are environmental friendly as they decompose quickly.
- They are only eco-safe alternative and do not have problematic residues.
- Development of resistance is less common in case of biopesticides.

Biological control of pest is increasing because of considerations of environmental safety and ecology. Biopesticides and bioinsecticides are welcomed by both farmers and consumers. Biological pest enemies such as predators (e.g., *Chrysoperia*), parasitoids (e.g., *Trichogramma*) are also considered as safe options to control pest.

Following are some examples of biopesticides and bioinsecticide:

- The fungi of *Trichoderma* spp. have proved useful for problems of many pathogens, including *Rhizoctonia solani, Sclerotium rolfsii, Sclerotinia sclerotiorum,* and *Pythium aphanidermatum.* They also can reduce the damage caused by *Botrytis cinerea, Pseuperonospora cubensis, Sclerotinia sclerotinia,* and *Sphaerotheca fusca* and thus important for protection of leaves.
- *Trichoderma harzianum* as nematode inhibitor, fungicide, and plant growth promoter.
- An alcoholic extract obtained from the plant *Albizzia lebbeck* (Fabaceae) along with *Bacillus thuriengiensis* delta-endotoxin acetone powder is used to kill lepidoptera insects very effectively even at very low dosage.
- *Streptomyces* strain with antimicrobial activity against phytopathogenic fungi. Novel strain of Streptomyces can inhibit capable of inhibiting the growth of a wide range of plant pathogenic fungi, including Rhizoctonia, Sclerotinia, Pythium, Fusarium, Curvularia and Alternaria.
- Use of plant essential oils is also promising. Many plants from families like Myrtaceae, Lamiaceae, Asteraceae, Apiaceae and Rutaceae are widely used to kill various pests from different ordrers like Lepidoptera, Coleoptera, Diptera, Isoptera and Hemiptera.
- Essential oils are used for repellent, fumigant, larvicidal and adulticidal activities against above insects.
- Plants containing essential oil like *Artemisia annua, Anethum sowa, Curcuma longa, Lippia alba* have potential for fumigant use. Many other compounds like eugenol, isoeugenol, cinnmate, menthol, safrol, d-limonene, carvones and 1, 8-cineole also have been well documented as fumigants and insect repellant.
- Compounds like cineole, geraniol and piperidine found in Bay leaves (*Laurus nobilis,* Lauraceae) possess repellent properties towards cockroaches.
- *Citrus aurantium* contain chemical named as Limonene is toxic to adult beanweevils (*Callosobruchus phasecoli*).
- Essential oils of *Artemisia* species have been reported for toxicity and repellent activity against different coleopteran beetles like *Sitophilus sp., Tribolium castaneum* and *Callosobruchus maculatus.*
- Some strain of *B. subtilis* inhibit the growth of several fungal pathogens including *Rhizoctonia soloni, Fusarium oxysporum, F. samitectum, Curvularia, Alternaria alternata, Colletotrichum acutatum, Colletotrichum capsici, Colletotrichum gloeosporioides, Corynespora, cassiicola,* and *Thielavia basicola in-vitro.*
- Trichogramma is genus of small polyphagous wasps that are used to control pest called as lepidopteron. Trichogramma is actually biological control of pest and can be considered as intergrated pest management. There are several species of Trichogramma

like *T. pretiosum, T. atopovirilia, T. carverae, T. brevicapillum, T. deion, T. exiguum, T. fuentesi, T. minutum* etc. These can be used to control other pests like cotton bollworm (*Helicoverpa armigera*), codling moth (*Cydia pomonella*), light brown apple moth (*Epiphyas postvittana*) and European corn borer (*Ostrinia nubilalis*) and also spruce bud moth (*Zeiraphera canadensis*).

- Nuclear Polyhedrosis Virus (NPV) is living virus used to control caterpillar named as *Spodopter litura* which is common pest grows on cotton, groundnut, pulses, cabbage, oil crops and roses.
- The seed oil from Custard apple (*Annona squamosa*) is used along with neem oil for control of the rice green leaf hopper pest *Nephotettrix virescens*.
- Shell oil of Cashew, *Anacardium occidentale* is used as insecticide.
- Seed oil and saponin from Mahua, *Madhuka latifolia* is used as insect repellant and insecticidal.
- Seed oil from *Pongamia pinnata* is used as insect repellant and insecticide.
- *Chrysoperla* is genus of green coloured lacewing insects common in North America and Europe. Larvae of these insects are predatory in nature and used to control aphids as biological pest control. Examples are *Chrysoperla mediterranea, Chrysoperla carne, Chrysoperla adamsi, Chrysoperla affinis, Chrysoperla argentina, Chrysoperla bellatule* etc.

QUESTIONS

1. Write in detail concept of biodynamic agriculture.
2. Explain concept of cow cat pit and biodynamic field spray.
3. What is organic farming? Write applications of organic farming.
4. Write Good Agriculutral Practices in cultivation of medicinal plants.
5. Which are different Good Collection Practices as per WHO?
6. What is pest? Give some harmful effects of chemical pesticides.
7. Explain role of plant secondary metabolites as pesticides with example.
8. Write a note on bioinsecticide with example.
9. Write a note on biopesticides with example.
10. Which are different plants used as natural pesticides?
11. Which are different examples of biopesticides and bioinsecticides?

Chapter...3

INDIAN SYSTEMS OF MEDICINE

Objectives

- To understand the basic principles of Ayurveda, Siddha, Unani, Homeopathy
- To understand preparation and evaluation of some Ayurvedic formulations

3.1 INTRODUCTION

There are several systems of medicine which are in practice worldwide. Allopathic system of medicine is recent system considered as Modern medicine systems. A group of diverse medical and health care practices and products that are not generally considered part of conventional medicine where alternative medicine indicates medicine used instead or in place of allopathic medicine is called as Complementary and Alternative Medicine (CAM). While Traditional Medicine (TM) is based on the theoris, experiences of indigenous people from different cultures. TM applies the knowledge, skills, practices of different cultures for the maintenance of health and in the prevention, diagnosis, improvement or treatment of physical and mental illness. For example, Ayurveda is traditional Indian system of medicine. China also has Traditional Chinese System of Medicine (TCM). There is one more term called as integrative medicine to describe combination of allopathic medicine with CAM that appears to be safe and have scientific base.

3.2 INDIAN SYSTEMS OF MEDICINE (ISM)

Indian civilization has rich tradition of various cultures. Indian system of medicine consists mainly 'Ayurveda', one of the oldest traditional systems of medicine still in use. Along with Ayurveda, other systems like Siddha, Unani and Homoeopathy also developed and flourished in India over the period. These all systems have unique blend, may be called as Indian System of Medicine. Ayurveda dates back to more than 5000 years also considered as Indian way of living. Siddha system was basically originated in southern part of India. Unani system as name indicated was originated in 'Yunan', country called as Greece today. Unani system was developed along with concepts of medicine called Tibb from Egypt and Mesopotamia. After contributions from Roman, Persian and Arab this system become developed. In eighth century, along with Mughal invasion, Unani system was introduced to India. Unani system along with traditional Indian system was flourished simultaneously. Today, Government of India has Central Council for Research in Unani Medicine (CCRUM) and this system is still in practice in India. Last two decades popularity of Indian system of medicine is increasing continuously. Government of India have department of AYUSH i.e. Ayurveda, Unani, Siddha and Homoeopathy to regulate traditional system of medicine. Ayurveda, Siddha and Unani systems of medicine have more than 90% formulations which are plant based.

Traditional System of Medicine (TSM):

According to World Health Organization (WHO), Traditional Medicine is the sum total of the knowledge, skills, and practices based on the theories, beliefs and experiences indigenous to different cultures, whether explicable or not, used in the maintenance of health as well as in the prevention, diagnosis, improvement or treatment of physical and mental illnesses. Examples of TSM include Traditional Chinese System of Medicine (TCM), Ayurvedic System of Medicine, Traditional African System of Medicine (TAM) or Traditional African Medical System (TAMS), Jamu (Indonesian Medicine System), Kampo (Japanese Traditional Medicine) and *Tibb-I-Islam* (Islamic Medicine). Conventional medicine system, also known as Western medicine system (popularly called as Allopathy) is considered as main stream system. 'Complementary' generally refers to using a non-mainstream approach together with conventional medicine. 'Alternative System' refers to using a non-mainstream approach in place of conventional medicine. Traditional medicine covers a wide variety of therapies and practices which vary from country to country and region to region. In some countries, it is referred to as "alternative" or "complementary" medicine (CAM). Examples of CAM include Medical Herbalism (Use of plant remedies or natural products), Homoeopathy, Aromatherapy, Flower Remedy, Naturopathy etc.

Table 3.1: Basics of Various Systems of Medicine

Criteria	Ayurveda (*Ayu-life; Veda-study*)	Siddha	Unani	Homoeopathy (*Homo-similar; pathos-study*)
Origin	India	South India	Yunan (Greece)	Germany
Period of origin	5000 BC	Pre-vedic period, Dravidian culture	1025 AD	200 years before date (Eighteenth century)
Historical person	Charaka, Sushruta	Siddhars, Agasthya	Hippocrates, Golen, Rhazes (al-Razi), Avicenna (Ibn Sena)	Samuel Hahnemann

Contd...

Historical books	Atharvaveda, Charaka Samhita, Sushruta Samhita	Tamil literatre	-	The Organon of Medicine
Main principle	'*Prana*'- the life energy or vital force; five element theory (earth, water, fire, air and space), Tridosha theory, Saptdhatu.	Five basic elements and humours - vatha, pitta and kapha and seven physical constituents	Hippocratic theory of four humours and Pythagorian theory of four proximate qualities, Umur-e-tabia	Like cures like, homoeopathic drug potentization, homeopathic drug proving, succession (minimal dose), single remedy at any one time
Cause of disease	Imbalance in Tridosha (vata, kapha, pitta), imbalance between mala and saptdhatu	Disturbed mind and body equilibrium	Imbalance between humours	Body's inability to cope with challenging factors such as poor diet and external environment
Diagnosis	Nadi, karma		Pulse, urine, stool and patient review	Detailed interview of patient
Treatment	Panchkarma, yoga	Deva *Maruthuvam*, (divine method); *Maanida Maruthuvam* (rational method); and *Asura Maruthuvam* (surgical method)	*Izalae Sabab* (elimination of cause), *Tadeele Akhlat* (normalization of humors), Tadeele *Aza* (normalization of tissues/organs), Polyherbal formulations and salts	Dilutions, trituration

Contd...

Formulations	Asava, Arishtha, Kwath, Avaleha, Churna, Gutika, Ghrita, Bhasma		Madar, fufal, Gilo, Kababchini, Karanj, Kulthi, Lodh, Qust, Sana, Tagar, Zeera, Siyah	Mother tincture, pills.
Important Plants	Amala, Ashwagandha, Guduchi, Sarpagandha, Shunthi,	Abini, Alari, Haikalli, Ratha polam, Gomathai	Polyherbal formulations and salts	Colchicum, Aconite, Nux vomica, Belladonna, Arsenic oxide, Arnica, Calcium carbonate.

3.2.1 Ayurveda

Origin: Ancient system of medicine originated in India.

Period of origin: Originated almost 5000 years before and still in practice throughout India and some other parts of world.

History: History of Ayurveda goes back to different Vedas or classical books, main contributors include Charak, Sushrut.

Historical books: Charak Samhita, Sushruta Samhita.

Basic principle: Vital energy called 'Prana' which activates body and mind. Ayurveda believes in different theories mainly five element theory and tridosha theory. Everything in universe is composed of five basic elements (*panch mahabhuta*) namely space, air (*vayu*), energy, liquid (*jala*) and solid. These five basic elements exist in every human body in the form of *vata*, *kapha* and *pitta* called *Tridosha*. Any one of the dosha, which is dominating in particular person called as Prakruti of that person. Human body is composed of seven elements called *saptdhatu* namely *rasa* (lymph), *rakta* (blood), *meda* (adipose tissue, fat), *mamsa* (muscle, flesh), *majja* (nervine tissue), *shukra* (reproductive tissue), *asthi* (bone).

Panch Maha-bhuta	Tridosha	Saptadhatu
Space	*Vatta*	*Rasa* (Lymph)
Air	*Kapha*	*Rakta* (Blood)
Energy	*Pitta*	*Meda* (Lipids)
Jal		*Mamsa* (Muscles)
Soloid		*Majja* (Nervine-tissue)
		Shukra (Reproductive tissue)
		Asthi (Bone)

Cause of disease: Imbalance between *tridosha*, *saptdhatu* and *mala* causes disease.

Diagnosis: Person who practices Ayurveda called Vaidya takes account of *Nadi* (pulse) and *prakruti, tridosha*. Based on this, different drug formulations and diet is advised. Basic diagnosis involves *mala*, *mutra*, tongue, thirst, eyes.

Formulations: Different formulations are available in Ayurvedic system of medicine like swaras, kalka, kwath, hima, phant. Other formulations are also available like churna, avaleha, asava, arishta, ghrita, sandhanakalpa, bhasma, mashi, parpati, vati.

Table 3.2: Important Plants and Their Uses

Botanical name	Ayurvedic Name	Family	Use
Acacia catechu	Khadira	Mimosaceae	Digestive
Adhatoda vasika	Vaasaka	Acanthaceae	Cough
Aegle marmelos	Bilva	Rutaceae	Diarrhoea
Aloe barbadensis	Ghritakumari	Liliaceac	Purgative
Azadirachta indica	Nimba	Meliaceae	Blood purifier
Bacopa monnieri	Braahmi	Scrophulariaceae	Memory enhancer
Centella asiatica	Mandukaparni	Umbelliferae	Rasayana, brain tonic
Cissus quadrangular	Asthisamhaara	Vitaceae	Fracture of bone
Curcuma longa	Haridra	Zingiberaceae	Cough, immunity booster
Ocimum sanctum	Tulasi	Labiatae	Immunomodulator
Piper longum	Pippali	Piperaceae	Bio enhancer
Piper nigrum	Maricha	Piperaceae	Respiratory disorders
Terminalia arjuna	Arjuna	Combretaceae	Cardio tonic
Terminalia chebula *Terminalia balerica*	Haritaki Bahera	Combretaceae Combretaceae	Constipation
Tinospora cordifolia	Guduchi	Menispermaceae	Rasayana
Zingiber officinale	Aardraka	Zingiberaceae	Emitic, appetizer

3.2.2 Siddha

The contributors of Siddha system, the Siddhars, of Tamil land, were yogis and seers and medical men of various combinations who developed this system. It is believed that there was a line of 18 siddhars, with Agasthya being the foremost. Large portion of Siddha knowledge is credited to Agasthya. The Siddhars were super human beings with different types of Siddhis or supernatural powers. They were considered as the greatest scientists of ancient times and the guardians of the world. They were men of great practical knowledge and wisdom. They had full awareness of the nature and activities of all the objects in this planet and of all times-past, present and future. Th Siddhars brought about the growth and development of Tamil medicine and its different branches like alchemy, medicine, yoga, kayakalpa (rejuvenation therapy), philosophy, astronomy, astrology, *varma, muppu, thokkanam* etc.

Origin: This system was originated in south India and believes in Bhakti and Yoga. The term Sidhha means achievement and the person who practice system are called Saint or Sadhu. The term 'Siddha' means achievement and 'Siddhars' were saintly personalities, who attained proficiency in medicine through practice of Bhakti and Yoga.

Period of origin: This is the system of pre-vedic period identified with Dravidian culture and it is largely therapeutic in nature.

Historical books: The literature of Siddha system is mostly in Tamil.

Main principle: In siddha system every individual is a microcosm of the universe. The human body consists of the five primordial elements and humours - vatha, pitta and kapha and seven physical constituents. Food is the basic building material of the human body and gets processed into humours, tissues and wastes.

Cause of disease: Disturbed mind and body equilibrium is main cause of disease. The equilibrium of humours is considered as health. When there is disturbance or imbalance, this leads to a disease according to Saint Thiruvalluvar in his *Thirukural.*

Diagnosis: Eight types of examinations are used for diagnosis. The identification of causative factors of diseases is done through pulse reading, colour of body, study of voice, urine examination, status of digestive system and examination of tongue. The diagnostic methodology in Siddha treatment is unique. Physician's acumen or skill is very crucial. The patient is examined with the help of pulse, skin, tongue, complexion, speech, eye, stools and urine.

Treatment: Three main types of medicines are used in this system. Mainly *Thaavaram* (herbal product), *Thaathu* (inorganic substances), and *Jangamam* (animal products) are considered as source of drugs. Mainly three types of treatments can be used like *Deva Maruthuvam* (divine method); *Maanida Maruthuvam* (rational method); and *Asura Maruthuvam* (surgical method). Medicines prepared from herbs like churanam, kudineer, vadagam are used. In surgical method, incision, excision, heat application, bloodletting, leech application etc. are practiced. Siddha treatment also includes purgation, emesis, fasting, steam, oleation and Yoga. There is also a branch of the traditional science that deals with injuries called *Varma* based on 100 vital points that are junctions of bones, tendons, ligaments, blood vessels and nerves called Varma points.

Formulations:

Siddha system uses medicines like *parpam, chenduram, guru, kuligai* prepared from mercury, sulphur and *pashanams*.

3.2.3 Unani

Unani system of medicine is called by various names in different parts of world such as Arab medicine, Greco-Arab medicine, Loniah medicine, Islamic medicine and also Oriental medicine.

Origin: This system is considered of Greek origin further spread to Persia (Iran), where it has been developed by Arabian physicians.

Period of origin: Time of origin is believed around 1025 AD. In 12th century this system has entered in India with Mughal Empire.

Historical person: The ancestries of this system go deep to the times of the well-known Greek philosopher Hippocrates who is credited with it. Aristotle Gelen (384 - 322 BC) Greek - Philosopher "Father of natural history" made valuable contributions to it. System further developed by Arabian and Persian physisions such as Rhazes (*al-Razi*), Avicenna (*Ibn Sena*) etc.

Main principle: Unani system follows Hippocratic theory of four humours and the Pythagorian theory of four proximate qualities. According to this system, the four humours are blood, phelgm, yellow bile and black bile while the four qualities are the states of living human body like hot, cold, moist and dry. They are denoted as earth, water, fire and air. The Greek ideas were put by Arabian physicians as seven working principles (Umur-e-Tabia) and included elements, temperaments, humours, organs, life, spirit, energy and actions. They assumed that these principles are responsible for the body constitution and its health, as well as, the diseased conditions. The theory postulates the presence of blood, phlegm, yellow bile and black bile in the human body. Each person has different and unique blend of these substances determines which his Mizaj (temperament).

Cause of disease: According to this system, imbalance the imbalance between humours is main cause of disease. Treatment id given accordingly. This abnormal humor results in pathological changes in the tissues teherby exhibiting the clinical manifestations.

Diagnosis: Detailed history of the patient is recorded in addition to his pulse, urine and stool examinations for diagnostic purpose. In the diagnosis, clinical features, i.e., signs, symptoms, laboratory features and Mizaj (temperament) are important.

Treatment: The Unani system of medicine aims at treating the cause of disease and not its symptoms. The drugs are mainly polyherbal formulations and salts. After diagnosing the disease, *Usoolellaj* (principle of management) of disease is determined on the basis of etiology in the following pattern: *Izalae Sabab* (elimination of cause), *Tadeele Akhlat* (normalization of humors), *Tadeele Aza* (normalization of tissues/organs)

Formulations: Madar, fufal, Gilo, Kababchini, Karanj, Kulthi, Lodh, Qust, Sana, Tagar, Zeera, Siyah.

3.2.4 Homoeopathy

Origin: Homoeopathy is relatively new system of medicine found by Samuel Hahnemann, a German Physician and chemist.

Period of origin: 200 years ago.

Historical person: Samuel Hahnemann is known as Father of Homoeopathy.

Historical books: 'The Organon of Medicine' by Samuel Hahnemann.

Main principle: Homoeopathy is based on few basic fundamental rules like '*Similae similibus curentur*' popularly known as law of simibus which literally means 'like cures like'. Minumum dose and single medicine at one time are other important aspects of homoeopathy.

Homoeopathic drug proving is the process in which new drug is given to healthy volunteer and symptoms are carefully noted. These symptoms generated in healthy volunteer are then compared with disease condition. Then according to this theory that drug can be used to treat that disease. For example, if onion is given to healthy person, it will produce tears in eyes and nasal congestion. So onion can be used for treatment of cold, which has similar symptoms. Another example of drug proving is cinchona. If cinchona is given to healthy person it produces fever like condition, which is almost similar as that of malaria. So cinchona can be used for treatment of malaria. Similarly Coffee, which is CNS stimulant, can be used to treat insomnia.

Cause of disease: According to homoeopathy, disease results from body's inability to cope with challenging factors like poor diet or environmental conditions. Signs and symptoms generated because of disease is nothing but bodies attempt to restore order. Body's own healing power (vital force) is important and it is stimulated by homoeopathic drugs.

Diagnosis: Diagnosis is done by asking different questions and taking patients detail history, physical, mental and emotional symptoms and comparing them with symptoms produced by drug in healthy individual.

Formulations: Formulation includes dilutions or trituration of various vegetable drugs, animal drugs, minerals and metals. Plants used mainly include Arnica, Belladonna, Marigold, Chamomile, Colchicum, Hemlock, Hyoscyamus, Hypericum, Ipecacuhna, Lycopodium, Opium, Ergot, Thuja, Aconite, Nux-vomica. It also contain salts like carbonates, arsenic oxide, barium carbonate, calcium phosphate, kalashisa, mercuric chloride, antimony tartarate, sulphur, copper, aluminium and phosphorus.

Homoeopathic drug potentization is a process of serial dilution which arouses or increases the inherent curative power of medicine.

Theory of dilution or succussion: Starting point of most of homoeopathic medicine is mother tincture or mother solution. Mother tincture is then diluted either by decimal method or centicimal method. In decimal method, one drop/ part of mother tincture is mixed with nine drops/ drops of diluents to get 1 X. Further one drop/ part from 1X is diluted by nine parts of diluents to get 2X potency. In centicimal scale, one part of mother tincture is diluted with 99 parts to get 1C. Further one part from 1C is mixed with 99 parts of diluents to get 2C potency. More the dilution, drug becomes more potent. Potencies of 24X or 12 C is diluted beyond that, Avogadro's number, so hardly containing molecule of original material. Homoeopaths believe that, the effect is due to 'memory of water' or imprints of original starting molecules on solvent. Homoeopathic remedies are so dilute that highly unlikely to cause adverse drug effect. However, recent clinical trials showed some mild adverse effect as compared to placebo.

3.3 PREPARATION AND STANDARDIZATION OF AYURVEDIC FORMULATIONS

Importance of Standardization:

Standardization is the process of setting quality parameters. Standardization gives rise to uniformity and consistency in quality of product. Properly standardized formulations are more effective with fewer side effects. Ayurvedic formulations are becoming more popular and enjoying widespread acceptance. However, with the increasing demands, rising concerns about safety are also becoming important. But at the same time, people want standardized and good quality of formulation. Due to the complex nature and intrinsic variability of the chemical constituents of Ayurvedic formulations, it is difficult to establish standardization parameters. Ayurvedic formulations, if standardized properly can have more security and increase the level of trust. Generally, Ayurvedic formulations have unique, traditional way of quality control but these formulations can also be standardized by using modern methods. Analytical protocols are available to ascertain consistency and quality of Ayurvedic formulations which is most welcoming towards safe and effective Ayurvedic formulations. The pharmacopoeial standards for Ayurvedic Formulations published by the Government of India, Ministry of Health and Family Welfare give certain physical parameters as standards for different formulations. However, these are not sufficient and there is a need to develop other additional methods for quality control based on modern analytical methods.

Table 3.3: Summary of Types of Ayurvedic Formulations

Formulation	Nature	Preparation	Standardization	Example
Arista	Liquid	Self-generated alcoholic preparations, prepared from **decoction of the raw drug** mixed with sugar to undergo fermentation.	Alcohol content	Ashokarista, Vidangarista, Draksharista, Arjunarishta, Dasamoolaarishtam, Amruthaarishtam, Kutajaarishtam, Balarishtam, Devadaarvaarishtam,

				Jeerakaarishtam, Khadirashtam
Asava	Liquid	Self-generated alcoholic preparations which are prepared from **juices of fresh plants** or water soaked dry drugs mixed with sugar to undergo fermentation.	Alcohol content	Lohasava, Kumariasava, Madhukasava, Drakshasav, Patrangaasavam
Bhasma	Solid	Fine powder of a metal or substance obtained by complete burning or incineration	Particle size, metal content	Swarn bhasma, Mukta bhasma, Naga bhasma, Tamra bhasma
Churna	Solid	Fine powder of drug or drugs	Particle size	Triphala churna, Mandukaparni churna, Rasnadi churna, Ashwagandha churna
Gutika	Solid	Pills prepared by triturating fine powder of drug with water or binder	Uniformity in weight, shape and size	Eladi gutika, Pranada gutika, Dugdha vati
Lehya	Semisolid	Sugar based preparation of drugs, prepared by boiling juice of the drug or its decoction.	Consistency	Chyavanprash, Draksavaleha, Vasavaleha

3.3.1 Asava and Arishta

Arishtas are made with decoctions of herbs in boiling water while asavas are prepared by directly using fresh herbal juices. These are unique liquid dosage forms that contain self-generated alcohol. Arishta (fermented decoction) and Asava (fermented infusion) are considered as a unique and valuable therapeutics in Ayurveda, due to their medicinal value, sweet taste and easy availability.

Preparation:

Asava and aristha are manufactured similarly with slight difference in starting material. Absolute cleanliness is necessary for manufacture of these preparations. Earthen pot used for fermentation should be old and properly cleaned. Fumigation with *Pipali Churna* should be done along with smearing with *Ghee*. According to Ayurvedic literature, self-generated alcohol acts as preservative so these preparations come without expiry date.

Preparation of Asava:

- The drugs mentioned in the texts are coarsely powdered and *Kashay* is prepared.
- *Kashay* is then filtered and kept in the fermentation pot.
- As per procedure, sugar or jaggery or honey are dissolved and added to solution after filtration.
- Finely powdered other drugs called as *Prakshep dravya* are added.
- *Dhataki Pushpa* which is dried flower of plant *Woordfordia fructicosa* is added at the end only.
- These flowers contain yeast, which brings about fermentation of sugar present.
- The mouth of the pot, vessel or barrel is covered with an earthen lid and the edges are sealed with clay-smeared cloth. Seven continuous layers of this cloth are used for covering.
- The pot is placed undisturbed in a heap of paddy to ensure fermentation. Temperature is maintained constant throughout entire period.
- During this period bubbling sound can be heard from pot because of releasing gas.
- After the specified period, the lid is removed, and the contents are examined to ascertain whether the process of fermentation called as *Sandhana* is completed.
- The fluid is first decanted and then filtered after two or three days to settle particles. If needed, this step can be repeated before bottling.

Preparation of Arishta:

- According to formula, jaggery or sugar are added to specific quantity of water.
- This mixture is boiled and cooled.
- After cooling, poured into the fermentation pot.
- Finely powdered drugs are added to this liquid.
- *Dhataki Pushpa* which is dried flower of plant *Woordfordia fructicosa* added at the end only while liquid is not hot.
- Further method of preparation of Arishta is same with preparation of Asava.

Standardization of Asava and Arishta:

Traditionally quality of Asava or Arishta is checked by absence of foam or froth. It should be clear sour tasting liquid.

Asava and arishta can be standardized with the help of following parameters:

Organoleptic characters: Colour, odour, taste, pH, foreign organic matter, ash value (total ash value, acid insoluble ash, water soluble ash, sulphated ash), extractive value (alcohol soluble extractive value and water soluble extractive value), moisture content, physical constant (melting point, boiling point, refractive index, optical rotation, specific gravity, solid content, alcohol content.

Chemical evaluation can be performed by using tests like a) Alkaloids - Dragandroffs test b) Glycosides - Molish test c) Flavonoids - Shinoda test d) Phenolic - Lead acetate test e) Tannins - Ferric chloride test f) Steroids - Salkowski reaction g) Amino acids - Ninhydrine test h) Carbohydrates - Fehling's test, Benedict test.

Toxicological parameters: It involves checking of parameters like pesticides residue, presence of heavy metal and microorganism.

Kumari Asava Compostion:

Kumari (*Aloe vera*), Haritaki (*Terminalia chebula*), Jatamansi (*Nardodtychys jatamansi*), Clove (*Syzygium aromaticum*), Long pepper, Chitrak (*Plumbago zeylanica*), Javitri (Myristica fragrance), Kakatshringi (*Pistacia chinensis*), Bibhitaki (*Terminalia belerica*), Pushkarmul (*Inula racemosa*), Loh Bhasma, Tamra Bhasma along with jaggery, honey and water.

Arjunarishta Composition:

Terminalia arjuna bark 4.80 kg, *Vitisvenifera* fruits 2.40 kg, *Madhuca indica* flowers 0.96 Kg, *Woodfordia fruiticosa* flowers 0.96 kg, Jaggery 4.80 kg, Water 49.152 L.

3.3.2 Gutika

Gutika is one of the simple Ayurvedic medicines like pill or tablet. Gutika is palatable and easy to consume, store and preserve. There are many examples of Gutika formulations in Ayurveda. Classical Ayurvedic text and Ayurvedic formulary of India (AFI) can be used to refer the formula for particular Gutika.

Preparation:

- First plant material is dried and made into fine powder.
- Other minerals, if mentioned in the formula are made into Bhasma in fine powdered form.
- In some cases, where mercury (*Parada*) and sulphur (*Gandhaka*) are mentioned, *Kajjali* (purified and consumable form of mercury and sulphur) is made first and other drugs are added to it, one by one.
- Mix the entire ingredients in mortar and pastel (Khalva). Triturate herb, bhasma or other ingredients.
- Mix prescribed fluid to above mentioned ingredients to form soft paste.
- Add any other liquid mentioned, if any.
- When mass will convert into soft paste, additional aromatic and flavoring materials, perfume can be added like *Kasturi, Karpura.*
- Triturate more to mix all the ingredients.
- Take non-sticky material while rolled to the fingers; make pills of required size by hand or pills making machine or automatic tablet punching machine.

- Dry the pill in shade or under sun according to requirement.
- Sugar or jaggery (*Guda*) or Guggulu (*Commiphora mukul*) or Babool (*Acacia arabica*) gum resin can be added as binder. In this case, binder should be added in liquid and then mixing is carried out.

There are different approaches for preparation of Gutika, like *sompakvidhi*, kwath along with other ingredients and mixture is patted 1000 times before manual rolling and preparation of Gutika by hand. In *suryapakvidhi*, quath and powder mixture is mixed and kept under sunlight. This process is repeated for several times before preparation of Gutika. In *analpakvidhi*, gentle heat is applied to form semisolid mass.

Standardization:

Traditional methods: Quality of Gutika can be checked by various parameters. Traditionally colour, odour, taste, size, and shape of Gutika can be checked.

Modern methods: Although Gutika is considered as traditional formulation, modern quality control and standardization parameters can be employed for it. Mainly Gutika can be evaluated for weight variation, disintegration test, hardness test, LOD, volatile oil content, total ash or even absorption of wavelength under UV spectrophotometer.

Physicochemical evaluation: Extractive value, pH, ash value, loss on drying can be used for standardization of Gutika.

Qualitative analysis: Phytochemical tests and alkaloid content, glycoside content or sugar content can be done.

Chromatography: TLC or HPTLC for content evaluation can be done.

Generally, Gutika have two years of shelf life, when stored in airtight containers. Some bhasma or mineral containing Gutika claims no expiry date. However, it should not loose original colour, smell, taste and form.When sugar, jaggery, salt or Kshara ingredients are used in Gutika, it should be kept away from moisture.

Examples:

Chandraprabha Vati, Eladi Gutika, Dhanwantaram Pills, Arogyavardhini Vati, Pushpadhanva Rasa.

Formula of Arogyavardhini Vati:

Picrorhiza Kurroa (Kutki) 50%, *Shuddha Guggulu* 10%, *Plumbago Zeylanica* (Chitrak) 10%, *Shilajit* (purified asphaltum) 7.5%, *Emblica officinalis* (Amla, Indian Gooseberry) 5%, *Terminalia bellirica* (Bibhitaki) 5%, *Terminalia chebula* (Haritaki) 5%, *Parad* Purified (*Shuddha Parad*) 0.5%, Purified Sulfur (*Shuddha Gandhak*) 0.5%, Loha Bhasma (*Lauh Bhasma*) 0.5%, *Abhrak Bhasma* 0.5%, *Tamra Bhasma* 0.5%.

3.3.3 Churna

Table 3.4: Types of Churna

Sr. No.	Name of Churna	Composition	Use
1.	Triphala Churna	*Phyllanthus emblica, Terminalia Belerica, Terminalia chebula*	Constipation, jaundice, anaemia, asthma, fever, chronic ulcers
2.	Trikatu Churna	*Piper nigrum, Piper longum, Zingiber officinale*	Cold, cough, appetizer, carminative, purgative
3.	Sitopaladi Churna	*Piper longum, Elettaria cardamomum, Cinnamomum zeylanicum*	Pleurodynia, intercostal neuralgia, coughs associated with bronchitis, supportive agent for allergy, viral respiratory infection, and in pharyngeal and chest congestion.
4.	Ajmodadi Churna	*Apium graviolens, Embelia ribe, Piper longum, Piper nigrum, Terminalia chebula, Anethum sova, Plumbago zylanica*	Carminative, antispasmodic, wormifuge

According to Ayurvedic system of medicine, Churna is defined as, "a fine powder of one or more drugs". Churna formulation is similar to powder formulations in Allopathic system of medicine. Now-a-day's churna is formulated into tablets in order to fix the dose easily and for convenience. These forms of medicament are prescribed generally because of their particle size. Smaller particle size of churna, better is the effect on body. Churna should be given with some other vehicle like honey, milk or sugar. This make administration of Churna easy and increased palatability also enhances therapeutic effect. Such vehicle is called as *Anupan* in Ayurveda.

Preparation:

- Plant material is collected and cleaned.
- Plant material is dried in shade or sun according to specific requirements.
- Dried material is pulverized and then sieved through mesh 60 or 80 according to drug.
- Finally, it is stored in well closed container on proper place.

Standardization:

Traditional method: The ideal Churna should be free flowing and without lumps or big particles. It should retain its potency for one year, if preserved in airtight containers. It should not change its colour, odour.

Modern method: Particle size, angle of repose, flow properties of Churna can be studied by using different modern analytical instruments.

Respective biological activity can be done to evaluate Churna. Apart from that pH, ash value, extractive value, moisture content, heavy metal, microorganisms, fibre content can be studied for standardization of Churna.

3.3.4 Lehya

Lehya is also known as or Avaleh one of the several groups of Ayurvedic formulations. It arises from Sanskrit root word *Lih Aswadane*, means it should be tasted with tongue. It is a semi-solid sugar based preparation. Lehya is prepared by using jaggery, sugar or sugar candy and boiled with prescribed drug juice or decoction. In some Lehya formulation, honey and ghee is also used as common ingredient. Generally, Lehya is supposed to be taken with some vehicle like water, goat milk, butter milk called as *Anupan*.

Preparation:

Lehya can be prepared by different ways. But following are some common points:

- First sugar is dissolved into liquid medium, which can be water or juice. Liquids used in preparation of Lehya may be decoction (*Kashay*) or expressed juice (*Swaras*) or hot infusion (*Phanta*). Different types of sweetening agents can be used like sugar, jaggery, sugar candy, honey etc.
- The liquid containing sugar is heated and concentrated till '*Paka*' stage. At this stage, concentrated semi-liquid will form into a thread when pressed between the thumb and index finger and released.
- Fine powder of drug is added into this mixture along with oil and ghee to get the semi-solid form. These are certain additives to increase potency of formulation called *Prakshep dravya* which can be herbal or metallic. Fat or oil added which works as *Sneha dravya*.
- Honey is added once the mixture is cooled. It is stirred further to get the appropriate semi-solid form.
- This is special formulation like medicated jam and should not be prepared overnight. Each avaleha need minimum seven days to one month to mature. After preparation it should be kept in proper place for maturation.

There can be two approaches for preparation of Lehya:

In first approach, juice or decoction is heated into a semisolid paste and after those fine powders of the *Prakshepa dravyas* are added. In the second approach, jaggery or sugar is mixed with water and heated till it becomes thick syrup followed by addition of prescribed drugs.

Precaution should be taken while addition of *Prakshepa dravyas*. *Prakshepa dravyas* should be added at the end when preparation is hot. *Sugandha dravyas* and *Madhu* (Honey) should be added after cooling.

Standardization of Lehya:

Traditional approach: Traditionally Lehya preparation is done like in-process quality control. While preparation of *Paka* or jaggery, it should pass some quality control tests like thread appearance of *Paka*, non-spreading of Paka when put in water, sinking in water. Finished Lehya product should stick to ladle, it should be non-spreading when placed on horizontal surface apart from this, colour, odour, taste are also checked to ensure good quality product.

Modern approach: As Lehya is polyherbal formulation, it is difficult to standardize by using modern instruments because of complex nature. Physico chemical parameters like Colour, odour, consistency and taste can be checked in order to determine quality of formulation. Also loss on drying, total ash value, extractive value and pH can be measured to determine quality of Lehya. Recently some research work is focused on standardization of Lehya by using chemical marker by HPTLC and HPLC is also under progress.

Analytical parameters which can be checked for Lehya are organoleptic properties (description colour, taste, odour, loss on drying, total ash, acid soluble ash, pH, total solid, fat content, identifications TLC/HPTLC, test for heavy metals like lead, cadmium etc. Apart from this, microbial contamination (Total bacterial count, Total fungal count), test for specific pathogen (*E. Coli*; *Salmonella* etc. pesticide residue (Organochlorine pesticides; organophosphorus pesticides etc.), test for Aflatoxins (B_1, B_2, G_1, G_2) also need to conducted for determination of quality.

Example:

Ashwagandhadi lehya contain Ashwagandha (*Withania somnifera*), *Elettaria cardamonum, Myristica fragrans, Glycyrrhiza glabra, Hemidesmus indicus* and *Cuminum cyminum*. Ashwagandhadi lehya is indicated in disorder of blood, cachexia, piles, psychosis, rejuvenating agent and aphrodisiac.

Other examples: Vachadhatryyadi Avaleha used to increase immunity.

3.3.5 Bhasma

Bhasma is a calcinated preparation in which the gem or metal is converted into ash after complete burning or incineration. Gems or metals are first purified in order to remove impurities. Then they are triturated with herbal extracts. The resultant mass is calcinated or burned to obtain the ashes.

'*Vibhuti*' (Sanskrit) and '*Thiruneeru*' (Tamil) are synonymous used for Bhasma. *Bhasmikaran* is a process by which a substance which is otherwise bio-incompatible is made biocompatible by certain *samskaras* or processes.

The objectives of *samskara* are: a) removal of harmful matters from the drug b) modification of unwanted properties of the drug c) conversion of some of the characteristics of the drug d) enhancement of the effect.

Various steps involved in the preparation of bhasma (bhasmikaran) are: 1) Shodhana-Purification, 2) Marana – Size reduction or powdering, 3) Chalan- Stirring, 4) Dhavana -

Washing, 5) Galan- Cleaning or filtering, 6) Putan- Heating, 7) Mardan- Triturating with mixing, 8) Bhavana- Coating with herbal extract, 9) Amrutikaran - Detoxification and 10) Sandharan - Preservation. Above mentioned steps can be selected depending upon type of metal. Sequence of these steps can be changed according to specific Bhasma. Details of *Bhasmikaran* process are as followsis elaborated in details in the following paragraphs.

Methods of Preparation:

Different types of bhasma are prepared by different ways depending upon metal or raw material involved. Preparation of bhasma involves two basic steps which are most common. However, some special type of bhasma may employ slight different approach.

- **Shodhana** (detoxification or purification) which can be done by washing of raw material (*Prakshalana*), trituration (*Mardana*), boiling with cow urine, milk, certain juice (*Swedana*), reduction of toxic properties by triturating with certain juice or decoction (*Bhavana*), roasting (*Bharjana*), heating and quenching (*Nirvapa*), melting of raw material and adding lime water or vegetable juice (Dhalana), distillation to remove impurity (*Patana*).
- **Marana** (incineration) which involves killing of metallic properties by several repeated steps.

Shodhana: The principle objective of shodhana is to remove unwanted part from the raw material and purification of metal. Metals obtained from ores may contain several impurities, which are removed by subjecting them to Shodhana process. Shodhana means purifying and making the product suitable for the next step i.e. Maran. Ayurveda classifies shodhana into a) General process can be (*Samanya Shodhana*) and b) Specific process (*Vishesh Shodhana*). General process for shodhana involves heating of metal and successively dipping or quenching into liquids like oil, buttermilk, cow's urine while metal is red hot. The procedure is repeated seven times or in certain cases thousand times. After heating and cooling successively, metal starts to lose its metallic properties. In certain cases, like specific process for shodhana for some metals a specific process is described for shodhana e.g. for purification of Jasad, the molten mass is poured in cow's milk 21 times.

Marana: Meaning of word Marana is killing. In this step, there is change in the chemical form or state of the metal. Because of this, metal lose its metallic characteristics and physical nature. Marana can be done with mercury, plants or sulfur. In short, after marana, metal can be converted into powder or other form suitable for administration. This step removes toxicity of metal used and make safe for consumption. Use of mercury is most controversial topic according to modern system of medicine, although considered as safe in Ayurveda. Bhasma prepared by using *Rasa* i.e. mercury is considered as the best quality while prepared using herbs are of better quality and those prepared using *Gandhak* (sulfur) is of inferior quality.

Chalan: Iron rod from specific plant is used for stirring hot metal. This process of stirring during heating the metal is called as chalan.

Dhavan: This step involves washing with water to remove the excess amounts of agents used in shodhana or marana stage to remove water soluble constituents.

Galan: The product is then sifted either through a fine muslin cloth or through sieves of suitable mesh so as to separate residual material larger in size.

Puttan: This is key step in preparation of bhasma. The term puttan means ignition or heating in special earthen vessel or pot. Generally shallowness of vessel is useful in heating the material faster and uniformly. After keeping the material on the shallow surface, other part is used as a lid, by placing it in an inverted position. Puttan can be of different types depending on nature of process like Chandraputta, Dhanyarashiputta, Suryaputta, Bhugarbhaputta, Agniptuta.

Toxicity:

Modern medical science finds that mercury is inherently toxic, and that its toxicity is not due to the presence of impurities. While mercury does have anti-microbial properties, and formerly was widely used in Western medicine, its toxicity does not warrant the risk of using it as a health product in most circumstances. The Centers for Disease Control and Prevention have also reported a number of cases of lead and mercury poisoning associated with rasa shastra containing Ayurvedic medicines.

Standardization of Bhasma (*Bhasma parikshas*):

Traditional method: The final bhasma is analyzed for quality by ancient parameters like colour (*Roopa*), taste (*Rasa*), touch (Sparsh), odour (*Gandha*) and smoke (*Dhoom*) described in Ayurvedic texts and the following observations:

1. ***Fineness test (Rekhapurnata):*** A pinch of bhasma is rubbed in between thumb and index finger. It buries in the lines of finger and very smooth then this test is passed.
2. ***Floating test (Varitara):*** Clean water is taken in a glass and allowed to standstill. A pinch of bhasma is sprinkled on the surface of water. It is observed that bhasma floats on the surface of the water.
3. ***Unama:*** This is continuation of the above test where in rice grain is placed on the surface of floating bhasma. It is observed that, the rice grain still floats.
4. ***Niswadu:*** A pinch of bhasma is tasted by the tongue and it should be tasteless.
5. ***Nishchandrata:*** A pinch of bhasma is taken and observed under bright sunlight. There should not be shining particles in the bhasma.
6. ***Nirdhumatva:*** A pinch of bhasma is sprinkled on the ignited charcoal and observed no fumes emerging out of it.
7. ***Apunarbhava:*** The process of bhasma preparation is irreversible, so bhasma cannot be again converted to metal. This is called as *Apunarbhava*. In case of Yashada Bhasma this test can be done as following method. *Yashada bhasma* is triturated with Guda (jaggery), *Gunja* (Abrusprecatorius), Tankana (borax), Madhu (honey) and Ghrita (ghee) one gram each and a paste can be prepared. This paste is kept in acrucible and sealing is done. It is heated upto 1000°C for one hour. After cooling, there should be any shining particles.

8. ***Niruttha:*** Yashada bhasma (5 g) and a silver piece (5 g) were kept in a crucible and after sealing, it is heated for one hour. After cooling, the silver pieces are weighed. There should not be any increase in the weight of the silver pieces which indicated the bhasma passed the test.

Apart from this, there are some special quality control tests like *Dahakatva* (burning / inflammation), *Amla Pareeksha* (acid test), scratch test, magnet test and crude test etc. depending upon type of bhasma.

Modern method: Analysis of bhasma can be done by various modern techniques like: X-Ray diffraction analysis, TLC analysis, Acid insoluble ash, Loss on ignition, Flame photometry, Inductive Coupled Plasma Atomic Emission Spectrometry (ICP-AES), Scanning Electron Microscopy (SEM), Inductively coupled plasma atomic emission spectroscopy, Atomic Absorption spectroscopy (AAS).

Table 3.5: Types of Bhasma and its Use

Bhasma	Metal used	Metal compound	Color of bhasma	Indication	Adverse effects of raw or improperly prepared Bhasma
Lauha	Iron (Fe)	Ferric oxide	Red dark brown	Anemia (Pandu), Oedema (Shotha), Tuberculosis (Rajyakshama), Skin disorders (Kushtha), Immunomodulator (Rasayana), intestinal parasites	Angina, urolithiasis, epilepsy, abdominal colic
Naga	Lead (Pb)	Lead oxide	Light red	Diabetis mellitus (Prameha), piles (Arsha), ulcer (Vrana), leucorrhoea (Pradar), oligospermia (Oligospermia), Urinary disorders, Malabsorption syndrome, tuberculosis	Fainting, edema
Rajat	Silver (Ag)	Argentous oxide, argentic sulfide, argenticoxide	Black	Alcohol poisoning (Madataya), emaciation (Kshaya), spleenomegaly (Plihodara), epilepsy (Apasmara)	Fever, constipation, body ache
Swarna	Gold (Au)	Aurous oxide, auric oxide	Violet red	Anemia (Pandu), Immunomodulator (Rasayana), Emaciation (Kshaya), cough (Kasa), Cardiac tonic (Hridya), Dyspnea (Swasa), tuberculosis, psychosis	Decrease bala (defense mechanism)

Contd...

Tamra	Copper (Cu)	Cupric oxide, cupric sulfide	Black	Anaemia (Pandu), Skin disorders (Kushtha), Worm infestation (Krumi), Obesity (Sthaulya), tuberculosis, cough	Vomiting, spasmodic pain
Vanga	Tin (Sn)	Stannic oxide	White/ greyish white	Worm infestation (Krumi), Vomiting (Vaman), Cough (Kasa), Dyspnea (Swasa), Anemia (Pandu), Diabetis mellitus (Prameha), leucorrhoea, genito urinary diseases	Vomiting, spasmodic pain
Yashada	Zinc (Zn)	Zinc oxide	White, reddish yellow	Ulcer (Vrana), Diabetis mellitus (Prameha), Anemia (Pandu), Eye diseases (Netrarog), Dyspnea (Swasa), leucorrhoea, genito urinary diseases	Vomiting, indigestion, hallucination
Parad	Mercury (Hg)			Anemia (Pandu), Nephritis, fever, Jaundice (Kamala), Emaciation (Kshaya), cough (Kasa), Cardiac tonic (Hridya), Dyspnea (Swasa), Immunomodulator (Rasayana)	Fainting, vomiting, diarrhoea, death

QUESTIONS

1. Explain in detail Ayurveda as Indian system of medicine.
2. Explain in detail Siddha as Indian system of medicine.
3. Explain in detail Unani as Indian system of medicine.
4. Write basic principle and working of homoeopathy.
5. Write in detail prepartaion and standardization of Ayurvedic formulation.
6. Differentiate Asava and Arishta with suitable example.
7. Write a note on standardization of Bhasma.
8. Explain method of preparation of Bhasma with suitable example.
9. Explain preparation and evalution of Asava and Arishta with example.
10. Write a note on gutika as Ayurvedic formulation.

UNIT-II

Chapter...4

NEUTRACEUTICALS

Objectives

- To learn about concept of neutarceuticals.
- To understand growth, scope, market scenario, products available in the market.
- To know about health benefits and role of nutraceuticals in various diseases.
- To understand details of herbs used as neutraceuticals.

4.1 INTRODUCTION

In ancient times, Hippocratus have explained importance of food 'Let food be your medicine and medicine be your food'. The word nutraceutical is a combination of two words 'Nutrient' and 'Pharmaceuticals'. The term nutraceutical was first coined by Dr. Stephen L. DeFelice, in 1989. The concept of nutraceutical first came into the picture during the survey conducted in Europe. As per survey consumer gave more emphasis on diet rather than exercise or hereditary factors to achieve a good health.

Neutraceuticals include wide range of products such as isolated nutrients, herbal products, dietary supplements and designer or genetically engineered foods and processed products such as cereals, soups and beverages etc. More number of people prefer to have nutrients in user friendly pharmaceutical dosage forms like tablets, capsules and others. Nutraceuticals have wide range of therapeutic applications such as cardiovascular ailments, anti-arthritic agents, to treat cold and cough, sleeping disorders, depression, digestion, cancer, osteoporosis, blood pressure, cholesterol control and diabetes etc.

4.2 DEFINITION OF NEUTRACEUTICALS

According to De Felice, nutraceutical can be defined as, "A food or a part of food that provides medical or health benefits, including the prevention and/or treatment of a disease".

The definition was further modified by Health Canada. According to Health Canada nutraceutical means 'a product prepared from foods, but sold in the form of pills, or powder or in other medicinal forms, not usually associated with foods and has a physiological benefit or provides protection against chronic diseases'.

Different countries use different nomenclature for neutraceuticals. The details are as follows:

- **Canada:** Neutraceuticals are known as 'Natural and non-prescription health products', The term covers naturally occurring substances obtained from plants, animals, microorganisms and marine sources and useful in restoring or maintaining good health.
- **USA:** They are called as 'Dietary Supplements' which cover products containing vitamins, minerals, herbs, amino acids and enzymes.
- **European Union:** They are known as 'Food Supplements' that cover concentrated sources of nutrients; substances with a nutritional or physiological effect.
- **Russia:** Neutraceuticals are called as biologically active supplements. The definition includes mineral substances, micro and macro elements; some amino acids; some mono and disacchardies; food fibres; microorganisms present in human body, vitamins etc.
- **Japan:** They are labelled as 'Foods with Health Claims', including food with nutrient function claims and food for specified health uses.
- **Australia:** They are known as 'Complementary medicines' which consist of herbal, vitamin, mineral and nutritional supplements.

4.3 CLASSIFICATION NEUTRACEUTICALS

The Neutraceuticals are mainly classified as follows:

1. **Dietary Supplements:** According to the United States, Dietary Supplement Health and Education Act (DSHEA) of 1994. A dietary supplement is defined as "the product taken by mouth that contains a dietary ingredient intended to supplement the diet". The dietary ingredients may include vitamins, minerals, herbs or botanicals, amino acids, and substances such as enzymes, organ tissues and metabolites. Dietary supplements are sold in the form of tablets, capsules, soft gels, gel caps, liquids or powders.
2. **Functional Foods:** Functional foods are products which can be consumed in the natural state rather than in liquid or capsule form. Functional food can modify function of body. These foods are either enriched or fortified, by a process called nitrification. According to Health Canada, functional foods are defined as "Ordinary food that has components or ingredients added to give it a specific medical or physiological benefit, other than a purely nutritional effect". Vegetables, rice, wheat, fruits, eggs, beef; meat get covered under this category.
3. **Medical Foods:** As per FDA, medical food can be defined as "food formulated to be consumed or administered internally under the supervision of a physician, and which is intended for the specific dietary management of a disease or condition for which distinctive nutritional requirements, on the basis of recognized scientific principles, are established by medical evaluation. In other words, Medical foods are not over the

counter products and should be administered under medical supervision. It can be administered orally or through tube feeding. These are designed to meet certain nutritional requirements for people diagnosed with specific illnesses.

Examples of medicinal foods are transgenic cows and lactoferrin for immunomodulation, oral vaccines, transgenic plants and health bars etc.

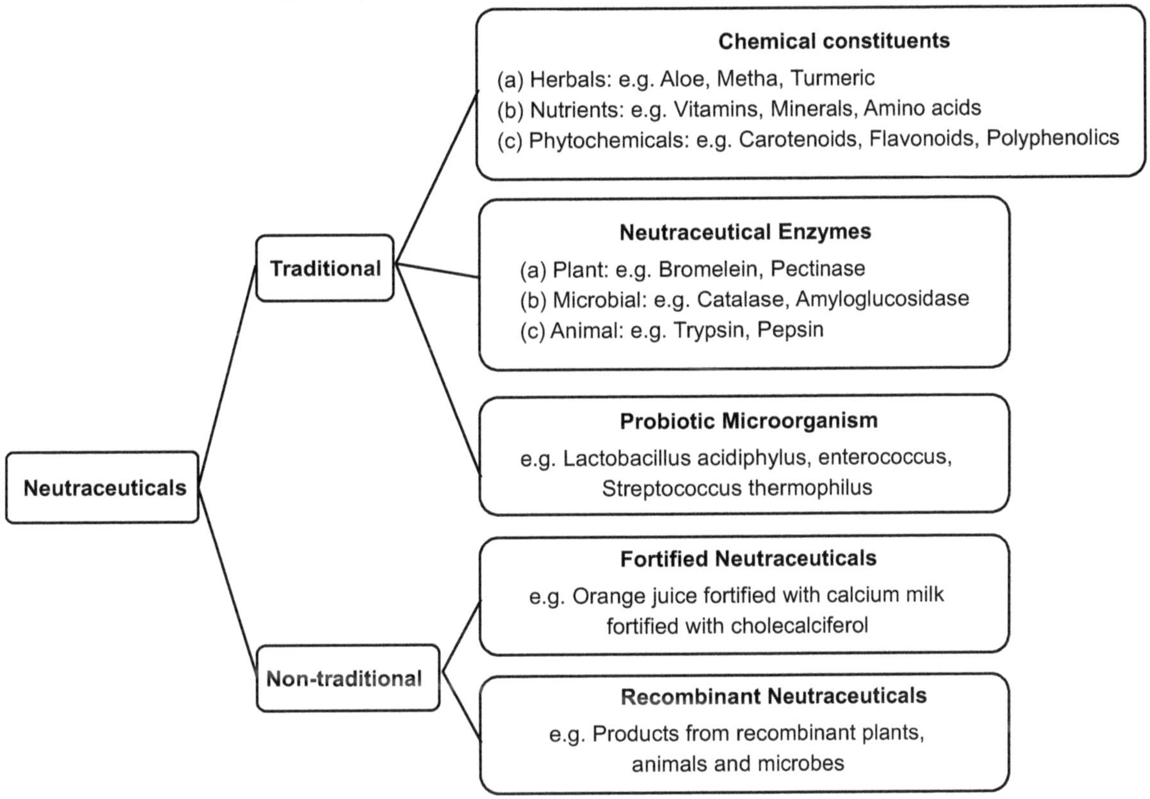

Fig. 4.1: Detail Classification of Neutraceuticals

Advantages of Neutraceuticals:

1. They are substances like food and not considered as drugs so have less or fewer side effects.
2. They are mainly used as preventive or prophylactic to improve medical condition.
3. They have natural ingredients, dietary supplement to balance diet discrepancies.
4. They enhance overall health and well being.
5. They are available without prescription means accessible and affordable.

Disadvantages of Nutraceuticals:

1. **Quality and regulation issues:** As compared to pharmaceuticals, nutracuticals are not regulated very strictly and directly. Some of the health claims made for nutrceuticals may not be scientifically validated. There is lack of proper regulation for nutraceuticals. Hence, there may be compromise on quality of raw material or method.

2. **Bioavailability:** Nutraceuticals may have poor bioavailability and data related to pharmacokinetic and pharmacodynamics may not be available in some cases.
3. **Placebo effect:** Body has mechanism to recover on its own. In such cases, consumers may not use nutraceuticals to treat ailments and may have placebo effect.
4. **Safety and Interactions:** Rarely, nutraceutical may have some side effects. As there is lack of appropriate regulations, there may be possible side effects, interaction with other drugs or may be ineffectiveness in treating disorders.

4.4 MARKET, GROWTH, SCOPE OF NEUTRACEUTICALS

Global Scenario:

Due to increased demand and relatively less stringent norms of quality control, many companies across the globe have entered into neutraceutical production. Amongst all countries US has the largest market for nutraceuticals, followed by Asia-Pacific and then Europe. Japan is the major consumer of nutraceuticals in the Asia-Pacific region. Indian neutraceutical market is also rapidly growing.

As more number of people prefers to consume properly formulated dosage form rather than crude extracts or powders, popularity of nutraceuticals is increasing. Hence, market for nutraceutical is rising continuously. By 2025, the global neutraceuticals market is expected to reach USD 578.23 billion, according report by Grand View Research, Inc. As per expert analysts, the nutraceuticals market will register a CAGR of close to 8% by 2023.

Along with India, demand for neutraceuticals is also growing in countries like Brazil, China, South Korea, Poland and Mexico, and hence the compound annual growth rate of the dietary supplement sector will exceed 9.7% from 2017 to 2025. As per this ASSOCHAM India report, the North American nutraceuticals market may grow at a compound annual growth rate of more than 7.8% up to 2024. Also in Brazil, due to growing demand for nutritional and nutraceutical products, the market is expected to reach a compound annual growth rate of 9.0% from 2017 to 2025. In other countries such as China, Japan and India and the Asia Pacific region, the market will rise at the fastest compound annual growth rate of 9.9% during the forecast period.

There are some reasons behind increase in global market demand for nutraceuticals:

1. The cost of medical treatment and hospitalisation has been increased. So focus of consumers is shifting towards health supplements and neutraceuticals as preventive or prophylaxsis.
2. There is great demand of micronutrients due to malnutrition status in developing countries like India.
3. Due to work culture, diet patterns and lifestyle is also changing with increased stress.
4. Women and senior citizens are also concerned about good digestive health. Also awareness about health supplements and neutraceuticals have been increased.

Indian Scenario:

India is also becoming a critical market for the global players in neutraceuticals. Nutraceuticals launched in India need FSSAI (Food Safety Standards Authority of India) permission. The various reasons are:

1. Fast growing economy.
2. Location of India on world trade routs.
3. Enhanced manufacturing facilities with good quality.
4. Low labour cost.
5. Strong technical and skilled personnel.
6. Ingredients, raw material widely available in low cost.
7. Sale of products through e-commerce and online marketing.
8. Enhanced set up and R&D facilities.
9. Commitment to world class infrastructure.

India accounted for a share of around 2% of the global market in 2015 but by 2022, this share will be increased to approximately 3%. Due to increase in life style disorders, consumers in India have become more concerned about health and fitness hence this provides a platform for nutraceuticals market to grow. So in near future, the Indian nutraceuticals market is forecasted to grow from a value of US $2.8 billion in 2015 to a value of US $8.5 billion by 2022 and to $18 billion in 2025. Every year there is 21% increase in market. Also as per report of ASSOCHAM India, the global nutraceuticals market is expected to reach $578.23 billion by 2025 at CAGR of 8.8%.

According to report 'Indian Nutraceuticals Market Outlook: Vision 2022' by ASSOCHAM India and RNCOS, the overall market is classified into two segments: Dietary Supplements and Functional Food & Beverages. Dietary supplements occupy the larger chunk of market around 65% in 2015. Also Functional food & beverages are expected to grow with a higher growth rate. This has happened due to the increasing visibility of such products in modern retail formats and promotional activities through media. Due to increased awareness and enhanced purchasing ability of consumers, the dietary supplements market is forecasted to reach a value of US $5.2 billion by 2022 from US $1.8 billion in 2015.

As per the report, Indian dietary supplements market is divided into vitamins and minerals, proteins, herbal supplements etc. Vitamins and mineral supplements can help to combat anxiety, stress, depression, bipolar disorder, autism, and trauma and also safeguard against nutritional deficiencies etc. In 2015, in India its market value was US$ 0.7 billion but now it is anticipated to grow and reach a value of US$ 2.1 billion by 2022. Herbal supplements, are dietary supplements which contains plant and its parts. In 2015, herbal supplements market in India was of US$ 0.6 billion. But now due to enhanced popularity of natural ingredients, the market is forecasted to reach a value of US$ 1.7 Billion by 2022. Proteins and amino acid market will reach to a value of US$ 1.09 billion by 2022 from US$

0.4 billion in 2015. The market for antioxidants and fatty acids was approximately US$ 0.1 billion in 2015 in India. Now, it is expected to reach a value of US$ 0.23 billion by 2022.

The market of functional foods and beverages will reach to a value of US $3.2 billion by 2022. The main reason of increase in demand of neutraceuticals is knowledge about wellness and health, is increasing along with expenditure on food by health conscious consumers. This is propelling the growth of market. As per report, The Indian Functional Foods and Beverages market is categorized into Functional Foods Market and Functional Beverages Market. The functional foods market occupies the major share of market that is about 70%. Functional foods contains constituents of natural origin and are used to improve wellbeing, prolong existence and prevention of chronic diseases. In 2015, its market value was US $0.7 billion but it is forecasted to grow to an approximate value of US $2 billion by 2022. Functional beverages include products such as Yakult, Ocean, Gatorade are available in the form of energy drinks, vitamin water, fortified milk and buttermilk etc. Its market is forecasted to reach an approximate value of US $1.1 billion by 2022.

- As per ASSOCHAM India and RNCOS report the market of neutraceuticals for nutritional deficiency will reach to US $4 billion by 2022. This will happen as 20% children in India suffer from malnutrition.
- The market of neutraceuticals for muscle building is forecasted to reach to US $3 billion by 2022 due to increase in number of health conscious people.
- According to research by Obesity Foundation India, more than 3% population in India is obese. Hence, the market of neutraceuticals for weight management will grow from US $ 0.4 billion in 2015 to US $1 billion by 2022.
- The market of anti aging neutraceuticals will reach to US $0.25 billion by 2022 from US $0.14 Billion in 2015.

Table 4.1: Types of Neutraceutical products available in the Market

Sr. No.	Products Available
1.	**Fortified/ Functional packaged food**
	Cornflakes, Oats
	PediaSure
	Sundrop
	Cheese, Nutrichoice biscuits, Tiger Glucose Biscuits
	Gemini, Sweekar
	Horlicks
	ActiPlus Dahi, CEREGROW, MILO, Baby & Me

Contd...

	Nutrela
	Sunfeast
	Choco Flakes, Corn Flakes, Oats, Power Vita
	Fruit & Vegetable Nutrifit
	Probiotics
	Cornflakes, Oats
	Dhara
	Amul products
2.	**Dietary supplements**
	Nutrilite Products
	Seacod Capsules
	Glucose – D
	Protinex
	Calcium Sandoz
	Herbal life Protein Powder
	Himalaya Pure Herbs
3.	**Functional beverages**
	Red Bull Energy Drink, Red Bull Sugar Free
	Minute maid juices
	Gatorade, Tropicana and Tropicana 100%
	Lucozade
	Cloud 9 Energy Drink
	Paper boat thandai, Chilli guava
	Aloevera Fibre Juice
	Fruit juices and Real and Real Active Brands

Sources:

1. Sector Capsule: Fortified/ functional packaged food in India by Euromonitor international dated 21 June 2017.
2. Sector Capsule: Vitamins and Dietary Supplements in India by Euromonitor International dated 19 September 2016.
3. India – Functional Drinks – Executive summary (Aug 2015) by Market Line; Sector Capsule: Sports Drinks and Energy Drinks in India by Euromonitor International dated 23 March 2017 and 7 April 2017 respectively.

Table: 4.2: List of Neutraceutical products with specific health benefits

Sr. No.	Brand Name	Constituent	Role
1.	Betatene	Carotenoids	Immune function
2.	Xangold	Lutein esters	Eye health
3.	Lipoec	Alpha lipoic acid Potent	Antioxidant
4.	Generol	Phytosterol	Coronary heart disease reduction
5.	Premium probiotics	Probiotics	Intestinal disorder
6.	Soylife	Soyabean phytoestrogen	Bone health
7.	Z-trim	Wheat	Zero calorie fat replacer
8.	Linumlife	Lignan extract flax	Prostate health
9.	Fenulife	Fenugreek, galactomannon	Control blood sugar
10.	Teamax	Green tea extract	Potent antioxidant
11.	Marinol	Omega 3 Fatty Acid, DHA (Docosahexaenoic Acid), EPA (Eicosapentaenoic acid)	Heart health protection
12.	Clarinol	Conjugated Linoleic Acid	Weight loss ingredient
13.	Cholestaid	Saponin	Reduce cholesterol
Source: Presnetation on https;//www/ slideshare.net/ArtiRThakkar/nutraceutical-march-april-2018-93319066)			

4.5 GENERAL HEALTH BENEFITS AND ROLE OF NUTRACEUTICALS

Nutraceuticals are useful in various diseases such as coronary heart disease, obesity, diabetes, cancer, osteoporosis, Parkinson's, Alzheimer's diseases, arthritis, sleeping disorders, cold, cough, digestion problems, osteoporosis, blood pressure, hyper cholesterol level, pain, and depression etc. According to research, they act by variety of mechanisms such as activation of antioxidant defenses, signal transduction pathways, gene expression related to cell survival, activation of cell proliferation and differentiation and by preservation of mitochondrial integrity.

The Health benefits of various types of Neutraceuticals are as follows:

1. Dietary fibers: Dietary fibers are the food material, which is not hydrolyzed by enzymes secreted by the GI tract, but can be digested by micro flora present in the gut.

Celluloses, hemicelluloses, gums and pectin, lignin, resistant dextrin and resistant starches are examples of dietary fibers. Chemically, these are carbohydrate polymers with a degree of polymerization not lower than 3. They may be soluble or insoluble in nature. Dietary fibers improve digestion and absorption of nutrients. Soluble fibre lowers serum LDL cholesterol, enhance insulin receptor binding activity and improve glucose tolerance. In colon, dietary fibre act as laxative by increasing water retention, transit time and hence bulk of fecal matter. These are also helpful to treat various disorders such as cardiovascular diseases, stroke, hypertension, diabetes, obesity, and certain gastrointestinal disorders and enhance immunity etc. The recent entry in market is FOS i.e. Fructooligosaccharides. FOS has various health benefits for lowering of cholesterol and improved digeston as well as immunity.

2. PUFAs: These are Poly Unsaturated Fatty Acids also called "essential fatty acids". These are vital for body's function and should be supplied externally through the diet. PUFAs are mainly omega-3-(n-3) fatty acids and omega-6-(n-6) fatty acids. The examples of omega-3-fatty acids are α-linolenic acid (ALA), eicosapentanoic acid (EPA) and docosahexanoic acid (DHA). ALA acts as the precursor of EPA and DHA. EPA and DHA are found mainly in fish. ALA is mainly present in flaxseed, soybeans, canola, walnuts and red/black currant seeds. Linoleic acid (LA), γ-linolenic acid (GLA) and arachidonic acid (ARA) are Omega-6-PUFAs. The vegetable oils like corn, safflower, soyabean and sunflower contains Linoleic acid. Animal products such as meat, poultry and eggs are main sources of ARA. PUFAs mainly help in brain development and show antiarrythmic, anti-thrombotic and hypolipidemic activities. They are helpful in maintainning cardiovascular health. They are also helpful to treat various disorders such as asthma, bipolar and depressive disorders, dysmenorrhea, and diabetes and improve pre-mature infant health etc.

3. Probiotics: Probiotics are live microbial feed supplement, which when administered in adequate amounts beneficial for host by improving intestinal microbial balance. It includes Lactobacilli, Gram-positive cocci such as *Lactococcus lactis, Enterococcus faecium Streptococcus salivarius spp, thermophilus,* and Bifidobacteria such as *B. bifidun, B. adolescentis*. Probiotics are used to treat various disorders such as lactose intolerance, acute diarrhoea, antibiotic-associated GI side effects, allergy, cancer, asthma, and infections of the ear, urinary tract etc. According to recent research probiotics also improve immunity and helps to fight depression.

4. Prebiotics: Prebiotics produces beneficial effects by selectively altering the composition or metabolism of the gut microflora. These promote the Lactobacillus and Bifidobacterial growth in the gut. These are chemically fructose based oligosacharrides. The various effects of the prebiotics are improvement in lactose tolerance, antitumor activities, toxins neutralization, and improvement of intestinal immune system, reduces constipation, anti hyperlipidemic effects.

5. Minerals: The health benefits of minerals are as follows:

Table 4.3: Health benefits of Minerals

Sr. No.	Mineral	Benefits
1.	Calcium	Important for bone and teeth, nerve, muscle and glandular function, blood clotting.
2.	Iron	For haemoglobin formation, energy production, and oxygen transport.
3.	Magnesium	For healthy functioning of nerve and muscle, essential for bone formation.
4.	Chromium	Energy formation from carbohydrate and fat, for treating diabetes.
5.	Phosphorous	For phosphorylation process, energy production, bone and teeth health, for genetic material.
6.	Cobalt	Important component of Vit. B_{12} and B_{12} coenzymes.
7.	Copper	For haemoglobin and collagen production, to produce energy functioning of heart, helps in Iron absorption.
8.	Iodine	Proper functioning of thyroid gland.
9.	Zinc	Essential for cell reproduction, for neonates, wound healing, sperm and testosterone hormone production.
10.	Selenium	Antioxidant, part of GPX enzyme, eliminates the toxic effects of reactive oxygen species, prevent cardiovascular diseases, chemo protective agent and immunomodulator.

6. Vitamins: Vitamin C, vitamin E and carotenoids are antioxidant vitamins. These have protective actions against oxygen free radicals. Hence, these are useful in degenerative diseases including cancer, cardiovascular diseases, cataracts etc. The details of health benefits of vitamins are as follows:

Table 4.4: Health benefits of vitamins

Sr. No	Vitamin	Function
1.	Vitamin A	Antioxidant, for growth and development, for healthy vision, skin and mucous membranes, to treat skin disorders, cancer.
2.	Vitamin B1	Important for neurologic functions, carbohydrate metabolism and for energy.
3.	Vitamin B2	Energy production and chemical processes of body, important for healthy eyes, skin and nerve function.

Contd...

4.	Vitamin B3	Formation of energy and maintenance of brain function.
5.	Vitamin B 6	Formation of essential proteins, convert proteins to energy.
6.	Vitamin B 12	Formation of genetic material, RBC, proper functioning of CNS, amino acids production, protein, fat and carbohydrate metabolism.
7.	Vitamin C	Antioxidant, useful for healthy bones, gums, teeth, skin and common cold helps in wound healing.
8.	Vitamin D	Helps in intestinal absorption of calcium, magnesium, phosphate. Immunomodulator, important for formation of bones and teeth.
9.	Vitamin E	Antioxidant helps in formation of blood cells, muscles, lung and nerve tissue, immunomodulator.
10.	Vitamin K	Important for blood clotting.
11.	Folic acid	For formation of RBC and genetic material of cell, important in pregnancy.
12.	Pantothenic acid	For synthesis of cholesterol, steroids, and fatty acids, helps in intraneuronal synthesis of acetylcholine.

7. Vitamin like compounds:

- **L- Carnitine:** Play vital role in oxidation of fatty acids, and oxidative phosphorylation.
- **Choline:** Regulates fat metabolism.
- **Inositol:** Important for transport of amino acid, potassium and sodium.
- **Taurine:** Plays important role in retinal photoreceptor activity, bile acid conjugation, WBC antioxidant activity, CNS neuromodulation, platelet aggregation, cardiac contractibility, sperm motility, insulin activity etc.

8. Polyphenols: These are group of secondary metabolites which have effects on various cellular processes such as apoptosis, platelet aggregation, gene expression, intercellular signalling etc. and hence can be useful to treat cancer and cardiovascular disorders. Also polyphenols have various therapeutic effects such as possess anti-inflammatory, anti-microbial, antioxidant cardioprotective activities, neuroprotective, chemopreventive agents and anti-diabetes etc.

9. Spices: Most of the spices are chemically terpenoids. They have various effects on human health such as chemopreventive, antioxidants, antiarthritic, antidiabetic, anticancer, anti-inflammatory, antimicrobial, immunomodulator, and are active against disorder of gastrointestinal tract, cardiovascular diseases, respiratory disorders, and metabolic diseases, reproductive, neural and other disorder.

The health benefits of various types of neutraceuticals are as follows:

Table 4.5: Health Benefits of Neutraceuticals

Sr. No.	Phyto Constituents	Source	Role
1.	**Carotenoids**		
	Lycopene,	Tomatoes, grape fruit, Guava, papaya, water melon	Reduces cholesterol levels, anti oxidants, avoid prostate cancer
	β-Carotene	Vegetables, fruits, oats, carrots, lutein, spinach, corn, avocado, egg yolk	Antioxidant
	Tocotrienol	Palm oil, grains.	Improves cardiovascular health, anticancer
2.	**Polyphenolic Compounds**		
	Flavonones	Citrus fruits	Anti oxidant & anticancer
	Flavones	Vegetables, soya	Anti oxidant & anticancer
	Curcumin	Turmeric	Anti-inflammatory and anticoagulant, antioxidant,
	Anthocyanidine and Catechin	Fruits, tea, babul pods, mustard cake, rapeseed	Antioxidants and anticancer
	Glucosinolates	Cruciferous vegetables	Cancer
3.	**Phytoestrogens**		
	Isoflavones	Legumes, beans	Lowers LDL cholesterol, antioxidants, anticancer
	Lignans	Vegetables, rye & flaxseed	Anticancer
4.	**Dietary fibers**		
	Soluble fiber	Legumes, oats, barley, fruits	Healthy digestive tract & have anticancer activity
	Insoluble fiber	Wheat, corn bran, nut	Healthy digestive tract, Anticancer activity
5.	Sulphides/Thiols	Cruciferous vegetables	Immunomodulator
6.	Omega 3 Fatty Acids	Fish & Flax seed	Vital for brain function, Reduce cholesterol disposition, controls inflammatory process

Contd...

7.	Monosaturated fatty acids	Nuts	Protect against cardiovascular diseases.
8.	Prebiotics/ Probiotics	Yogurt, other dairy and non-dairy products	Important for gastro-intestinal health and systematic immunity.
9.	Polyols, Sugar alcohols (xylitol, sorbitol)	Fruits	Reduce the risk of dental carries
10.	Saponins	Soybean, liquorice, lucerne, chick peas	Antihyperlipidemic, Anticancer activity

(**Soruce:** Riyaz Ahmed Khan et.al. The pharma Intovation Journal 2014).

Commonly Used Herbs with their Therapeutic Effects:

Table 4.6: Therapeutic effects of herbs

Sr. No.	Plant name	Therapeutic effects
1.	*Aloe barbadensis, Liliaceae* Aloe	Antiulcer, anthelmintic, wound healing
2.	*Andrographis paniculata,* Acanthaceae Kalmegh	Respiratory tract infection
3.	*Artemisia annua,* Asteraceae Artemisia	Antimalarial
4.	*Cassia senna,* Leguminosae Senna	Laxative
5.	*Allium sativum, Amaryllidaceae* Garlic	Arteriosclerosis, Lowers cholesterol, cardio protective
6.	*Capsicum annum, Solanaceae* Red pepper	Antioxidant, stimulant
7.	*Cymbopogon citrates,* Poaceae Lemon grass	Stomach ache, carminative
8.	*Curcuma longa, Zingiberaceae Turmeric*	Inflammation, indigestion, antioxidant
9.	*Glycyrrhiza glabra, Fabaceae Liquorice*	Anti-inflammatory, expectorant
10.	*Plantago ovate, Plantaginaceae Psyllium*	Laxative Anti-inflammatory, congestion

Contd...

11.	*Phyllanthus emblica, Phyllanthaceae Amla*	Diuretic, anti ageing, antidiabetic agent
12.	*Zingiber officinale, Zingiberaceae Ginger*	Indigestion, antioxidant
13.	*Eugenia caryophyllus, Myrtaceae clove*	Dental analgesic
14.	*Matricaria chamomilla, Asteraceae chamomile*	Wound healing, indigestion, insomnia
15.	*Swertia chirata, Gentianaceae chirata*	Antidiabetic, migraine

(**Source:** Ruchi, et al: Role of nutraceuticals in healthcare: A review).

4.5.1 Benefits and Role of Nutraceuticals in Cancer Prevention

Cancer is becoming a major health problem due to enhanced life expectancy, growing urbanization, environmental changes and change in lifestyle and diet patterns. Cancer is a major cause of death worldwide. As per research, it is estimated that one-third of all cancer deaths can be prevented by change in life-style pattern including diet. Cancer treatment is very expensive, so neutraceuticals having chemo preventive effects can be employed. Chemoprevention means the substances which are used to prevent, suppress or reduce the process of carcinogenesis. There are many evidences that foods having relatively low carbohydrates and rich in fibres, vitamins, minerals, proteins, essential fatty acids are useful in cancer treatment. Neutraceuticals are also helpful in reducing toxicity of drugs, chemotherapy, radiations and assist to live better life.

Use of nutrceuticals stared in late 1960 with some vegetables and fruits have shown inhibition of tumours in laboratory animals. Further research on retinoids gives rise to new term called 'cancer chemoprevention'. Cancer chemoprevention is different from cancer chemotherapy means use of cytotoxic agents. Several studies have demonstrated that use of carotene rich food, vitamin E, Vitamin C and many more compounds in foods benefit to fight cancer. There are more than 600 different compounds from natural origin which may have benefit in prevention of cancer.

Plant contains a variety of therapeutically active constituents such as micronutrients, polyunsaturated fatty acids, glucosinolates, polyphenols, phytoestrogens, phytosterols, lignans, terpenes, phytates etc. Various studies have showed that phytoconstituents such as curcumin (turmeric), capsaicin (green chilies), resveratrol (grapes), epigallocatechin gallate (green tea), gingerol (ginger), genistein (soya beans), caffeic acid phenyl ester (propolis from honey bee), sulforaphane (cruciferous vegetables), silibinin, indole-3-carbinol (cabbage) , tangeretin (citrus species), apigenin (tea, cabbage, garlic), lycopene (tomatoes), emodin (aloes), allicin and diallyl sulfide (garlic), quercitin (*Rhododendron cinnabarium*), anethole (fennel, camphor), β-carotene has anticancer activity.

What is cancer?

When there is accumulation of multiple sequential mutations and alterations in nuclear and cytoplasm molecules, the process is called as Carcinogenesis. There are three phases of carcinogenesis mainly initiation, promotion and progression.

Initiation: In this phase, carcinogen rapidly binds to the target and causes DNA damage.

Promotion phase: During this phase, tumor promoters (mitogens) induce clones of initiated cells to expand. It is reversible but there is functional loss of regulatory proteins and cellular check points which are important for proliferation and apoptosis.

Progression: In this phase, cells are completely altered phenotypically and genotypically causing irreversible macroscopic changes. Promotion and progression phases continue for many years.

Mechanism of Action of Nutraceuticals Against Cancer:

Several nutraceuticals may act by different mechanisms and may have overall synergy effect. American Cancer Society has recommended five to seven servings of vegetable or fruits daily. Nutrient, micronutrient, food additives like antioxidant, non-nutritive molecules like coumarin, alkaloids may have beneficial effect in prevention of cancer. Benefits of nutraceuticals can be seen at cellular level where cancer cells originate. At cellular level, nutraceuticals help for cell differentiation, proliferation, signal transduction, cell cycle, and enzyme expression. At organism level, tumor angiogenesis inhibition, prevention of invasion and metastasis can be tackled with certain nutrceuticals.

- Neutraceuticals acts as antioxidants and anti-inflammatory. They inhibit the signaling pathways related to redox mediated transcription factors.
- Some nutraceuticals like ascorbic acid, tocopherol, phenols are inhibitors of carcinogen formation.
- They act by modulating endocrine system, immunological cascades and inflammatory enzymes.
- They also alter DNA repair and cleavage process.
- They protect against lipid peroxidation.
- Neutraceuticals suppress mutagenic activity of carcinogens; suppress cell proliferation and induce cancer cells apoptosis.
- In very low concentration, they regulate the process of gene expression.
- They help to reduce cachexia in cancer patients. Cachexia means alteration in carbohydrate, lipid and fat metabolism resulting bad life quality and poor survival of patients. Neutraceuticals are helpful to regulate metabolism in such patients.
- They enhance the function of natural killer cells and tumour necrosis factor and thus help to fight malignancy.

Phytochemicals Effective Against Cancer:

These are secondary metabolites which contains hydroxyl group attached to benzene ring. Human diet contains more than 8000 polyphenolic compounds present in tea, coffee, cocoa, vegetables, fruits, wine and cereals etc. They act by suppressing initiation of carcinogenesis process and suppress progression of cancer.

1. Polyphenolic compounds: These are secondary metabolites which contains hydroxyl group attached to benzene ring. Human diet contains more than 8000 polyphenolic compounds. They act by suppressing initiation of carcinogenesis process and suppress progression of cancer.

(a) Epigallocatechin 3 gallate is example of polyphenolic compound present in green tea. It has prominent antitumour properties. It suppresses inducible nitric oxide synthase (iNOS) expression and hence inhibits nitric oxide production.

(b) Resveratrol is another example of poplyphenolic compounds which are used in treatment of cancer because of its antiproliferative action. Resveratrol is a stilbenoid, present in skin of grapes, blueberries, peanuts etc. Grape seed proanthocyanidins are used to prevent lung cancer, prostate cancer, blood cancer and cutaneous squamous cell carcinoma.

(c) Flavonoids: Flavonoids can affect the mRNA levels of genes important in cell cycle control and apoptosis. They interact with enzymes related to DNA topology. Some flavonoids like genistien modulate topoisomerase II activity. It has strong estrogen agonist activity and inhibite growth activity of breast cancer cells. **Genistein** and related isoflavones are helpful in cancer of stomach, bladder, lung, and blood by inhibiting chemically induced cell growth and development. Flavonoid **Quercetin**, also has anticancer effects. It initiates cell apoptosis, prevent carcinogenesis, and inhibit melanoma, growth, invasion of cancer. Quercetin regulates phases of the cell cycle mainly G(1), S, G(2), and M and inhibit the expression of specific oncogenes and genes. It also up-regulate the expression of several tumour suppressor genes. As per one study, Quercetin inhibited the growth of PC-3 and DU-145 prostate cancer cell line. **Apigenin** flavones are potent anticancer agents found in chamomile tea, cabbage, garlic, french peas and guava etc. It act by several mechanisms such as inhibition of MAPK activity, stimulation of the p53- p21/waf response pathway, inhibition of IkB kinase activity, inhibition of transcriptional activation of COX-2 and inducible nitric oxide synthetase (iNOS) etc.

(d) Phytoestrogenes are special group of compounds containing isoflavonoids, flavonoids, stilbenes, and lignans and have property to bind estrogen receptors. These are used to treat diseases such as cardiovascular disease, osteoporosis, cancer of the breast, endometrium, prostate, colon, rectum, stomach and lung etc. Example of phytoestrogenes with anti tumor activity are puerarin *(Pueraria lobata)*, formononetin (clovers), fenugreek and Black cohosh *(Actaea racemosa* syn., *Cimicifuga racemosa)*, glabridin and glabrene *(Glychirriza echinata)*.

(e) Soy protein consists of genistein and daidzein. Soya proteins reduce the levels of luteinizing hormone (LH), follicle stimulating hormone (FSH) and progesterone. It protects from breast cancer or prostate cancer. Equol, a metabolite of daidzein inhibit benign and malignant human prostate epithelial cells. Genistein and daidzein also modify cytokine production. They reduce proliferation of ovarian cancer cell and also used to treat acute leukemias.

(f) Blueberries, blackberries and strawberries are polyphenolic compounds and are good antioxidants. These are effective in the prevention of development of cancer cells. Many studies suggested that berries interrupt the activities of proteins involved in the oncogenesis and hence promote normal gene expression and growth of healthy cells.

2. Vitamins and Minerals: Vitamins A, C, E and trace elements like selenium can prevent cancer. Ascorbic acid reported to induce apoptosis through cell cycle arrest, activates the apoptosis factors and interferes with iron uptake in cells. Ascorbate (Vitamin C) act as an electron donor in redox reactions. The oxidative stress plays a major role in the mechanism of ascorbate toxicity in tumor cells. Various *in-vitro* and *in-vivo* studies have showed that ascorbate can also be combined with chemotherapeutic drugs to get desired effects. Appropriate dose of supplements like β-carotene, vitamin C, vitamin E and zinc, calcium and vitamin D reduces the chances of bladder cancer, breast and skin cancer. Selenium protects against prostate cancer, colorectal cancer, ovarian cancer and papillary thyroid cancers. Vitamins and minerals are antioxidant in nature. They act by modulation of immune function, by inhibiting N-nitrosamine formation or by cell-to-cell interactions and by modulation of the enzyme activity. Thus, they protect DNA damage from the free radical attack. Vitamins and minerals inhibit cells differentiation and growth by inhibition of protein kinase C activity; prostaglandin E1- stimulated adenylate cyclase activity, expression of c-myc, H-ras, and a transcription factor (E2F), and induction of transforming growth factor-β and p21 genes. Vitamins enhance the anti-tumor effects of x-ray irradiation, chemotherapeutic agents, and hyperthermia and also reduce toxic effects of anticancer drugs.

3. Curcumin: It is chemopreventive in nature. It induces apoptosis in malignant cell lines by suppressing cellular signaling pathways. It suppresses tumour growth by disrupting the activity of several enzymes required for growth and proliferation of cells. Curcumin can affect the expression of genes that contribute to carcinogenesis by inhibiting the activation of transcription factors. It acts as Anti-neoplastic agent causing cell-cycle arrest and induces apoptotic signals. Being the potent inhibitor of TNF-α, curcumin suppresses cancer cell proliferation. Curcumin is useful in treatment of colon, stomach, lung, breast, and skin cancers etc.

4. Capsaicin: It is a pungent principle obtained from red chili peppers of Capsicum genus of Solanaceae family. It induces apoptosis which is regulated by Bcl-2 and the protein phosphatase calcineurin. It is used to treat ovarian carcinoma, mammary adenocarcinoma and promeyelocytic leukemia (HL-60). It inhibits growth and induces apoptosis of cancer cells by inhibiting plasma membrane NADH oxidase activity.

5. Gingerol: Gingerol oleoresin isolated from Ginger (*Zingiber officinale* Family: Rosaceae) is commonly used dietary supplement. It has many therapeutic effects such as antiinflammatory, analgesic, antihepatotoxic, antipyretic, and cardiotonic effects. Being antioxidant in nature, it inhibits phospholipid peroxidation induced by the $FeCl_3$ – ascorbate system. It also suppresses generation of superoxide anion by inhibiting xanthine oxidase.

6. Lycopene: Lycopene is present in Tomatoes (*Lycopersicon esculentum* Family: Solanaceae) has antioxidant properties. It suppress the insulin like growth factor–I (IGF-I) receptor signaling, cell cycle progression, reduces the binding capacity of AP-1 transcriptional complex and inhibits proliferation of cells. It also decreases activation of NFkB. It is used to treat prostate cancer, gastric cancer, breast cancer, liver and lung cancer etc.

7. Chestnut: Chestnut is antioxidant in nature and is used to treat gastric cancer, and mild prostate cancer and breast cancer. The flesh and inner shell of chestnut, uncooked chestnuts and processed chestnut have antioxidant effects.

8. Ginseng: It is used to treat various cancers such as blood, colon, liver, breast and lung being antioxidant in nature.

9. Cruciferous vegetables: Dietary fiber rich cruciferous vegetables like broccoli, cabbage, cauliflower, Brussels sprouts, turnip, collard, mustard etc. are used in treatment of cancer. They have chemopreotective effects against colorectal cancer, breast cancer and lung cancer etc.

Table 4.7: Mechanism of action of some nutraceuticals

No.	Mechanism of Anticancer Effect	Example
1.	Immune stimulants	Astragalus, bromelain, eleutherococcus, ganoderma, ginseng, glutamine, melatonin, polysaccharopeptide (PSP), Polysaccharide Krestin (PSK), shiitake
2.	Directly acting	Apigenin, arctigenin, boswellic acid, centella, curcumin, EGCG, emodin, EPA/DHA, flaxseed, genistein, daidzein, garlic, hypericin, luteolin, monoterpenes, parthenolide, quercetin, resveratrol, selenium, vitamin A, vitamin D_3, vitamin E
3.	Indirect acting	anthocyanidins, butcher's broom, horse chestnut, proanthocyanidins, vitamin C
4.	Compounds that induce apoptosis	Vitamin D_3, vitamin A, boswellic acids, curcumin, EPA, Flavonoids (including apigenin, luteolin, genistein, quercetin, EGCG), garlic, hypericin, monoterpenes, resveratrol, selenium, Vitamin C, Vitamin E

Cond...

5.	Compound that inhibit protein tyrosine kinase	Curcumin, emodin, flavonoids (including apigenin, luteolin, quercetin, genistein, and EGCG), hypericin, parthenolide
6.	Inhibition of vascular permeability, antiangiogenic activity	Anthocyanidins, Butcher's broom, *Centella asiatica*, Horse chestnut, proanthocyanidins
7.	Anti-oxidant	Glutamine, Glutathione-enhancing compounds (i.e., most antioxidants), Selenium, Vitamin C, Vitamin E
8.	Immunostimulants	*Astragalus membranaceus, Eleutherococcus senticosus, Ganoderma lucidum, Panax ginseng,* Shiitake *(Lentinus edodes),* mushroom polysaccharides

4.5.2 Benefits and Role of Nutraceuticals in Prevention of Cardiovascular Diseases

Cardiovascular diseases are most common cause of death worldwide. Fortunately, most of the cardiovascular diseases can be avoided with change in lifestyle especially diet and exercise. On this background, nutraceuticals are critically important. Mediterranean diet rich in various phytonutrient is successful in low cardiovascular deaths in those countries. 'French paradox' include low incidence of cardiovascular diseases despite of high fat diet, smoking and wine consumption. This clearly shows nutraceuticals and dietary factors have major role in preventing cardiovascular ailments as nutraceuticals are rarely used in emergency.

Diseases related to heart and blood vessels are known as cardiovascular diseases (CVDs). Many of these are related to a process called atherosclerosis. In atherosclerosis artery walls get damaged due to oxidized low-density lipoproteins (LDL) causing inflammation of arteries and also plaque formation takes place on their walls. Thus, arteries become narrow and there is resistance to blood flow. If blood clot formation takes place, it leads to heart attacks. Cardiovascular diseases (CVDs) are major cause of deaths and are growing health concern. It is responsible for 17.3 million deaths annually worldwide, which means 30 per cent of all global deaths. The factors responsible for development of CVDs are family history, hypertension, raised serum cholesterol, diabetes, life style factors, smoking, diet and lack of exercise etc. It is proposed, by 2030 about 23.6 million people will die due to CVDs (WHO 2012). India is also becoming global capital of diabetes and cardiovascular diseases. In India about 50 per cent patients of CVDs die due to Coronary heart Diseases. Different types of CVDs are Arrhythmia, Angina, Coronary artery disease (CAD), Heart attack, Heart failure, Peripheral artery (arterial) disease, Stroke, Blood clotting disorders and Atherosclerosis etc. Neutraceuticals play vital role in prevention and treatment of CVDs.

Neutraceuticals Act by following Mechanisms:

- Nutraceuticals act by different ways to help in cardiovascular problems. Nutraceutical may increase force of contraction and even may have effect on conductivity, helps in atrial fibrillation. Some, like Onion, Arjuna increase force of contraction and even have diuretic effect to lower blood pressure.
- Edema and systemic congestion can be cleared by using some nutraceuticals. Cinchona alkaloids like quinine have good affect on arrhythmia and stability of heart. Cardiac glycosides have positive ionotropic effect.
- Nutraceuticals reduces LDL cholesterol levels by forming micelle with bile salts (as it contains cholesterol). Some have thrombolytic and antiplatelet effects.
- Because of anti-inflammatory and antioxidant effect, they inhibit formation of free radicals.
- Nutraceuticals have fibrinolytic activity and thus reduce artery plaque. During coagulation fibrin clots are formed which are cut by plasmin enzyme and are cleared by kidney and liver.
- Some nutraceuticals improve microcirculation, antidiuretic effects and thus clears edema.

Table 4.8: Different diseases and possible phytotherapy

Sr. No.	Disease	Symptoms	Herbal Drugs	Mechanism
1.	Heart failure	Chest pain, irregular heart	Foxglove - *Digitalis purpurea* (Scrophulariaceae) Hawthorn- *Cratagus oxycanthoides, C. monogyna* (Rosaceae) Arjuna- *Terminalia arjuna* (Combretaceae)	Increase myocardial contractility and force of contraction.
2.	Venous insufficiency	Swelling, systemic congestion	Bilberry- *Vaccinium myrtillus* (Vacciniaceae) Butcher's broom - *Ruscus aculeatus* (Liliaceae) Ginkgo- *Ginkgo biloba* (Ginkgoaceae) Horse Chestnut- *Aesculus hippocastanum* (Hippocastanaceae)	Increase blood circulation, increase in microcirculation, decrease in vascular permeability and help in varicose vein.

Contd...

3.	Atherosclero-sis	Plaque in blood vessel	Garlic - Allium sativum (Liliaceae)	Antiplatelet effect, prevent oxidative damage to endothelial cells of blood vessels, hypolipidemic activity, antithrombotic activity
4.	Hypertension	Increase in blood pressure	Sarpagandha *Rawolfia serpantina* (Apocynaceae)	Centrally acting blood pressure lowering effect

Phytochemicals effective Against Cardiovsacular Diseases:

1. Curcumin: It is a major component of turmeric *(Curcuma longa)*. It has various therapeutic activities such as anticarcinogenic, antiinflammatory, antioxidative, antibacterial, hypoglycemic, and hypocholesterolemic etc. Curcumin has enhancing effects on LDL receptor, HMG-CoA reductase, and farnesyl diphosphate synthatase. It stimulates rate of cholesterol catabolism and liver X alphareceptor (LXR) expression by enhancing hepatic cholesterol-7–hydroxylase. Curcumin reduces oxidation of LDL-C by enhancing hepatic superoxide dismutase (SOD) and glutathione peroxidase (GSHPX). It significantly decreases serum lipid peroxides, increases in HDLC, and decreases total serum cholesterol level. Hence, it acts as anti-hyperlipidemic. Curcumin prevent cardiac hypertrophy, heart failure modify genetic expression involved in cholesterol homeostasis. It improves functioning of heart and blood vessels and has membrane stabilizing effects. It is good antioxidant hence, it helps to avoid oxidative injury.

2. Coenzyme Q10 (Ubiquinone): Coenzyme Q10 (CoQ10) is an antioxidant naturally produced in the body, present in the heart, kidney, pancreas and liver. It is mainly found in meat and seafood.

- It takes part in various activities such as free radical scavenger, mitochondrial energy production, regeneration of vitamins E, C and A, inhibition of oxidation of LDL, membrane phospholipids, DNA, mitochondrial proteins, lipids, reduction of total cholesterol, triglycerides, sugar levels, raises HDL-C and protects from ischemic reperfusion injury.
- Low level Coenzyme Q10 leads to hypertension, CHD, hyperlipidemia, Diabetes, and atherosclerosis.
- Various studies have proved that CoQ10 is linked with improvements in functional factors of heart such as ejection fraction, stroke volume and cardiac output, and reduces major adverse cardiovascular events (MACE), improves HF symptoms caused due to aging.

- CoQ10 inhibits lipoprotein oxidation in the vessel wall and cell adhesion molecules. Thereby it avoids formation of atherosclerotic lesions.
- CoQ10 reduces BP which is major factor of CVDs.
- Coenzyme Q10 has protective action against ischemia- reperfusion injury caused during coronary artery bypass graft (CABG) surgery. It avoids myocardial damage caused ischemia-reperfusion injury by increasing ATP concentration, enhancing antioxidant capacity, reducing oxidative damage and reducing cardiomyocyte apoptosis.
- CoQ10 can be beneficial if included in conventional angina therapy.
- The dose of 100-300 milligrams of CoQ10 per day is recommended to avoid endothelial dysfunction and atherosclerosis.

3. Flavonoids: These are class of polyphenolic compound having antioxidant potential. Flavonoids are mainly present in onion, apples cruciferous vegetables, black grapes, red wine, grapefruits, cherries, berries and herbs etc. Flavonoids block the angiotensin-converting enzyme (ACE), thus reduces blood pressure. It blocks cyclooxygenase enzyme that breaks down prostaglandins and hence prevents platelet aggregation. They also have protective effects on the vascular system and tiny capillaries.

Isoflavonoids show cholesterol lowering activity by altering thyroid status, enhanced bile acid excretion, up-regulate LDL receptors and thus reducing cholesterol absorption rates. Hypercholesterolaemia leads to cardiovascular diseases. Being scavenger of peroxyl radicals they inhibit of lipid peroxidation. The consumption of soya proteins may also lower the risk of CVDs.

Flavonoids persuade the expression of phase-2 detoxification proteins and thereby reduce oxidative stress. As per study conducted by Davison et al. (2008) it was observed that flavanol-rich cocoa reduced insulin resistance by 0.31% ($P < 0.05$), diastolic blood pressure by 1.6 mm Hg and mean arterial blood pressure by 1.2 mm Hg ($P < 0.05$). Flavonoids present in cocoa reduces blood pressure, serum LDL-C levels and increase HDL cholesterol. Thus, it is cardioprotective in action.

The consumption of black tea reversed endothelial vasomotor dysfunction in patients with coronary artery disease as showed by Duffy et al (2001). Flvonoids present in tea acts by various mechanisms such as suppress free radicals, protect mitochondrial damage, and suppress hyperglycemia. Thus, they reduce hypertension and improve cardiac hypertrophy.

Also Egallate present in green tea reduces gastrointestinal cholesterol absorption. Different mechanisms like interfering emulsification, digestion and micellar solubilization of lipids, upregulation of hepatic LDL receptor, stimulation of FA synthase and paroxonase, inhibition of HMG-CoA reductase, enhancement of energy expenditure, and reduction in LDL oxidation.

4. Dietary fibers: The consumption of fiber rich food significantly reduces the risk of CVDs. Soluble fiber (gums, fruits) helps to lower blood fat and maintain blood sugar level. Water insoluble fibers such as cellulose, hemicelluloses pass into the digestive tract and trap cholesterol, toxins etc. As per different studies fibers present in vegetables, fruits, Fenugreek seeds, Psyllium husk, Guar gum, pectin, buckwheat seeds, can reduce the LDL levels. These fibers bind cholesterol, bile acids, and disrupt the enterohepatic cycle. Also Bile acid biosynthesis needs cholesterol and hence blood cholesterol levels can be reduced. Due to presence of fibers and folate, corn protects against heart diseases. It maintains the homocysteine. Homocysteine is responsible for damage of blood vessel, heart attack, stroke, or peripheral vascular disease.

5. **Plant sterols:** these are natural compounds found in vegetable oils, nuts, seeds, legume, fruits, vegetables and grains. E.g. sitosterol, campesterol and stigmasterol. It should be consumed 150 to 400 mg/day. Stanols are the saturated plant sterols found in avocados, pumpkin seeds, cashews, rice bran etc. Both plant sterols and stanols help to reduce serum cholesterol levels by suppressing intestinal absorption of cholesterol. Hence, sterols are useful in preventing coronary heart diseases.

6. **Nuts:** Nuts contains mono- and poly-unsaturated fatty acids, dietary fiber, phytosterols, and polyphenols etc. Nuts reduce levels of LDL cholesterols and thus reduce the risk of CVDs.

7. **Omega 3 fatty acids:** Omega 3 fatty acids such as eicosapentanoic acid (EPA) and docosahexanoic acid (DHA) protect against CVDs. As per various studies it can be predicted that Omega 3 fatty acids reduces platelet aggregation, blood viscosity, plasma fibrinogen levels, PF4, and thromboglobulin and increase capillary flow. Thus, it can be used to treat CVDs. Omega 3 fatty acids reduce triglycerides levels and have antiarrythmic effects. Various research studies have proved that small intake of fish per week would reduce the risk of nonfatal Myocardial infarction by 27 % and death from CVD by 17 % as fish contains Omega 3 fatty acids. As per National and international guidelines, person should consume at least 250 mg/day Omega 3 fatty acids for maintenance of good cardiovascular health.

8. **Rice bran:** It lowers the level of LDL and increases the level HDL and hence protect against heart disease.

9. **Probiotics:** Probiotic bacteria inhibit cholesterol synthesis and enhance cholesterol metabolism. This action is due to short-chain fatty acids produced during carbohydrate fermentation carried out by these bacteria. Probiotics reduce total cholesterol, triglycerides and LDL. They act by various mechanisms such as coprecipitation and deconjugation of lipids with bile salts, assimilation of cholesterol into the cellular membrane and with microbes. Probiotics are also antioxidant in nature.

10. **Soy Proteins:** Soy products are rich in polyunsaturated fatty acids, fibre, vitamins and minerals etc. Soy proteins decrease the micellar content and absorption of lipids. It inhibits angiotensin converting enzyme (ACE) and thereby reduces systolic and diastolic BP. According to one study, it was observed that intake of 30-50 g soy per day, reduce total cholesterol (TC), LDL-C, and TG and enhance increase in HDL-C.

11. **Polyphenols:** Polyphenols include number of phytoconstituents such as flavonoids, phenolic acids, stilbenes and lignans etc. food like fruits, vegetables, cereal and legumes, and

beverages are main sources of phenolic compounds. Polyphenols improve HDL-C levels. Polyphenols act as anti-atherosclerotic agent by decreasing LDL oxidation; improving endothelial function, increasing nitric oxide release; modulation of inflammation and improvement of antioxidant status; protection against myocardial ischemia and platelet aggregation.

Resveratrol (RES) (3, 5, 4 tri-hydroxy-stilbene), is a polyphenol, found in grapes, berries and red wine. Various studies have showed that Resveratrol improve skeletal muscle and vascular function, inhibiting LDL-C oxidation, and thereby retards atherosclerosis. It has cardioprotective effects exerted by various mechanisms such as retarding cardiac fibrosis, improvement in cardiac remodelling, enhancing endothelial, diastolic and systolic functions, and myocardial energy metabolism. It also inhibit endothelial apoptosis, endothelial activation and vascular inflammation, and improves the endothelial function. It reduces oxidative stress, activates eNOS, improves calcium cycling and inhibit hypertrophic gene expression. Hence, it has protective effects, cardiac hypertrophy and heart failure.

12. Spirulina: Spirulina (Cyanobacterium) is a type of blue green algae rich in protein, vitamins, minerals, carotenoids and phycocyanins etc. It shows alterations in blood lipid profiles. It reduces TC and LDL-C.

13. α-Tocopherol: It is vitamin E and is fat soluble antioxidant. Being antioxidants it reduces cholesterol, inhibits cancers and manages diabetes. It suppresses the activity of enzyme hydroxy-3methyl-glutaryl-CoA(HMG-CoA reductase) involved in cholesterol synthesis.

14. Vitamin D (Calciferol): Vitamin D protect against atherosclerosis by inhibition of macrophage cholesterol uptake, foam cell formation, reducing vascular smooth muscle cell proliferation, and avoiding expression of adhesion molecules to endothelial cells.

15. Carnitine and L-carnitine: These are naturally occurring amino acids which play critical role in energy production. It is documented that L-carnitine supplementation avoids myocardial infarction, progression of heart failure, ventricular dysfunction, ischemia-reperfusion injury, cardiac arrhythmia and myocardial cell damage and death due to CVD. L-Carnitine acts as cardioprotective agents by facilitating transport of long-chain fatty acids into the mitochondrial matrix, reducing oxidative stress, inflammation and necrosis of cardiac myocytes. L-carnitine also regulates calcium influx, maintains endothelial integrity, regulates intracellular enzyme release and membrane phospholipid content for sustained cellular homeostasis.

16. Garlic: Garlic acts as cardioprotective agent by lowering lipids, through both inhibition of fat absorption and suppression of hepatic cholesterol synthesis. Garlic acts as antihypertensive agent by angiotensin-converting-enzyme inhibitor effect, calcium channel blocking activity, reducing catecholamine sensitivity, improving arterial compliance, increasing bradykinin and NO etc.

17. Sesame: Various studies have indicated that Sesame lowers serum glucose, LDL–C, increases HDL, reduces oxidative stress markers, lowers BP, reduces inflammation etc.

18. Vitamin C: It is antioxidant, thus it helps to prevent atherosclerosis by inhibiting endothelial dysfunction, vascular smooth muscle proliferation, and reduce oxidized LDL cholesterol.

19. Carotenoids: Carotenoids are used for immune enhancement and for reducing the risk of cancer, CVD and cataract. They reduce oxidative stress and blood markers of inflammation. Various studies have showed that intake lots of fruit and vegetables containing avoid risk of CVD.

4.5.3 Benefits and Role of Nutraceuticals in Prevention of Diabetes

Numerous plants and nutraceutical agent lower blood glucose level by different mechanisms. Diabetes Mellitus is a complex metabolic disorder characterized by abnormally high levels of blood glucose which is due to insulin resistance, impairment in insulin signaling, destruction of β-cell dysfunction, abnormal glucose and lipid metabolism, sub-clinical inflammation and increased oxidative stress etc. There are two types mainly: Type 1 diabetes (Insulin dependent diabetes mellitus) which can occur in 5% population and is an autoimmune disorder. Another is type 2 diabetes (Non- Insulin dependent diabetes mellitus) which can affect about 95% population, and is associated with obesity. Gestational diabetes occurs in pregnancy. It is estimated to affect 4.4% of total population of world by 2030. Type 2 diabetes can be controlled by modification in diet and nutraceuticals. Use of Nutraceuticals rich PUFAs, Probiotics, Prebiotics, fibres, vitamins, polyphenols and spices etc. can lower the risk of developing diabetes and help to control sugar level.

Phytochemicals Effective Against Diabetes:

- **Vitamins:** Vitamin C being antioxidant in nature (ascorbic acid) scavenges reactive oxygen species and thus reduces protein glycation. Vitamin E also has protective action against type 2 diabetes. Biotin (member of B complex) is effective against diabetes. It acts by stimulating liver glucokinase activity, increasing insulin production, and enhaning glucose uptake in muscle cells.
- **Calcium and Vitamin D:** Appropriate levels of calcium and vitamin D suppresses secretion of parathyroid hormone (PTH), hence help to conserve insulin sensitivity, improve glucose tolerance and prevent diabetes mellitus. Vitamin D alters the balance between intracellular and extracellular calcium in β cells thereby decreases insulin resistance and increases insulin secretion. Vitamin D is immunomodulatory and anti-inflammatory agent. It reduces the inflammation of pancreatic islets and decreases the autoimmune insulinitis. Vitamin D deficiency is also observed in obese patients with type 2 diabetes. As per study, it is observed that infants taking appropriate amount of vitamin D have less chances of developing Type 1 Diabetes. Few randomized controlled trials have indicated that combined calcium and vitamin D treatment reduces the risk of type 2 diabetes. Vitamin D and calcium enhances function of β-cell of pancreas.
- **L-carnitine:** It is vitamin like compound, present in mammalian plasma mainly in skeletal and cardiac muscles. L-carnitine helps in fatty acid transport across the inner mitochondrial membrane into the matrix for β-oxidation, detoxification of potentially

toxic metabolites, regulation of the mitochondrial acyl-Co A/CoA ratio, and stabilization of cell membranes. It avoids accumulation of short- and medium-chain fatty acids in mitochondria. It promotes insulin sensitivity, affects oxidative metabolism of glucose and lowers lipid. L carnitine helps to fight with oxidative stress and insulin resistance of skeletal muscles. Carnitine prevents diabetic ketoacidosis by enhancing break down fatty acids and binding acyl residues.

- **Omega-3 fatty acids:** Omega 3 fatty acids supplement lowers triglycerides, VLDL-cholesterol, inflammatory markers and blood pressure. It also avoids insulin resistance. Hence, it is helpful in treatment of type 2 diabetes.
- **CoQ10:** As per clinical study it was observed that CoQ10 improves insulin resistance, loweres glucose and fasting insulin levels.

Minerals:

Chromium increases insulin sensitivity and improves glucose tolerance in patients with type 2 diabetes. Chromium improves insulin receptor-mediated signalling and potentiates its action. It regulates reactions involving phosphorylation/dephosphorylation which are important for insulin binding to receptors. Chromium regulates activation and inhibits termination of insulin receptor-mediated responses, which in turn influence glucose utilization by peripheral tissues. Thus, it regulates glucose levels.

Magnesium is involved in glucose oxidation and glucose transport across cell membranes. It enhances insulin secretion; improves insulin sensitivity and peripheral glucose uptake. Magnesium intake lowers the levels of fasting insulin. It helps to preserve adipocyte insulin sensitivity. Zinc and antioxidants prevents the damage of retina due to oxidative stress.

Manganese, zinc and iron catalyses the breakdown of the superoxide anion into oxygen and hydrogen peroxide to water. Thus, it protects β cells from oxidative stress.

- **α-Lipoic acid:** Ischemic injury to retina occurs due to diabetes is major cause of visual loss. α-Lipoic acid have protective action on retina injury. It is antioxidant in nature. It enhances insulin sensitivity. It also improves insulin resistance. It lowers blood glucose levels by inhibiting mammalian pyruvate dehydrogenase kinase. Various studies have shown that α-Lipoic acid has protective effects on acute symptoms and disease progression indiabetic neuropathy.
- **Phytoestrogens:** Phytoestrogens and soy proteins reduce adipose tissue and improve glucose uptake.
- **Dietary Fibers:** Because of formation of viscous solutions and gelling properties, soluble dietary fiber increases insulin sensitivity and reduces postprandial glucose levels. Also various studies have demonstrated that consumption of insoluble fibres may reduce the risk of diabetes by 21%.
- **Berberine:** It is active constituent of the ancient Chinese herb *Coptis chinensis* Franch which is used to treat diabetes. It decreases in HbA_{1c}, fasting plasma glucose, post-

prandial glucose, and plasma triglycerides as per various clinical studies. Berberin increases insulin receptor expression and improves glucose utility. It suppresses intestinal disaccharidases (sucrase and maltase) and reducing the intestinal glucose absorption. Other benefiary effects of Berberine includes reduction of serum cholesterol, triglyceride, LDL-C, systolic and diastolic blood pressures etc.

- **Curcumin:** Curcumin, active principle of turmeric, directly interacts with cyclooxygenase-2 (COX- 2), DNA polymerase, lipoxygenase (LOX), glycogen synthase kinase 3b (GSK-3b), and cytokines (TNF-a). It interacts indirectly with several transcription factors, activator protein1 (AP-1), b-catenin, signal transducer and activator of transcription (STAT) proteins, and peroxisome proliferator – activated receptor c (PPARc). All these factors are related to obesity-induced insulin resistance and chronic inflammation. Hence, it has role in prevention of Diabetes.

Herbs used in Diabetes Treatment:

The details of herbal drugs used to treat diabetes are as follows:

Table 4.9: Details of herbal drugs used to treat diabetes

Sr. No.	Botanical Name of Plant	Common Name	Role in Curing Diabetes
1.	*Names Italics Acacia arabica (Lam.) Muhl.* Fabaceae	Babul	Enhances release of insulin from pancreatic β cells.
2.	*Aegle marmelos (L.) Correa* Rutaceae	Bel	Stimulation of glucose uptake enhanced insulin secretion decreases the elevated glucose and glycosylated haemoglobin levels.
3.	*Allium cepa L.* Liliacaeae	Onion	Hypoglycemic effects and potent antioxidant activity.
4.	*Aloe vera (L.) Burm. f.* Liliaceae	Aloe	Control carbohydrate metabolizing enzymes so maintains glucose homeostasis and stimulates insulin.
5.	*Artemisia pallens Wall. Ex DC.* Compositae	Davana	Inhibits glucose re-absorption or increase in peripheral glucose utilization.
6.	*Azadirachta indica A.Juss.* Meliaceae	Neem	Inhibits action of epinephrine on glucose metabolism, increases utilization of peripheral glucose and altering the serum cortisol concentration.

Contd...

7.	*Andrographis paniculata Nees* Acanthaceae	Kalmegh	Hypotriglycaeridemic effect and antioxidant activity.
8.	*Brassica juncea* Brassicaceae	Mustard	Increases the concentration of hepatic glycogen and glycogenesis and suppressed the activity of glycogen phosphorylase and gluconeogenic enzymes, reduces glycogenolysis and gluconeogenesis.
9.	*Cassia auriculata L.* Leguminosae		Suppresses gluconeogenesis and enhance utilization of glucose through increased glycolysis, alpha-glucosidase inhibitory hence act as Hypoglycemic agent.
10.	*Caesalpinia bonducella* Caesalpiniaceae	Fever Nut	Antihyperglycemic, increases the release of insulin.
11.	*Coccinia indica* Cucurbitaceae	Kundru	Inhibit glucose-6-phosphatase and fructose-1, 6-bisphosphatase enzymes and thus suppress glucose synthesis. Enhances enzyme glucose-6-phosphate dehydrogenase and hence glucose oxidation.
12.	*Eugenia jambolana* Myrtaceae	Jambhul	Increases insulin release, alters hepatic and skeletal muscle glycogen content and hepatic glucokinase, hexokinase, glucose-6-phosphate and phospho-fructokinase levels.
13.	*Gymnema sylvestre* Apocynaceae	Gurmar	Increases secretion of insulin, regenerates islet cells, increases utilization of glucose and enhances activities of enzymes responsible for utilization of glucose, increases phosphorylase activity, decreases gluconeogenic enzymes and sorbitol dehydrogenase, inhibit glucose absorption from intestine.
14.	*Moringa oleifera* Moringaceae	Drum stick	Causes hyperglycemia and dyslipidemia.

Contd...

15.	*Momordica charantia* Cucurbitaceae	Bitter gourd	Increasing hepatic glycogen, hypoglycaemic.
16.	*Ocimum sanctum* Labiatae	Tulsi	Cortisol inhibiting hence lowers blood glucose levels.
17.	*Lagenaria siceraria* Curcurbitaceae	Bottle gourd	Reduces LDL C levels, decrease in fasting glucose and total cholesterol.
18.	*Linum usitatissimum* Linaceae	Flax seeds	Inhibit lipid peroxidation and antioxidant.
19.	*Trigonella foenum-graecum* L. Leguminosae	Fenugreek	Reduces plasma glucose and increases insulin receptors.
20.	*Emblica officinalis* Euphorbiaceae	Amla	Reduces total cholesterol (TC), low-density lipoprotein (LDL), triglyceride (TG), Hypoglycemic agent.
21.	*Murraya koenigii* Rutaceae	Kadhipatta	Increases hepatic glycogen concentration and decreases in concentration of glycogen phosphorylase and gluconeogenic enzymes.
22.	*Vigna mungo* Dicotyledonae	Black gram/Black lentil	Prevent insulin resistance, control blood sugar level due to low glycemic index.
23.	*Camellia sinensis* Theaceae	Green tea	Reduces plasma glucose.
24.	*Pterocarpus marsupium* Papilionaceae	Vijaysar	Hypoglycaemic agent.
25.	*Tinospora cordifolia* Menispermaceae	Guduchi	Potent hypoglycaemic activity.

(**Source:** Ruchi, et al.: Role of nutraceuticals in health care: A review)

4.5.4 Benefits and Role of Nutraceuticals in Prevention of IBD and Other GIT Diseases

GIT related diseases are becoming very common now-a-days because of various reasons. Irritable bowel syndrome (IBS) is disease of GIT, may be associated with pain in ilium, diarrhoea and/ or constipation. This can be treated with bulk laxatives and carminative drugs. The most common natural remedy for GIT problem is peppermint or some other essential oils. Some tropane alkaloids like atropine, hyocine may also have beneficial effect in these conditions. An inflammatory bowel disease (IBD) is idiopathic, chronic and relapsing inflammatory disorders of Gastrointenstinal tract including Crohn's disease (CD) and ulcerative colitis (UC). UC is a mucosal or submucosal inflammation of mainly the rectum and occasionally involve colonic area. CD is regarded as a transmural inflammation of the ileum, colon, or any other part of the gastrointestinal tract. It forms granulomas, fistulas, and strictures in the intestine. IBD can occur due to immune deregulation, altered intestinal microflora, oxidative stress, defects in the gastrointestinal mucosal barrier and increased permeability which leads to inflammation. Then inflammatory molecules cross the epithelial barrier and form crypt abscesses. It stimulates release of cytokines. In IBD, balance between pro-inflammatory cytokines, such as TNF-α, IFN-γ, interleukin (IL)-1, IL-6, and IL-12 and anti-inflammatory cytokines, which includes IL-4, IL-10, and IL-1 etc. get disturbed. It causes inflammation and tissue damage. The disease is characterised by symptoms like diarrhoea, nausea, abdominal pain, fatigue, rectal bleeding, weight loss, anxiety. Types of IBD are Constipation predominant (IBS-C), diarrhoea-predominant (IBS-D), and IBS with predominant irregular (mixed diarrhoea/constipation) bowel habits (IBS-M). IBD affects 10 % to 20 % of world population. Along with IBD other gastrointestinal problems includes ulcers, constipation, hemorrhoids, an fissures, perianal abscesses, anal fistulas, perianal infections, colitis, and colorectal cancer etc. Current therapies of IBD are based on steroidal, non-steroidal drugs and biological agents. But the treatment is expensive and has many adverse health effects. So treatment based on natural products is in great demand. Use of appropriate food and neutraceuticals plays crucial role in treatment of IBD.

Table 4.10: Role of Neutraceuticals in Inflammatory Bowel Disease (IBD)

Sr. No.	Name of disease	Symptom	Nutraceutical or Treatment
1.	Diarrhoea	Sudden watery stool	ORS or rice water with salt.
2.	Constipation	Frequency of bowel movement is less the once in 2-3 days	Bulk laxative Isapgol - *Plantago ovata* Linseed – *Linum usitatissimum* Wheat bran - *Triticum aestivum* Osmotic laxative Stimulant laxative Senna - *Cassia senna* Frangula - *Rhamnus frangula, R. purshiana.*
3.	Gastritis	Inflammation of stomach	Chamomile- *Matricaria recutita.*
4.	Ulcer	Heartburn, pain in stomach	Liquorice- *Glycyrrhiza glabra.*
5.	Dyspepsia	Nausea, pain, heartburn	Arentian- *Gentiana lutea* Wormwood-*Artemisia absinthum.*

Contd...

6.	Nausea, Vomiting	Vomiting, dizziness, sweating, vertigo	Ginger- *Zingiber officinale* Hyoscine.
7.	IBS	Alternating diarrhoea and constipation	Peppaermint- *Mentha Piperita* Umbelliferous fruits- Caraway - *Carum carvi* Fennel - *Foeniculum vulgare.*

Phytochemicals Effective Against GIT Disorders:

- **Dietary Fibers:** Fiber improve intestinal transit and decrease constipation being bulking agents. IBS patients are recommended to include soluble fibers in diet.
- **Gas producing foods:** IBD can be treated with gas producing food such as alcohol, apricots, bananas, beans, caffeine, carrots, celery, onions, raisins and wheat germ etc.
- **Curcumin:** Curcumin obtained from *Curcuma longa*, family: Zingiberaceae can be used to treat various GIT disorders. It acts as anti-inflammatory agent and reduces mucosal injury by inhibition of nuclear factor NF-kB and pro-inflammatory cytokines. Curcumin heals peptic ulcers by preventing peroxidase inactivation and enhancing free radical scavenging activity.
- **Glutamine:** Glutamine is a precursor for nucleotide synthesis, serves as a substrate for hepatic gluconeogenesis. It provides energy to GI epithelial cells, lymphocytes, fibroblasts and reticulocytes etc. Glutamine supplements helps to improve mucosal and plasma glutathione concentrations, improve GI function and decrease markers of lipid peroxidation. Less concentration of Glutamine causes degeneration of the mucosa, diarrhoea, and growth failure.
- **Zinc:** Zinc deficiency causes ulcerations, inflammatory infiltration, oedema of the jejunum, leads to poor absorption of dietary fats, with accumulation of lipids, impairs sodium and water balance and causes intestinal tract damage by free radicals. Zinc supplements improve markers of intestinal permeability and reduce diarrhoea.
- **Probiotic:** Probiotics are living microorganisms like species of lactobacilli or bifidobacteria. They maintain good health by improving balance in intestinal microflora. They avoid damage of pathogens on intestinal flora by competing for receptor sites on the intestinal surface, producing antibiotic substances, enhancing host immune defences and competing pathogens for intraluminal nutrients. Probiotics also strengthen defence mechanism by strengthening intestinal tight junctions, increasing mucous secretion, enhancing motility, and producing protective nutrients etc. Various studies have showed that probiotics can prevent IBD, colitis and other GI disorders. Probiotics can reduce the chances of occurrence of colon cancer. By lowering pH level in the colon probiotics limits the growth of pathogens. Probiotics inhibit inflammation by modulating the NF-κB signalling pathway, inflammatory cytokines, and the regulatory T cell response.

Probiotics have protective effects like prevention of colonic shortening, lowering of liver and thymus weights, and prevent spleen enlargement. Various clinical studies have indicated that probiotics have protective effects against diseases such as Rotavirus infections, Antibiotic-associated diarrhoea, Necrotizing enterocolitis, infantile allergic dermatitis, microbe-induced gastroenteritis and Traveller's diarrhoea etc.

- **Prebiotics:** Prebiotics are defined as, "non-digestible polysaccharides like oligosaccharides and insulin which stimulates growth and activity of specific species of bacteria in the colon." Breast milk, a prebiotic facilitates the preferential growth of bifidobacteria and lactobacilli in the colon. Prebiotics have various beneficiary effects such as improvement in bowel function, increased mineral absorption, altered lipid metabolism, and a reduced risk of colon cancer. They enhance bioavailability and absorption of calcium, magnesium, iron and zinc. They also reduce fasting insulin and triacylglycerol concentrations. They produce anti-inflammatory effects by decreasing pro-inflammatory cytokines such as, IFN-γ, IL-17, and TNF-α.
- **Vitamins:** Fat soluble vitamins A and D have protective action against IBD. Patients with GI disorders show deficiency of Vitamin A and D. Vitamin D produces protective effects by down regulating pro-inflammatory cytokines like IL-6, IL-21, TNF-α, and IFN-γ and by stabilizing the intestinal barrier. Vitamin D increases the level of IL-10, IL-6 and inhibites the proliferation of T cells. Vitamin A supplementation has protective effect against IBD. It acts by increasing the proliferation of mitochondrial transcription factors NFR-1 and TFAM and preventing intestinal tissue damage. Vitamin K protects against IBD and maintains bone health in patients.
- **Fatty acids:** Omega 3 fatty acids reduce the levels of iNOS, COX-2, TNF-α, LTB_4, and IL-1β and hence have protective effects against various GI disorders. Omega 3 fatty acids when administered with arachidonic acid (AA) decreased TNF-α and IL-6 and increased PPAR γ. Thus, have protective effects against colitis. Short chain fatty acids (SCFAs) such as acetate, propionate, and butyrate are beneficial for patients with colitis. Butyrate increases production of regulatory T cells (Tregs) and enhances levels of IL (Interleukin) - 10 and IL (Interleukin) - 12.Thus, avoids damage of intestinal mucosa. Fatty acids such as Acetate and propionate inhibit the expression of immune-related genes and inflammatory mediators, such as NF-κB and IL-6.

Table 4.11: Role of different phytochemicals/herbs against various GI disorders

Sr. No.	Herbs or Phytochemicals	Role
1.	Aloe *Aloe vera*, Liliaceae	Prevent stress-induced gastric ulceration by enhancing collagen synthesis and fibroblast activity.
2.	Garlic *Allium sativum*, Liliaceae	Gastro protective effects due to antioxidant nature.

Cond...

3.	*Coriolusversicolor, Polyporaceae*, Mushroom	Protective effects against IBD by reducing TNF-α, IL-1β and IL-6.
4.	*Cordiceps militaris, Clavicipitaceae* mushroom extract	Prevent IBD by decreasing epithelial damage, suppressing iNOS and TNF-α mRNA expression.
5.	Pomegranate extract *Punica granatum, Lythraceae*	Decreased the expression of TNF-α, COX-2, IL-4, and STAT6.
6.	Cranberry *Vaccinium oxycoccos*, Ericaceae	Protect against IBD by Modulating NF-κB and IL-1β signalling, prevent colon shortening.
7.	Ginger *Zingiber officinalis, Zingiberaceae*	Protect mucosa by decreasing the level of pro-inflammatory cytokines.
8.	Green algae	Protect colon tissue damage by Down regulating IFN-γ and IL-4 and decreasing pro-inflammatory cytokines.
9.	Apple *Malus pumila, Rosaceae*	GIT protective effects by reducing COX-2 and TNF-α and Recovering transglutaminase protein.
10.	Resveratrol	Suppress NF-κB and TNF-α.
11.	Cardamonin	Reduced iNOS, NF-κB, TNF-α, COX-2, and caspase-3.
12.	Flavonoids	Protect gastric mucosa by interfering both with gene expression and receptor-regulated signaling pathways of inflammation.
13.	Salai Guggulu *Boswellia serrata, Burseraceae*	Preserve intestinal epithelial barrier and inhibit oxidative and inflammatory damage.
14.	Kalmegh *Andrographis paniculata*, Acanthaceae	Reduce the transcriptional activity of NF-κB and decrease secretions of pro-inflammatory cytokines such as TNF-α and IL-6.
14.	Mastic *Pistacia lentiscus, Anacardiaceae*	Effective against IBD by inhibiting TNF-α and stimulating macrophage migration inhibitory factor (MIF) activity.

4.6 DIFFERENT HERBS USED AS HEALTH FOOD

(1) ALFALFA

Synonym: Lucerne, Alfalfa weevil, Buffalo herb.

Biological Name: It consists of entire herb of *Medicago sativa Linn*, family Leguminosae.

Geographical Source: Alfalfa is mainly obtained from the Mediterranean and southwest Asia. It is mainly produced in USA and cultivated in Europe, Middle-East, Africa, South America and Australia.

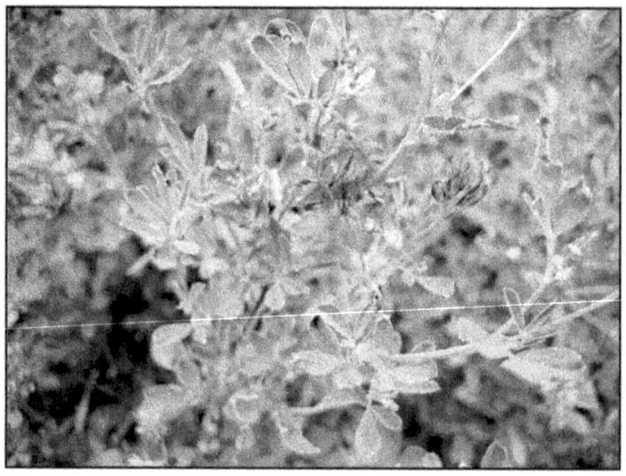

Fig. 4.2: Herb of *Medicago sativa Linn*

Description:

Alfalfa is perennial legume with three to twelve years life. The palnt has deep root, erect or decumbent stems up to 1 m in height, glabrous or hairy in the upper parts. It has trifoliate laeves with obovate leaflets, 10-45 mm long and 3-10 mm broad. It bears 5 to 40 yellow, blue or purple flowers. Fruits are curly pods with 2-8 seeds.

Constituents:

It contains most of the vitamins but it is high in vitamin K, contains vitamin C, Thiamin, Riboflavin and minerals like calcium, potassium, phosphorous, iron, copper, manganese, magnesium, and folate. It consists of following phytoconstituents:

Alkaloids: Asparagines, trigoneline, stachydrine, and l-homostachydrine.

Amino acids: Medicanine, lysine, arginine, histidine, tyrosine, phenylalanine, methionine, aspartic acid, glutamic acid, asparagine, serine, alanine, threonine.

Coumarins: Myrsellinol, scopoletin, esculetin, 4-coumaric acid.

Flavonoids: Quercetin, myricetin, luteolin, apigenin, chrysoeriol, tricin, 4'-O-[2'-O-E-feruloyl-O-β-glucuronopyranosyl (1→2)-O-β-lucuronopyranoside] apigenin, 7-O-β-glucuronopyranosyl-4'-O-[2'-O-E-feruloyl-O-β-glucuronopyranosyl(1→2)-O-β-glucuronopyranoside] apigenin, 7-O-β-glucuronopyranosyl-4'-O-[2'-O-p-E-coumaroyl-O-β-glucuronopyranosyl(1→2)-O-β-glucuronopyranoside] apigenin, 7-O-{2-O-E-feruloyl-[β-glucuronopyranosyl(1→3)]-O-β-lucuronopyranosyl(1→2)-O-β-glucuronopyranoside} apigenin, O-glycosyltransferases, medicarpin, coumestrol, sativan, vestitol, formononetin.

Phenolic compounds: p-hydroxybenzoic acid, vanillic acid, p-coumaric acid, ferulic acids, salicylic acid, sinapic acids, caffeic acid, hesperetin, naringenin, chlorogenic acid, tannic acid and heterosides.

Phytoestrogens: Coumestrol, genistein, formometin, diadzein and biocanine A etc.

Saponins: Soyasapogenols, hederagenin, medicagenic acid, Ara-Glc-Ara-hederagenin, soyasapogenol A, soyasapogenol B, soyasapogenol E, bayogenin glycoside etc.

Coumarins: Myrsellinol, scopoletin, esculetin, 4-coumaric acid.

Phytosterols: β-sitosterol, stigmasterol.

Volatile components: Terpenes, limonene, linalool, trans ocimene, furanoids, nonadienal, 2-methyl 4-pentenai, benzaldehyde, ethyl benzaldehyde, alcohols, butanol, hexanol, octanol, pentan-3-ol, 3-methylbutanol etc.

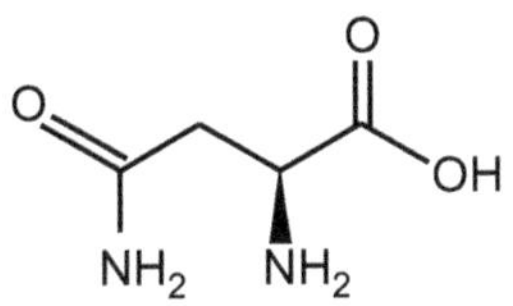

Asparagin

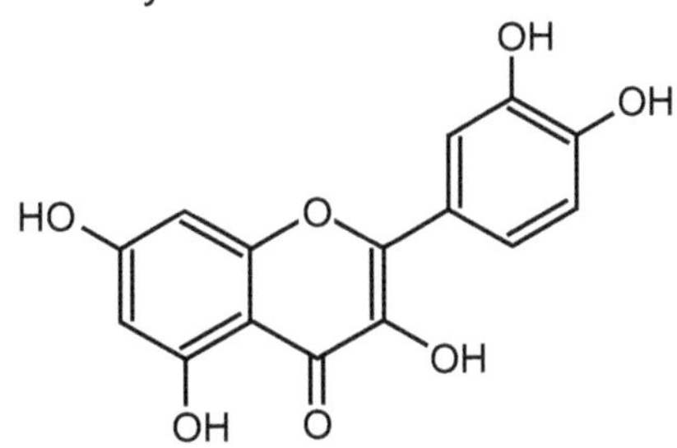

Quercetin

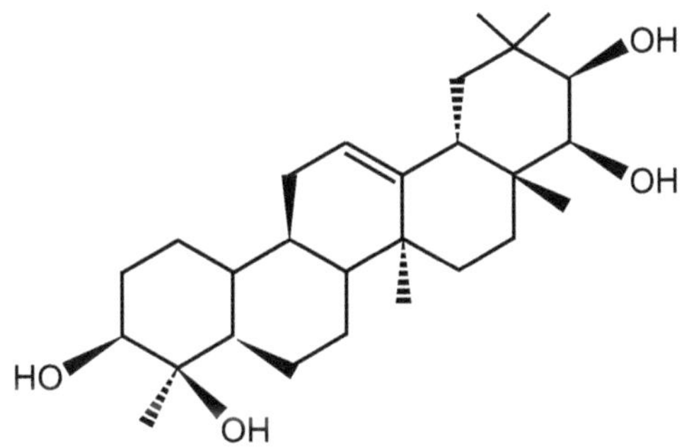

Soyasapogenol A

Chemical constituents of Alfalfa

Health Benefits of Alfalfa:

Alfalfa is used to treat various disorders such as kidney , bladder and prostate disorders, treating menopausal symptoms, high BP, asthma, rheumatoid arthritis and stomach upset.

- Alfalfa roots and leaves have shown antibacterial activity against *Corynebacterium michiganense, Corynebacterium insidiosum and Agrobacterium tumefaciens.* It also possesses antifungal and nematicidal activity.
- It is used to treat kidney stones, fever, gravel, dysuria and to relieve fluid retention and swelling.
- Alfalfa decreases intestinal absorption and increase fecal excretion of cholesterol without changing levels of HDL. It is antiatherosclerotic agent. It reduces accumulation of cholesterol in liver. It also reduces serum cholesterol, low-density lipoprotein (LDL) cholesterol and apolipoprotein B.
- It possess estrogenic activity and used in treatment of hormone-related cancers.
- It exerts antidopaminergic action and also shows immunomodulatory action.
- Polysaccharides from alfalfa show anti HIV activity.

- It exhibits antioxidant and cerebroprotective effects.
- It potentiates the action of aminopyrine N-demethylase, a liver drug metabolizing enzyme.
- It helps to maintain function of digestive system, nutrition balance in human body, and prevents osteoporosis and aging.
- It has been found to reduce basal plasma glucose concentrations, also potentiates insulin secretion and action, hence it is used to treat diabetes.
- Alfalfa can be used in treatment of peptic ulcers, polycystic ovaries, as a tonic after blood loss, anemia, urinary and bowel problems, scurvy, secondary hypothyroidism and Herpes simplex viral infection.
- It is beneficial in arthritis, cardiovascular disorders, convalescence, debility, in protein allergies and GI upset.

Recommended Dosage: 5 to 10 g of the dried herb can be taken 3 times daily. Dose of 40 g of heated seeds can be taken by mouth 3 times daily.

Side Effects: Use of Alfalfa is safe in adults. But long-term use can cause autoimmune disease called lupus erythematosus.

Special Precautions: Avoid the use of Alfalfa in pregnancy and lactation because of its oestrogen like action. It should not be taken in persons having autoimmune disorders like lupus erythematosus, multiple sclerosis as it can worsen the symptoms. Use of Alfalfa should be avoided in Hormone-sensitive conditions such as breast cancer, uterine cancer, ovarian cancer and endometriosis.

(2) CHICORY

Synonyms: Hindubar, Kasni, Indyba, Belgium endive.

Biological Name: It consists of dried roots of *Cichorium intybus* L. Asteraceae.

Geographical Source: The plant commonly grows in Africa, Europe, Australia, Northern America and Southern America Europe and Asia.

Description:

Chicory plant is erect, rough and more or less glandular herb. The herb flowers in summer. Flower are brilliant bluish-purple having radial symmetrical bloom. It has large-dandelion-shaped leaves near the base of the stem and small lanceolate too blong-shaped leaves along the length of the stem. Leaves have dentate margin.

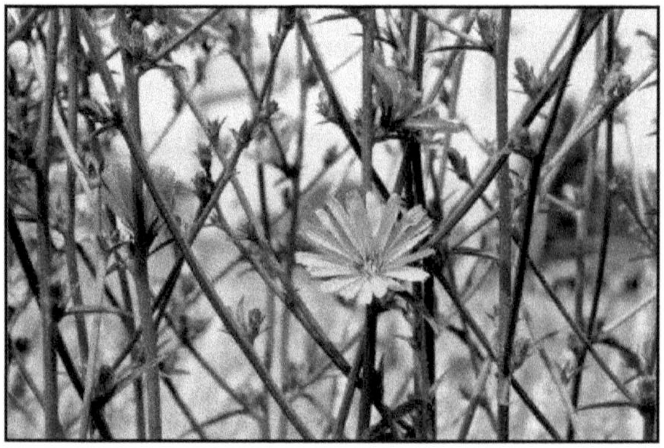

Fig. 4.3: Herb of *Cichorium intybus*

Chemical Constituents:

Fresh chicory root contains 68 % inulin, 14% sucrose, 5% cellulose, 6% protein, 4% ash, and 3% other compounds. The root extracts showed presence of volatile oils, fatty acids, alkaloids, triterpenes, flavonoids, latex, tannins and saponins, pyrazines, benzothiazoles, aldehydes, aromatic hydrocarbons, furans, phenols, organic acids, 2-acetylpyrrole, furfural, phenyl acetaldehyde, phenyl acetic acid and vanillin. Roots of Chicory also have harman and norharman alkaloids, flavone dervatives, saccharides, anthocyanins, sesquiterpenes lactone germacrene and vitamins.

Chicory seeds shows presence of amino acids like arginine, histidine, isoleucine, leucine, lysinemethionine, cysteine, phenylalanine, tyrosine, threonine, valine, serine, glutamic acid, glycine, alanine, aspartic acid, and proline. Seeds contain minerals such as phosphorus, potassium, calcium, magnesium, sodium, iron, copper, zinc, manganese, molybdenum, selenium, strontium and cadmium.

Seeds contains 18 α 19 β-20(30)-taraxasten-3-β,21-α-diol (cichoridiol), 17-epi-methyl-6-hydroxyangolensate (intybusoloid), lupeol, friedelin, β-sitosterol, stigmasterol, betulinic acid, betulin, betulinaldehyde, syringic acid, vanillic acid 6,7-dihydroxycoumarin, methyl-α-D-galacto pyranoside.

Leaves, flowers, shoots contains inulin, fructose, choline, resin, chicoric acid (dicaffeoyl tartaric acid), esculetin, esculin (esculetin-6-glucoside), cichoriin, umbelliferone, scopoletin and 6,7-dihydrocoumarin, sesquiterpene lactones and their glycosides.

Chicory plant shows presence of sesquiterpene lactones mainly lactucin, lactucopicrin, 8-desoxy lactucin, guaianolide glycosides, including chicoroisides B and C, sonchuside C etc.

Caffeic acid derivatives like chiroric acid, chlorogenic acid, isochlorogenic acid, dicaffeoyl tartaric acid are also present in plant.

Chicory shows presence of *volatile constituents* such as Octane, Octen-3-ol, 2-Pentyl furan, (2E, 4E)- Heptadienal, 1,8-Cineole, Benzene acetaldehyde, n-Nonanal, Camphor, (2E, 6Z)-Nonadienal, (2E)-Nonen-1-al,n-Decanal, (2E, 4E)-Nonadienal, n-Decanol, (2E, 4Z)-Decadienal, n-Tridecane, (2E, 4E)-Decadienal, β-Elemene, (E)-Caryophyllene, β-Ylangene, Geranyl acetone, (E)-β-Farnesene, allo-Aromadendrene, dehydro Aromadendrene, β-Ionone, Pentadecane, trans-β-Guaiene, (2E)-Undecanol acetate, Sesquicineole, (2E)- Tridecanol, n-Hexadecane, Tetradecanal, Tetradecanol, 2-Pentadecanone, (E)-2-Hexylcinnamaldehyde, Octadecane, n-Nonadecane, (5E, 9E)-Farnesyl acetone, n-Eicosane, n-Octadecanol and n-Heneicosane etc.

Sixty four phenolic acids and flavonoids were extracted from different types of Chicory which includes hydroxycinnamic acid derivatives including 8 mono- and dicaffeoylquinic acids, 3 tartaric acid derivatives, 31 flavonol and 2 flavone glycosides and 10 anthocyanins.

Other constituents present in chicory are 5-p-Coumaroylquinic acid, Quercetin-3-Oglucuronide-7-O-(6-O malonyl)-glucoside, Kaempferol-3-O-glucosyl-7-O-(6–O malonyl)-Glucoside, Dimethoxy cinnamoyl shikimic acid, Kaempferol-3-O-sophoroside, Isorhamnetin-

7-O-(6-O-acetyl)-glucoside, 5-O-Feruloylquinic acid, Dicaffeoyltartaric acid (chicoric acid), Kaempferol-7-O-glucosyl-3-O- (6-malonyl)- glucoside, Delphinidin-3-O- (6-O-malonyl)-glucoside-5-O-glucoside, Cyanidin-3,5-di-O-(6-O-malonyl)- glucoside, Cyanidin- 3- O-(6-O-malonyl)-glucoside, Petunidin-3-O-(6-O-malonyl)-glucoside, Cyanidin, Cyanidin-3-O-galactoside, Cyanidin-3-O-glucoside, Cyanidin-3-O-(6-O-acetyl)-glucoside, Malvidin-3-O glucoside, Pelargonidin-3-O-monoglucuronide, 4-O-Feruloylquinic acid, Apigenin-7-O-glucoside, Chrysoeriol 3-O-glucoside, Tricin-3-O-glucoside, 1,3-dicaffeoylquinic acid, 1,4-Dicaffeoylquinic acid, 3,4-Dicaffeoylquinic acid, Quercetin-7-O-galactoside, Quercetin-3-O-(6-O-malonyl)-glucoside, Quercetin-7-O-glucoside, Quercetin7-O-glucuronide, Quercetin-7-O-(6-O-acetyl)-glucoside, Kaempferide glucuronide, Kaempferol-7-O glucoside, Kaempferol-7-O-rutinoside, Quercetin-7-O-p-coumaroylglucoside etc.

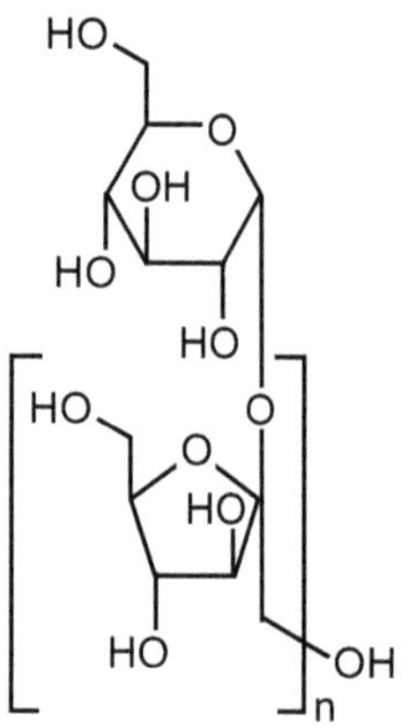

Inulin

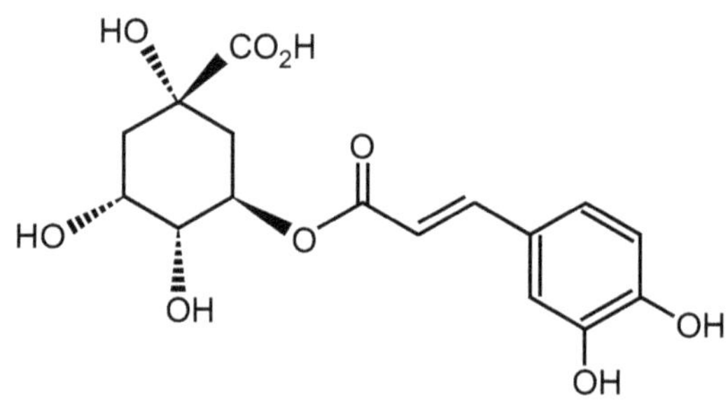

Chlorogenic acid

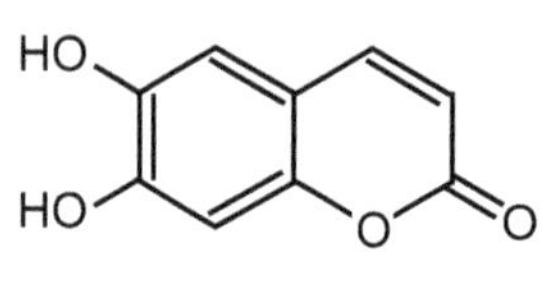

Esculetin

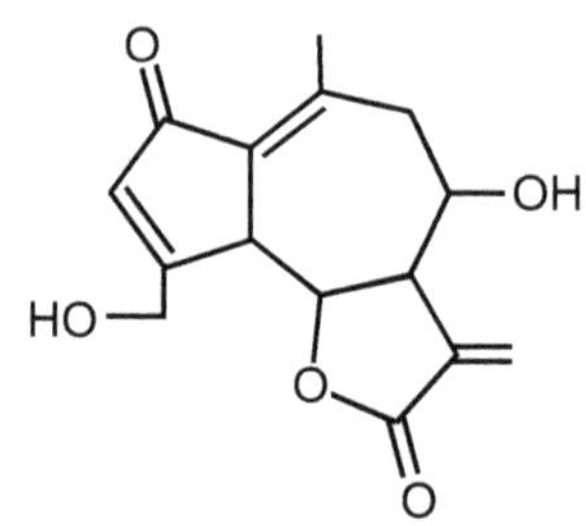

Lactucin

Health Benefits of Chicory:

- Traditionally chicory is used for the treatment of diarrhoea, prostate and other reproductive organ disorders, pulmonary disease and cough, cancer, hangover, for purification of biliary tract, liver diseases, as spasm, GIT disorders, in sore throat, hemorrhoids, tuberculosis, abdominal cramps, deafness, rashes and as laxative etc.
- Chicory exhibit hepatoprotective effects by suppressing the oxidative degradation of DNA in the tissue debris.
- It helps to reduce blood glucose, total cholesterol (TC) and triglycerides (TG) levels.
- Being inhibitor of COX-2 protein expression chicory acts as anti-inflammatory agent. It also has analgesic and sedative effects.

- It acts as antioxidant, immunomodulatory agent and has potent wound healing activity.
- It has gastroprotective effect and maintains good health of gastrointestinal tract.
- Chicory inhibits oedema and leukocyte infiltration in pancreatitis tissue. Hence, acts as pancreas protective agent.
- By inhibiting protein tyrosine phosphatase 1B (PTP1B) it exhibits effect on energy homoeostasis.
- It produces vasorelaxation and inhibits platelet aggregation hence acts as cardioprotective agent.
- Chicory inhibits mast cell-mediated immediate-type allergic reactions.
- It can be used to treat prostate cancer, breast cancer, leukemia and colon cancer etc. It is potent antiproliferative and cytotoxic agent.
- It has antimicrobial effects against *Escherichia coli, Staphylococcus aureus, Bacillus thuringiensis, Bacillus subtilis,* and *Salmonella typhi.* It also possesses antifungal effects.
- Chicory has anti-obesity effect and improves lipid metabolism.
- It has anthelmintic and anti-protozoal effects.

Recommended Dosage: 3-5 g root powder can be administered with 150-250 ml water.

Side Effects and Toxicity: Chicory is safe for human use. It may cause slight sensitization of skin.

(3) GINGER

Synonyms: Adrak, African ginger, Amomum zingiber, Ardraka, Black ginger, Cochin ginger.

Biological Name: It consists of fresh and dried rhizomes of *Zingiber officinale* Roscoe, belonging to Zingiberaceae.

Geographical Source: Tropics of the south and south-eastern Aasia. Ginger is cultivated in China, Nepal, US, India, Bangladesh, Taiwan, Jamaica, Nigeria. India is the largest producer of ginger.

Description: Ginger is herbaceous rhizomatous perennial plant. It is about 1 m tall having upright shoots sprout from the rhizome at the base of the plant. Rhizomes are aromatic, thick lobed, fleshy, pale yellow having ring-like scars. Plant has green, long leaves with sheathing bases, tapering at the apex. The flowering spikes originate from the rhizomes and when the plant matures they become dry.

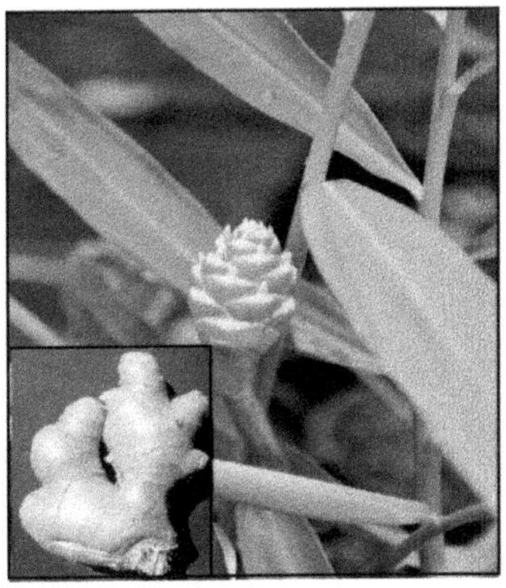

Fig. 4.4: Plant of *Zingiber officinale* Roscoe

Chemical Constituents: Ginger consists of volatile and non-volatile compounds. The volatile oil of ginger is a mixture of over 24 constituents, mainly monoterpenes like phellandrene, carnphene, cineolc, citral, and borneol and sesquiterpenes like zingiberene, α-curcumene, β-bisabolene, (-) β-sesquiphellandrene and (E, E)-α-farnesene etc. Zingiberol is main aromatic principle of ginger. Other constituents of volatile oil includes α-pinene, camphene, 6-methyl-5-hepten-2-one, myrcene, α-and β-phellandrene, limonene, 1,8-cineole, linalool, borneol, α-terpineol, citronellol, neral, geraniol, geranial, bornyl acetate, 2 undecanone, citronellyl acetate, α-copaene and geranyl acetate etc.

The main pungent non-volatile principle of ginger is gingerols, a phenolic compound. Other non-volatile principle of ginger are 6-, 8- and 10-gingerol, 1,7-bis-(40-Hydroxy-30-methoxyphenyl)-3,5-heptadione, adenine, 1-Dehydro-3-dihydro-[10]-gingerdione, Acetoxy-6-dihydroparadol, [4]-Isogingerol, 5-Methoxy-[6]-gingerol, Methyl diacetoxy-[4]-gingerdiol, and other derivatives of gingerols, 6-, 8-and 10-shogaol, Paradol and its derivatives, β-sitosterol palmitate, isovanillin, glycolmonopalmitate, hexacosanoic acid 2,3-dihydroxypropyl ester, maleimide-5-oxime, p-hydroxybenzaldehyde and 1-(omega-ferulyloxyceratyl) glycerols etc. When subjected to heat or alkali treatment, gingerols are converted into shogaols by dehydration and or to the compound zingerone after heat or alkali treatment. The shogaols is more pungent than gingerols. The pungency of dry ginger is mainly due to shogaols.

Fresh ginger also contains nutrients such as protein, fat, minerals, fibers, carbohydrates, lipids, protease, iron, calcium, magnesium, sodium, zinc, manganese, potassium and phosphorous. Vitamins such as thiamine, riboflavin, niacin and vitamin C etc. are also present. It also contains 1-2% volatile oil, 5-8% resinous matter, starch and mucilage.

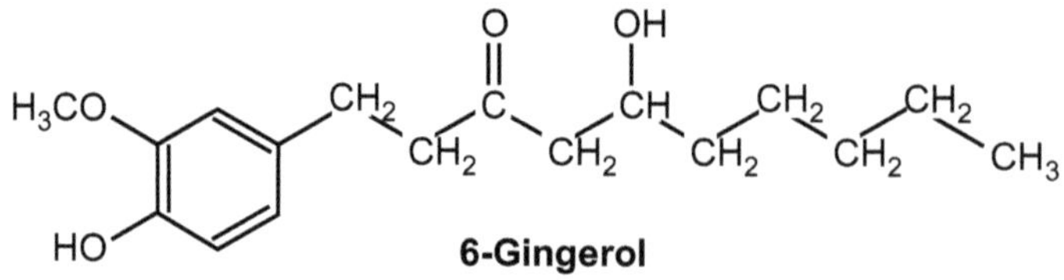

6-Gingerol

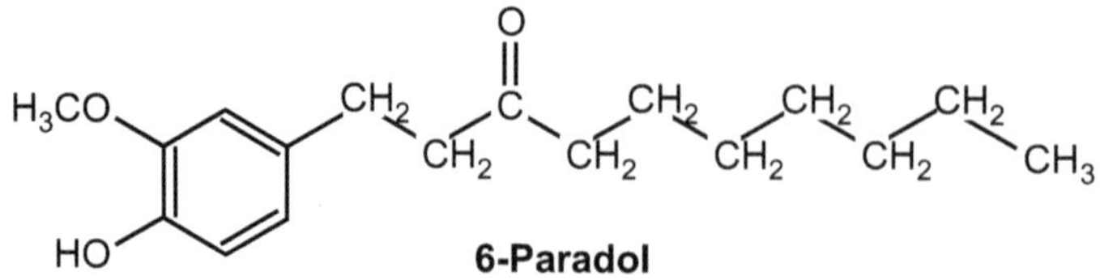

6-Paradol

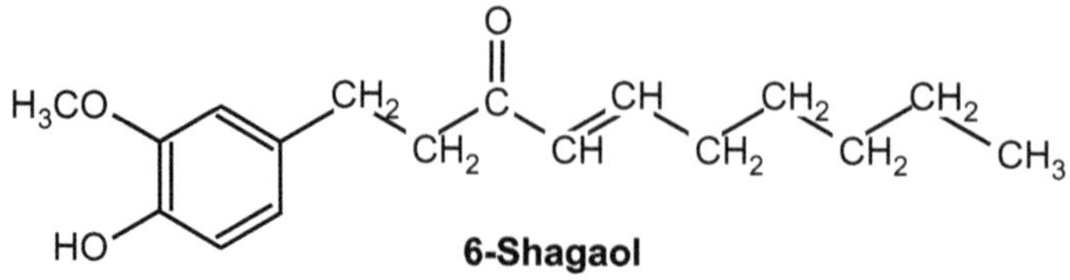

6-Shagaol

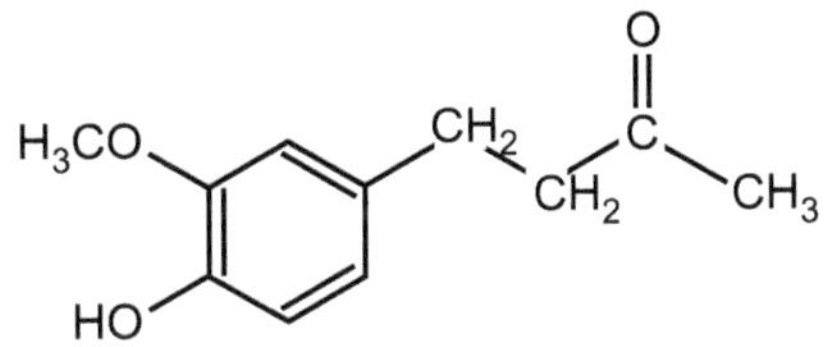

Zingerone

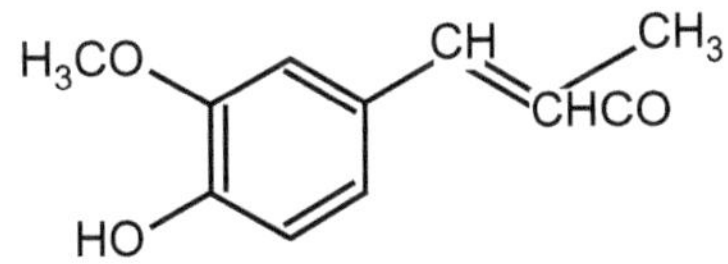

Dehydrozingerone

Health Benefits of Ginger:

- Traditionally ginger is used to treat indigestion, tastelessness, loss of appetite, flatulence, intestinal, biliary colic, nausea, vomiting, allergic reactions, acute and chronic cough, common cold, fever, allergic rhinitis, sinusitis, acute and chronic bronchitis, respiratory troubles, pain, headache, backache, muscular pain, toothache and swelling gums etc.
- It prevents morning sickness and motion sickness.
- It has antimicrobial activities against various bacterias such as *Staphylococcus aureus, Escherichia coli, Salmonella typhi, Bacillus cereus, Klebsiella pneumoniae and Pseudomonas aeruginosa.* Also possesses antifungal activity against two strains of Candida albicans (PTCC 5027 and ATCC 10231).
- Ginger is used to treat type I diabetes by increasing insulin levels and decreasing fasting glucose levels. It also improves insulin sensitivity and impaired insulin signaling.
- It also decreases serum cholesterol, serum triglyceride and blood pressure.
- It also possesses neuroprotective effects. It accelerates brain anti-oxidant defence mechanism, down regulates the MDA levels and increases GSH, SOD, CAT, GPx, GST levels etc.
- Ginger acts as hepatoprotective agent by reducing plasma SOD, hepatic MDA, serum AST and increasing plasma protein levels.
- It has Larvicidal activity against round worm *Angiostrongylus cantonensisa* which causes eosinophilic meningitis. Larvicidal activity is also reported against Anisakis *simplex Adese aegypti* and *Culex quinquefasciatus.*
- Ginger can be used to treat colorectal, gastric, ovarian, liver, skin, breast and prostate cancers. It can act by different mechanisms such as inhibition of proliferation, induction of apoptosis, and suppression of NFκB and heme oxygenase (HO) expression. It also inhibits angiogenesis.
- Ginger can inhibit platelet aggregation.
- Ginger has antiserotoninergic and 5-HT_3 receptor antagonism effects hence can be used to treat nausea, vomiting or morning sickness during pregnancy.
- It has anti-inflammatory and analgesic effects as reduces prostaglandin synthesis and inhibits NFκB, TNF-α, COX-2 expression. It also has analgesic and antipyretic activity.
- Antioxidant properties of ginger improve body's defence mechanism. It scavenges reactive oxygen species (ROS), free radicals, peroxides and prevent oxidative stress.

- Ginger has anti helmintic property and is antigenotoxic agent.
- Ginger reduces levels of fatty acid synthase and adipocyte-specific fatty acid binding protein thereby acts as antiobesity agent.
- Ginger restores renal functions, reduce lipid peroxidation and enhance the levels of glutathione, superoxide dismutase and catalase. Hence, it has renoprotective activity.
- By increasing mucin secretion, it prevents formation of gastric ulcers.
- It exhibit cardioprotective effects by inhibiting blood clotting, lowering cholesterol, exhibiting positive inotropic action and reducing blood pressure.

Dosage: Varies from 250 mg to 1 g as per disease condition. E.g. For migraine 500 mg by mouth every 4 hours; 1-4 g per day for nausea; for osteoarthritis 170 mg extract is given by mouth thrice a day; for motion sickness 1 g taken by mouth 30 minutes to 4 hours before travel.

Side Effects: Ginger is relatively safe for human use but can produce mild side effects such as heartburn, diarrhoea, extra menstrual bleeding, skin rash and stomach discomfort. Ginger should be administered cautiously in patients taking antihypertensive medication, antidiabetic drugs and anticoagulants.

(4) FENUGREEK

Synonyms: Methi, Metha.

Biological Name: It consists of herb of Trigonella foenum-graecum L, of family Fabaceae.

Geographical Source: It can be cultivated in Asia, Europe, Africa, America and in some parts of Australia. In India, 80 % production of fenugreek occurs in Rajasthan.

Description: Fenugreek herb is aromatic, 30-60 cm tall, annual herb. It has roots bearing nodules. Leaflets are 2-2.5 cm long, oblanceolate or oblong, toothed. Flowers are 1-2 in number, axillary, sessile and are white to yellow coloured. It has calyx with linear teeth. Pod has a long persistent beak, often falcate, contains 10-29 seeds, without transverse reticulations. Seeds are solid-rhomboidal, hard, pebble-like, yellowish brown-light brown colour, with characteristic spicy odour, bitter and mucilaginous taste.

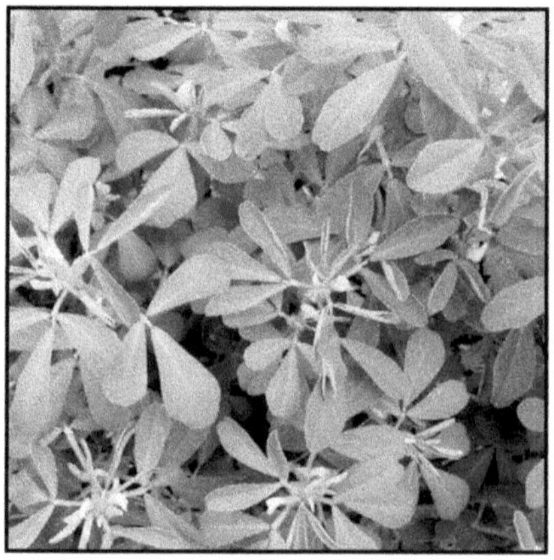

Fig. 4.5: Herb of *Trigonella foenum-graecum L*

Chemical Constituents:

- Fresh Fenugreek leaves contain ascorbic acid, β carotene, fibers, Galactomannan and calcium.

- It contains steroids like diosgenin and sapogenins. Other Steroidal sapinogens present in fenugreek are yamogenin, smilagenin, sarsasapogenin, tigogenin, neotigogenin, gitogenin, neogitogenin, yuccagenin and saponaretin etc.
- Fenugreek consists of saponins such as graicunins, fenugreen B, fenugreekine, trigofoenosides A-G.
- Alkaloides: Major alkaloid is Trigonelline. Other alkaloids are Trimethylamine, Neurin, Choline, Gentianine, Carpaine and Betain.
- Seeds contains flavonoids like vitexin, tricin, naringenin, quercetin, tricin -O-β-d-glucopyranoside. Other phenolic compounds are scopoletin, coumarins, p-coumaric acid, phytolexins, chlorogenic acid etc.
- Stolone furanone is volatile principle present in fenugreek.
- It contains amino acids such as Isoleucine, 4-Hydroxyisoleucine, Histidine, Leucine, Lysine, L-tryptophan, Argenine.
- The seed contain minerals like calcium, phosphorus, iron, sodium and potassium. Seeds also contain vitamins like carotene, thiamine, riboflavin, nicotinic acid and folic acid etc.

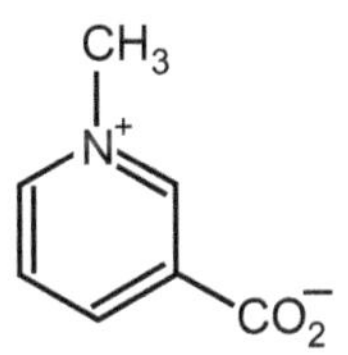

Trigonelline

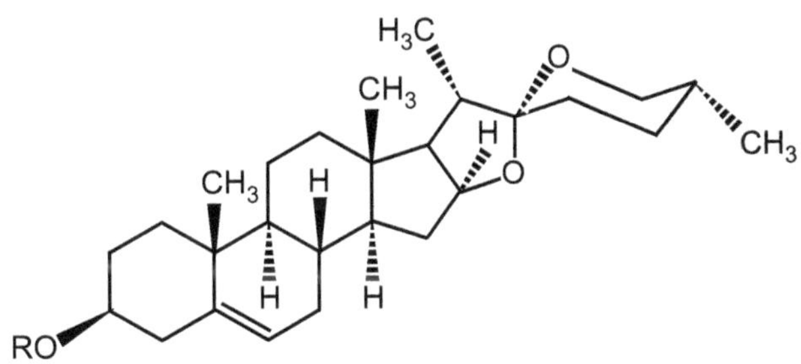

R = H

Diosgenin

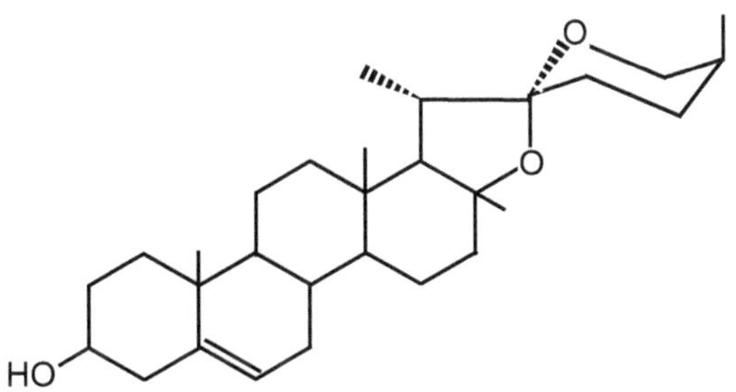

Yamogenin

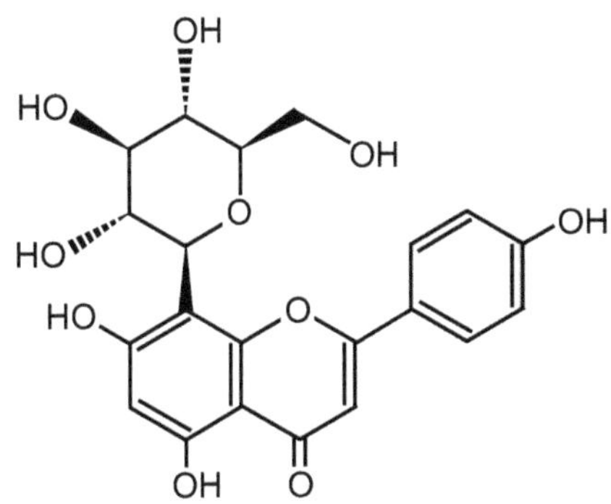

Vitexin

Chemical constituents of Fenugreek

Health Benefits of Fenugreek:

- It acts as preservative and flavouring agent. Traditionally fresh fenugreek leaves are used to treat indigestion, flatulence and a sluggish liver. Leaves are good hair growth promoter and treat dandruff.
- Traditionally, it can be used in digestive problems such as loss of appetite, upset stomach, constipation, gastritis, painful menstruation, menopause, polycystic ovary syndrome, arthritis, poor thyroid function and obesity.
- It prevents atherosclerosis and reduces levels of cholesterol and triglycerides.
- Seeds are used to treat sore throat. Fenugreek seeds increase the flow of milk. It has soothing effect on skin so used to treat eczema or skin disorders. It is applied as a warm poultice in muscle aches and gout pain. Seeds are used to remove kidney stones.
- Due to presence of Galactomannan and amino acids, fenugreek shows antidiabetic activity. It stimulates pancreatic β-cell, delays gastric emptying and inhibits of glucose transport. It also increases insulin secretion and insulin receptors. Hence, it reduces levels of glucose.
- Fenugreek acts as antihyperlipidemic agent. It increases faecal bile acid and cholesterol excretion due to presence of saponin which can form large micelles. Fibres in fenugreek seeds reduces the rate of hepatic cholesterol synthesis.
- Fenugreek inhibits mammary hyperplasia, hence use to prevent breast cancer. Flavonoids present in fenugreek induce apoptosis in cancer cells, so it can be used in treatment of lung cancer, colon cancer, prostate cancer, stomach cancer, brain tumor, head and neck squamous carcinoma and cervical cancer etc. It also stimulates action of macrophages.
- Fenugreek seeds have anti-secretary action, reduce mucosal injury and have effects on mucosal glycoproteins. So they can act as antiulcer agent.
- Fenugreek has hydroxyl radicals (OH) scavenging activity and inhibit hydrogen peroxide-induced lipid peroxidation. This antioxidant effects are due to presence of polyphenolic compounds.
- It exhibits antiinflammatory, analgesic and antipyretic effects.
- Fenugreek regulates hyperthyroidism. It has Anthelmintic and immunomodulatory activity.
- It possesses antifertility activity. It reduces sperm concentration, reduces plasma androgen and increases concentration of progesterone in females.
- It is diaphoretic, decongestant, relieves cold, bronchial complaints, influenza, asthma, constipation, sinusitis, pneumonia, sore throat, hay fever and is blood purifier.
- Fenugreek can be used in treatment of kidney disorders, beriberi disease, mouth ulcers, boils, bronchitis, cellulitis, tuberculosis, chronic coughs, chapped lips, baldness, Parkinson's disease, and heart burn.

Recommended Dosage:

- For diabetes: 5-100 g of powdered fenugreek seed once or twice per day 4 days to 3 years or 1 g extract /day.
- For dysmenorrhoea: 1800-2700 mg of powdered seeds three times daily for the first 3 days of menstruation, followed by 900 mg three times daily for remaining days.

Side Effects: Fenugreek may increase the risk of bleeding. It can cause numbness, facial swelling, breathing difficulty and fainting in some patients. It can cause dizziness, diarrhoea gas, nasal congestion, uterine contractions and hypoglycemia.

Fenugreek should be administered cautiously in patients taking antihypertensive medication, antidiabetic drugs and anticoagulants.

(5) GARLIC

Synonyms: Lasuna, Lashan, Lahsun

Biological Name: It consists of bulbs of Allium sativum family Liliaceae. It has two varieties *A. sativum var. sativum,* called as softneck garlic, and *Allium sativum var. ophioscorodon,* also known as hard neck garlic.

Geographical Source: It is distributed in Central Asia, Southern Europe, USA and India. It can be cultivated all over the world.

Description: It is bulbous perennial herb, similar to onion. Plant consists of underground bulbs which are rounded, composed of up to 15 smaller bulblets known as cloves. Cloves and bulbs are covered by a whitish or pinkish membranous coat. Cloves are held together by a basal plate. The stem is tall, erect and flowering with pink or purple flowers. Leaves are sword-shaped, leaves attached to an underground stem. Hard neck varieties produce a flower stem while soft neck variety does not produce it. Garlic has strong pungent smell due to organosulphur compounds.

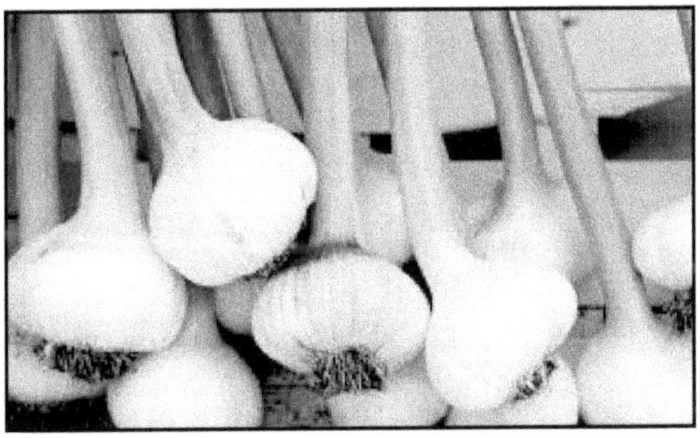

Fig. 4.6: Bulbs of Allium sativum

Chemical Constituents: The main sulphur containing compound present in garlic is glutamyl cysteins. It hydrolyzed to form alliin. When garlic is crushed alliin reacts with the enzyme alliinase to form allicin. Chemically Allicin is a diallyl thiosulfinate. Allicin has strong odour and is therapeutically active. Allicin is also highly unstable, get oxidized easily and gets broken down to sulfur compounds such as diallyl sulfide (DAS), diallyl disulfide (DADS), diallyl trisulfide (DATS), ajoene, and hydrogen sulphide. Garlic shows presence of Germanium, Magnesium, Selenium, Zinc, Vitamin A, C and volatile oil. It also consists of 65% water, 28% carbohydrate, 2.3% organosulphur compound, 2% proteins, 1.2% free aminoacids, 1.5% fiber, 0.15% lipids, 0.08%, phytic acid, 0.07% saponins.

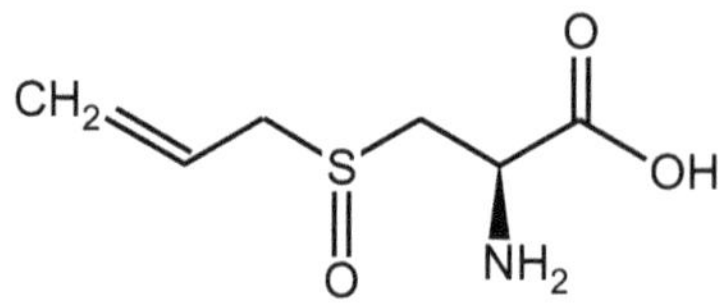

Alliin

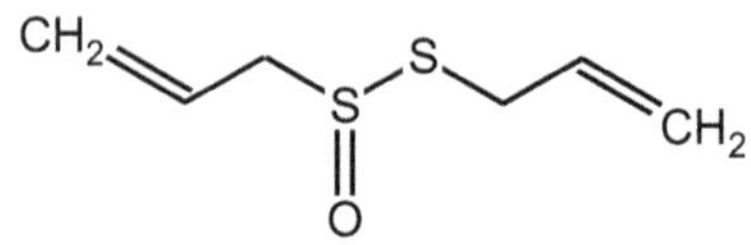

Allicin

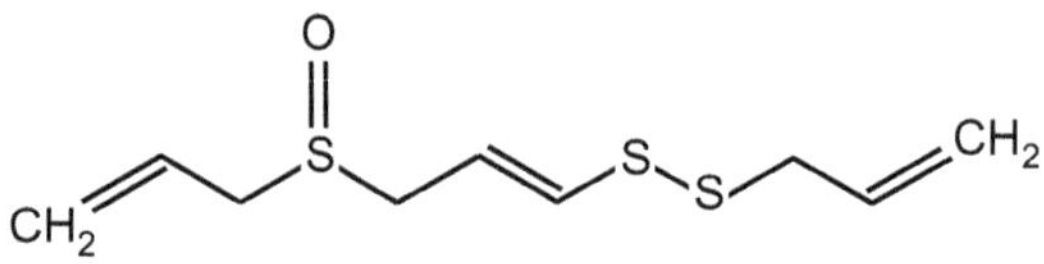

(E)-ajoene

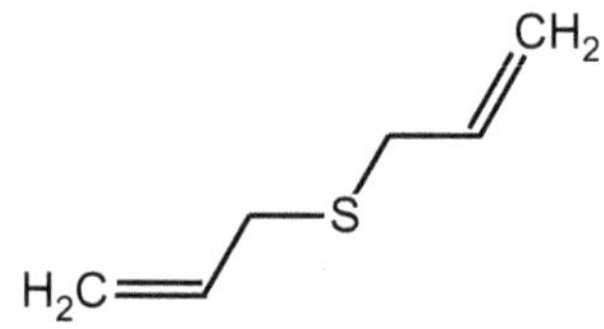

Allyl sulfide

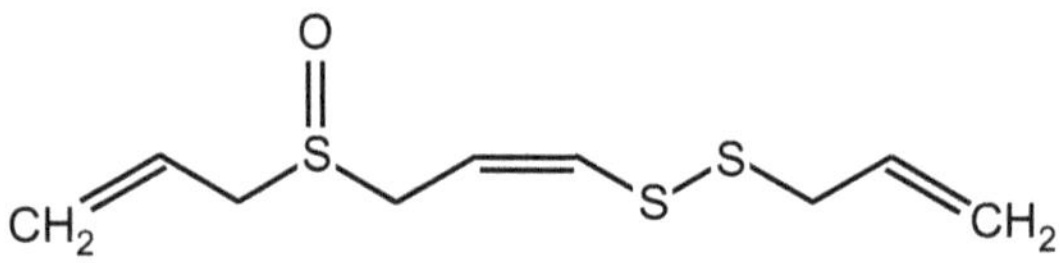

(Z)-ajoene

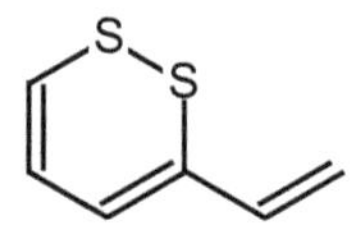

1,2-vinyldithiin

Health Benefits of Garlic:

- Garlic is used in treatment of high blood pressure, high cholesterol, Angina pectoris coronary heart disease, heart attack and atherosclerosis. It can improve blood circulation, acts as blood thinner. Thus, garlic protects against cardiovascular diseases.
- It is anticancer agent and used to prevent cancers like colon cancer, rectal cancer, stomach cancer, breast cancer, prostate cancer, bladder cancer, and lung cancer. It arrests cell cycle of cancer cells. Also inhibits inflammation by altering cytokines and inhibiting NFkB.
- It is used in various disorders like fever, coughs, headache, stomach ache, sinus congestion, gout, rheumatism, hemorrhoids, asthma, and bronchitis, shortness of breath, high blood pressure, high blood sugar, and snakebites.
- Garlic oil can prevent earache and ear infection.
- It is antibacterial, antifungal, antiparasitic, antiprotozoan and antiviral agent. Garlic is effective against the organisms responsible for cholera, dysentery and enteritis, paratyphoid disease, putrefactive intestinal bacteria, streptococcus and staphylococcus bacteria and typhus disease. Garlic is effective against viruses such as coxsackievirus species, herpes simplex virus types 1 and 2, influenza B, para-influenza virus type 3, vaccinia virus, vesicular stomatitis virus, human immunodeficiency virus type 1 and

human rhinovirus type 2 etc. It exhibited anti-parasitic activity against human intestinal parasites such as *Entamoeba histolytica, Ascaris lumbricoides* and *Giardia lamblia* etc.

- It has good wound healing activity by correcting angiogenesis
- Garlic acts as immunomodulator by fighting infection, improving resistance to infection, enhancing the activity of white blood cells and T-helper cells (natural killer cells), protecting cell membranes and preventing DNA from damage.
- It is effective against various GI disorders such as chronic stomach and intestinal catarrh, digestive infections, colic, flatulence, nausea, worm infection, ulcers etc.
- It possesses hepatoprotective effect. It lowers cholesterol, increases HDL's, lowers homocysteine levels, regulates liver and gallbladder activity, stimulates production of detoxifying enzymes which neutralize carcinogens and environmental toxins etc.
- It has diuretic effect which is beneficial in treatment of rheumatism, gout, arthritis, hidropesia, and oedemas.
- It has neuroprotective effect, so used to prevent Alzheimer' disease.
- Garlic is useful in dropsy, urinary infections, and fluid retention.
- It has various applications in treating respiratory tract disorders such as asthma, chronic bronchitis, colds, coughs, breathing difficulty, tuberculosis and sinusitis etc.

Recommended Dose:

- Whole garlic clove - 2-4 g/day fresh,
- Dried garlic - 600-900 mg daily
- 4 g in 150 mL of water infusion can be given per day
- Tincture in ratio 1:2 in 95 % alcohol, 40 drops up to six times per day.

Side Effects: It produces side effects such as upset stomach, bloating, bad breath, body odour, headache, and fatigue, loss of appetite, muscle aches, vertigo, and allergic asthmatic reaction. It can also cause skin reactions and bleeding disorders.

Interactions:

- Garlic potentiates the action of antiplatelet medications like aspirin, dipyridamole, indomethacin etc.
- It may lead to bleeding disorders when used with blood thinners like Aspirin.
- Blood sugar levels should be monitored when garlic is taken with antidiabetic medications.
- Garlic may reduce blood levels of anti HIV drugs.
- Garlic potentiates the action of antihyperlipidemic drugs like atorvastatin, lovastatin etc. It also increases action of antihypertensive drugs like captopril, enalapril etc.

(6) HONEY

Synonyms: Madhu, Madvika, Kshaudra, Saradha, Makshika.

Biological Source: Honey is produced from the nectar of flowers by *Apis mellifera*. Honey bees convert nector of flower into honey by processes called regurgitation (spitting the nectar from mouth of one honey bee to other) and evaporation using enzymes present in their gut. It is stored as primary food. It is golden amber coloured liquid.

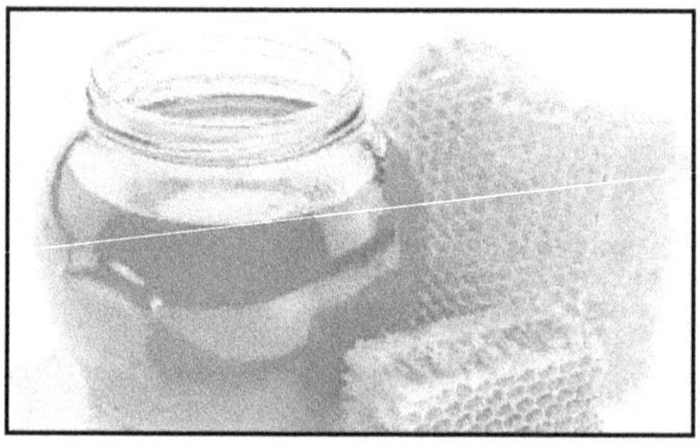

Fig. 4.7: Honey

Geographical Source: Honey is produced in India, Mexico, Iran, Romania, Republic of Korea, New Zealand, Poland and Kenya.

Properties:

- Honey is viscous hygroscopic liquid. It's colour differ depending on age, botanic source and storage environment. It crystallises upon storage.
- **Composition:** Honey is a mixture of sugars and water. It consists of fructose 38.5 %, glucose 31% and small amount of disaccharides, trisaccharides and oligosaccharides and 17.1 % water. Other nutrients present in honey are 18 essential and non-essential amino acids, vitamins, minerals and enzymes.
- Vitamins like B_2, B_4, B_5, B_6, B_{11} and vitamin C, and minerals such as calcium, iron, zinc, potassium, phosphorous, magnesium, selenium, chromium and manganese are present in honey.
- Amino acids like Proline, lysine, phenylalanine, tyrosine, glutamic and aspartic acid etc. are present in honey. Honey shows presence of enzymes such as enzglucose oxidase, invertase, diastase (amylase), catalase, and acid phosphatase.
- Honey possesses particular flavour and antimicrobial properties because of presence of organic acids like gluconic acid, butyric, acetic, formic, lactic, succinic, malic, citric, oxalic and pyroglutamic acid.
- It shows presence of flavonoides such as apigenin, pinocembrin, pinobankcin, kaempferol, quercetin, galangin, chrysin, acacetin and hesperetin etc.
- It shows presence of phenolic acids such as ellagic, caffeic, p-coumaric, and ferulic acids etc.

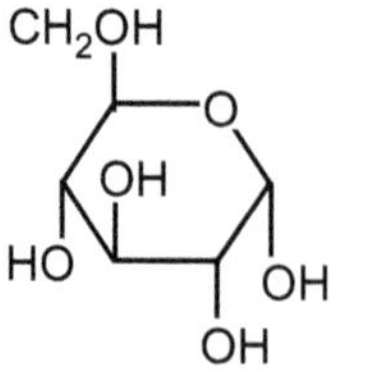

Glucose

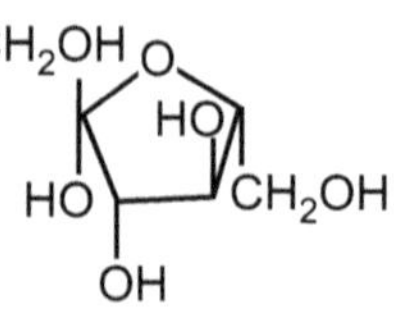

Fructose

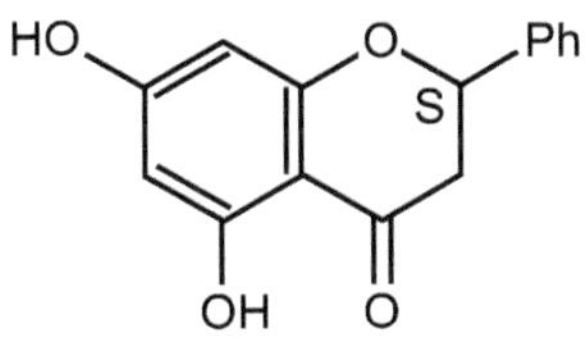
Pinocembrin

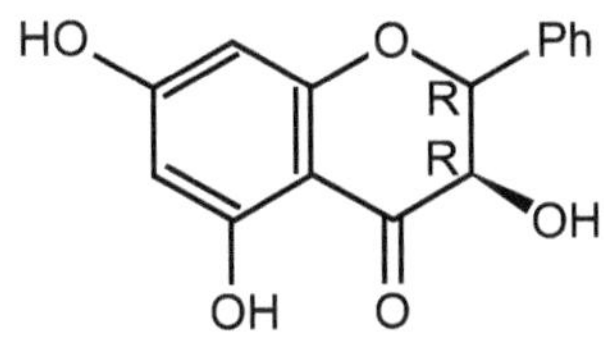
Pinobanksin

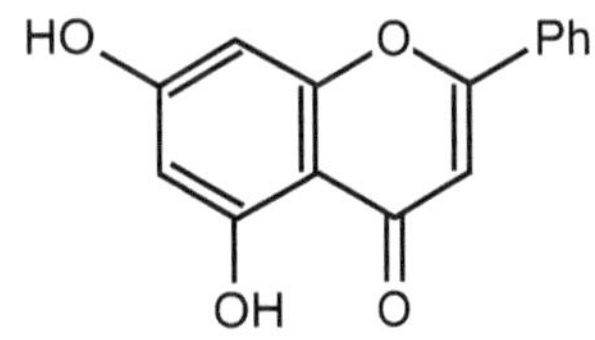
Chrysin

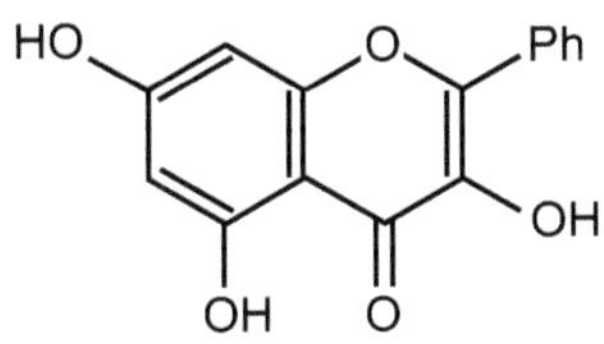
Galagin

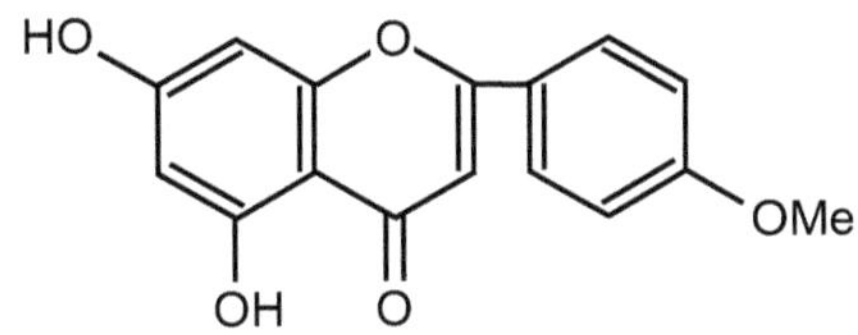
Acacetin

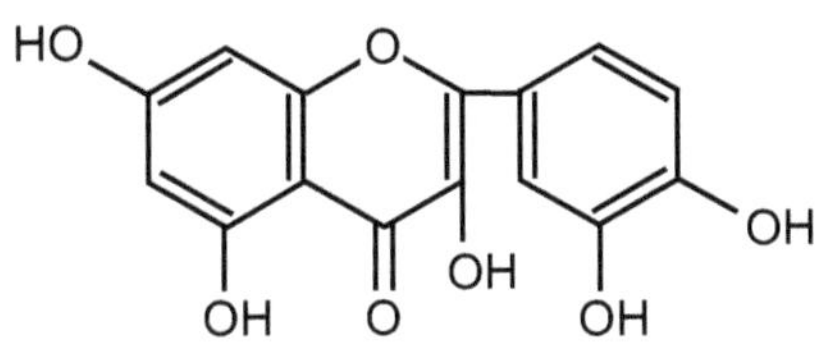
Quercetin

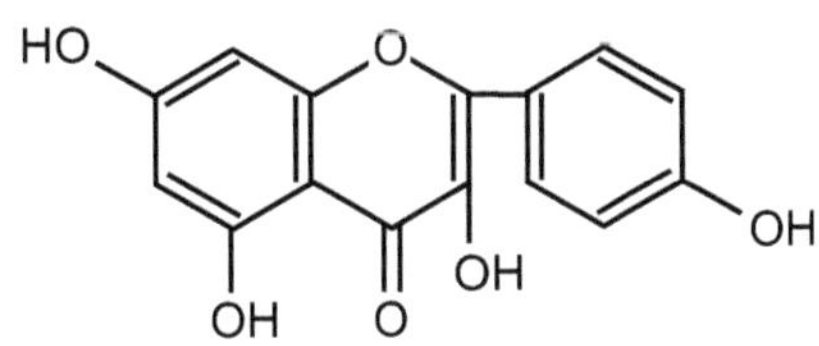
Kaempferol

Chemical constituents of Honey

Health Benefits of Honey:

- Traditionally honey is useful for eyes and good vision, balances kapha, reduce toxicity, stops hiccups, for bleeding disorders, urinary tract disorders, diabetes, skin diseases, worm infections, bronchial asthma, cough, diarrhoea, nausea, vomiting, and for wound healing.
- It relieves constipation, stomach pain; nasal congestion, mouth sores, burns and for obesity.
- Honey is used in treatment of gastrointestinal infection such as gastritis, duodenitis and gastric ulceration, diarrhoea and gastroenteritis. It inhibits attachment of bacteria to gut cells by forming coat around bacteria or alter bacterial electrostatic charge or hydrophobicity. Also it has antibacterial effects. It possesses cytoprotective effects hence protect against peptic ulcers.
- Honey acts as anti-inflammatory agent by reducing the activities of cyclooxygenase-1 and cyclooxygenase-2. It also decreases concentrations of prostaglandin E2, prostaglandin F2α, and thromboxane B2.
- Due to presence of phenolic compounds honey acts as potential antioxidant.
- Honey stimulates tissue regeneration, reduces inflammation hence it possesses potential wound healing effects.

- Honey stimulates insulin secretion, decrease blood glucose levels, increases hemoglobin and also lowers lipids, homocysteine levels and C-reactive protein levels. It has lower glycemic index. All these aspects make honey as powerful antidiabetic agent.
- It exhibited antibacterial activity against bacteria such as *Bacillus anthracis, Corynebacterium diphtheriae, Haemophilus influenzae, Klebsiella pneumoniae, Listeria monocytogenes, Mycobacterium tuberculosis, Pasteurella multocida, Yersinia enterocolitica, Proteus species, Pseudomonas aeruginosa, Acinetobacter spp., Salmonella diarrhoea, Salmonella typhi, Serratia marcescens, Shigella dysentery, Staphylococcus aureus, Streptococcus faecalis, Streptococcus mutans, Streptococcus pneumoniae, Streptococcus pyogenes,* and *Vibrio cholerae* etc.
- Honey acts as antifungal agent against Aspergillus, Penicillium, and Candida albicans. It also acts as antiviral agent.

Side Effects: Honey produced from nectar of Rhododendrons is unsafe. Honey is safe when administered to adults or children over one year age.

Recommended Dose: 1–2 tsp of honey can be taken daily.

(7) AMLA

Synonym: Amlaki, Indian gooseberry, Emblic myrobalan.

Biological Source: It consists of fresh and drired fruits of *Emblica officinalis Gaertn* or Phyllanthus emblica belonging to family *Euphorbiaceae*.

Geological Scource: Amla is native to tropical and subtropical regions. Mainly it is found in central and southern India, Pakistan, Bangladesh, Sri Lanka, Southern China, the Mascarene Islands and Malaysia.

Description: Amla is medium sized deciduous tree, with thin greenish-grey bark having small thin irregular flakes. Leaves are feathery linear-oblong, with a rounded base and obtuse or acute apex, subsessile, light green coloured and pinnate margin. Amla fruits are spherical or globular, drupaceous, fleshy with slight conic depression on both apexes. Mesocarp is yellow and endocarp becomes yellowish brown at maturity. Fruit has six ridges and six trigonous seeds. After ripening, fruits become astringent or bitter and extremely acidic.

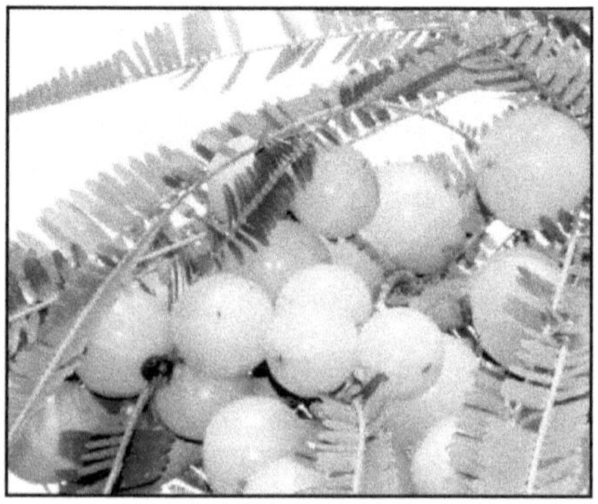

Fig. 4.8: Plant of Phyllanthus emblica

Plant bears greenish yellow, unisexual flowers in axillary fascicles. Plant has 4 to 6, smooth, dark brown seeds.

Chemical Constituents:

Plant shows presence of hydrolysable tannins like emblicanin A and B, punigluconin, pedunculagin etc. Plant is rich in phenolic compounds like apigenin, gallic acid, ellagic acid, chebulinic acid, quercetin, chebulagic acid, corilagin, isostrictiniin, methyl gallate, luteolin etc. Glutamic acid, proline, aspartic acid, alanine and lysine amino acids are present in plant.

Leaves of amla plant contain gallic acid, chebulic acid, ellagic acid, chebulinic acid, chebulagic acid, amlic acid. Alkaloids like phyllantine and phyllantidine are presnt.

Seeds shows presence of fixed oil, phosphatides and a small quantity of essential oil. Different fatty acids present in seed are linolenic acid (8.78%), linoleic (44%), oleic (28.40%), steric (2.15%), palmitic (2.99%) and miristic acid (0.95%) etc.

Barks are rich in leukodelphinidin, tannin and proanthocyanidin.

Amla plant roots contains ellagic acid and lupeol. Fruit pulp contains gallic acid 1.32%, tannin, gum 13.75%; albumin 13.08%; crude cellulose 17.08%; mineral matter 4.12% and moisture 3.83%.

Amla consists of chromium, zinc, copper, manganese etc. It is rich source of Vitamin C.

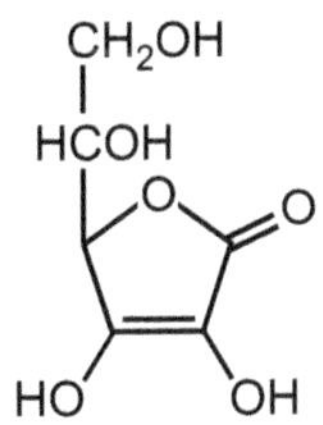

Vitamin C

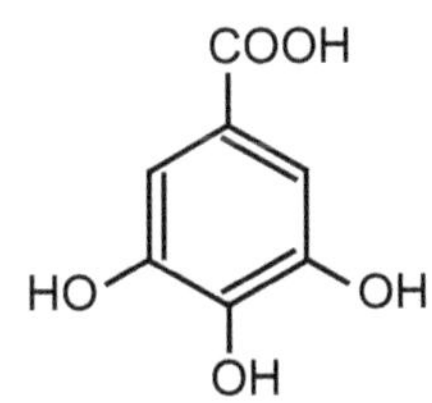

Gallic acid

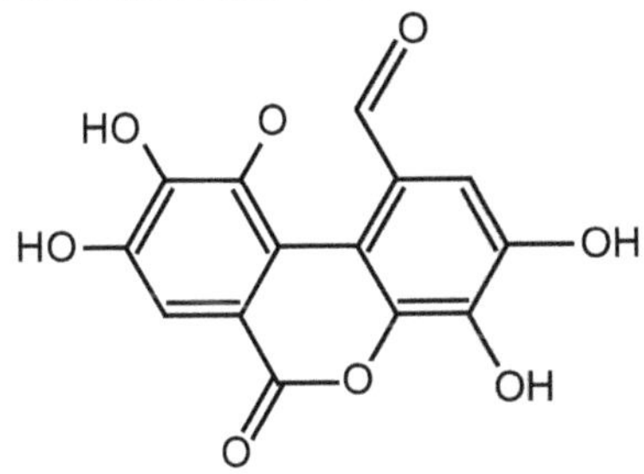

Ellagic acid

Chemical constituents of Amla

Health Benefits of Amla:

- Traditionally amla is used as rejuvenative herbs to build lost vitality and vigor. It is tonic for heart and brain. It is useful in conditions like fever, hemorrhage, diarrhoea and dysentery, fever, constipation, eye diseases, dental problems and rheumatism.
- Amla balances tridoshas. It is used for weight loss, source of vitamin C, antiaging agent, skin disorders and burning sensation etc.
- It acts as anabolic, antibacterial, anti-inflammatory, analgesic, hair growth promoter, and immunomodulator.
- Amla shows antifungal activity against *Fusarium equiseti* and *Candida albicans.*
- It acts as insecticidal or cytotoxic agent.
- Amla contains polyphenolic compounds. So it acts as potent inhibitor of lipid peroxide formation and scavenger of hydroxyl, nitric oxide and superoxide radicals. Hence, it exhibits antioxidant effects.
- Due to antioxidant nature amla inhibits the production of advanced glycosylated proteins formed due to oxidative stress. It reduces lipid peroxidation, improve albumin and adiponectin levels. Hence, it is used to control diabetes.
- It can prevent hyperthyroidism and gastric ulcers.
- It possesses larvicidal, insecticidal and mosquitocidal activity.
- It shows immunomodulatory effects by inhibiting apoptosis, DNA fragmentation and restoring IL-2 and γ-IFN production.

- It exhibited hepatoprotective effects by reducing elevated levels of collagen-hydroxyproline and inhibiting the induction of fibrosis.
- It reduces gastric motility and inhibits PGE2-induced enteropooling thereby acts as antidiarrhoeal agent.
- It is used as antitussive agent by exhibiting antiphlogistic, antispasmolytic, antioxidant and mucus secretary property in airways.
- Amla reduces serum cholesterol, TG, phospholipid and LDL levels. Hence, it is antihyperlipidemic agent.
- Amla induces apoptosis and inhibit cell cycle regulating enzymes so it can be used in cancer treatment. Antiproliferative effects are also observed due to polyphenolic compounds present in amla.
- Amla possesses cardioprotective, radioprotective and antidepressant effects.
- Amla also inhibit HIV-Reverse Transcriptase (HIV-RT).
- Amla possesses antimutagenic effects and also shows wound healing activity by enhancing cellular proliferation at the wound site.

Recommended Dose: Powder of fruit can be taken 1-3 g daily.

Side Effects: It is safe for human use. It should be administered with caution in patients of diabetes, bleeding, liver disorders etc.

(8) GINSENG

Synonyms: American ginseng, Asiatic ginseng, Chinese ginseng, Korean ginseng, Tartar root, Western ginseng.

Biological Source: It consists of dried roots of plant Panax ginseng (Renshen, Chinese ginseng) belongs to family Araliaceae. Other species consists of *Panax quinquefolium* (*Xiyangshen*, American ginseng), *Panax notoginseng* (*Sanqi*) and *Panax japonicas* (Japanese ginseng).

Geographical Source: Ginseng is native to China, Korea and Russia.

Description: Ginseng is deciduous perennial plant. There are two forms, red and white ginseng. It grows well in shade. The leaves are five-fingered, compound with five pointed and toothed leaflets. Plant bears tiny white or greenish-yellow flowers form single, ball-like cluster, red berries, and a yellowish-brown root. Thick roots show human-like shape.

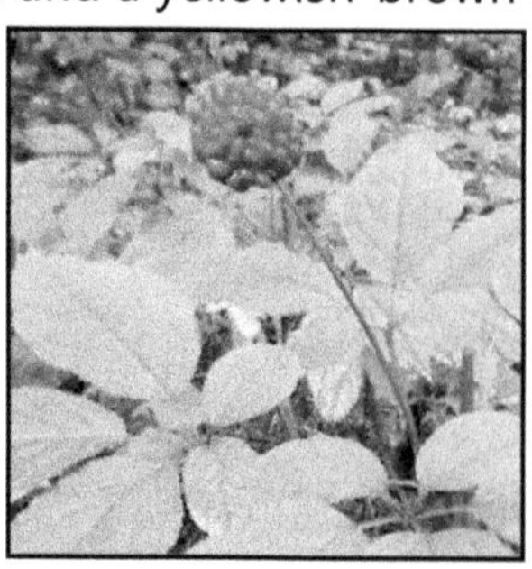
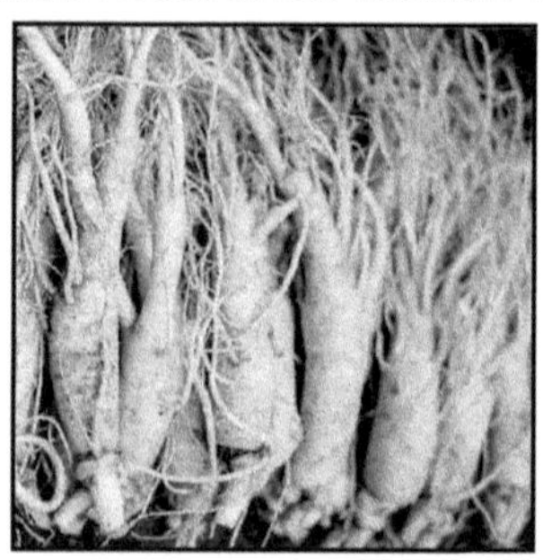

Fig. 4.9: Plant of *Panax ginseng*

Chemical Constituents:

- Major constituents of ginseng are ginsenosides which are triterpene glycosides or saponins. Ginsenosides are denoted as Rx, where x is the retention factor (Rf) of spots observed on TLC plant from bottom to top (polarity decreasing from index "a" to "h"). Ginsenosides are a dammarane skeleton having 17 carbons in a four-ring structure with various sugar moieties like glucose, rhamnose, xylose and arabinose attached to the C-3 and C-20 positions. Plant consists of more than 30 ginsenosides classified mainly into two categories:
  1. 20(S)-protopanaxadiol (PPD) like Rb1, Rb2, Rb3, Rc, Rd, Rg3, Rh2, Rs1.
  2. 20(S)-protopanaxatriol (PPT) like Re, Rf, Rg1, Rg2, Rh1.
- Main difference in PPD and PPT is PPDs contains carboxyl group at the C-6 position. Plant consists of rare ginsenosides, like ocotillol saponin F11 (24-R-pseudoginsenoside) and pentacyclic oleanane saponin Ro (3,28-O-bisdesmoside).
- Berry of ginseng contains indole alkaloid, ginsenine, βsitosterol, 20 (R)-protopanaxatriol, daucosterine and 20(R) -ginsenoside-Rg3, isoginsenoside-Rh (3), ginsenoside -Rb(1), -Rb(2), -Rc, -Rd, -Re, - Rg(1), -Rh(1), -Rh(2). Berries consists of 11 saponins mainly 20(R)-dammarane-3β, 12β, 20, 25-tetrol (25-OHPPD); 20(R)-dammarane-3β, 6α, 12β20, 25-pentol (25-OH-PPT); 20(S)-protopanaxadiol (PPD); daucosterine, 20(S)-ginsenoside-Rh(2) (Rh(2)); 20(S)- ginsenoside-Rg(3) (Rg(3)); 20(S)-ginsenoside-Rg(2) (Rg(2)); 20(S)-ginsenoside-Rg(1) (Rg(1)); 20(S)- ginsenoside-Rd (Rd); 20(S)-ginsenoside-Re (Re); and 20(S)-ginsenoside-Rb(1) (Rb(1)).
- Seeds of ginseng showed presence of new dammarane-type triterpene ketone, two dammarane-type and lupane-type triterpenes, an aromatic oligoglycoside, three sterol glycosides, and three dammarane-type triterpene oligoglycosides (ginsenosides Rd, Re, and Rg(2))etc.
- Red and white ginsengs are almost similar by chemical nature. Only partly deglycosylated saponins such as ginsenosides Rh1, Rh2 and Rg3 are present in Red variety. Presence of such saponins is due to steaming process carried out to prepare red variety from white variety. It also contains ginsenosides Ra1, Ra2, Ra3, Rf2, Rg4, Rg6, Rk1 etc.Two minor saponins present in red ginseng, are ginsenosides Rs1 and Rs2. Red variety shows presence of new dammarane glycosides mainly ginsenosides Rg5, Rh4, Rs3 and Rf2 h.
- Ginseng also contains Polyacetylenes like panaxydol and ginsenoynes A–E.
- It consists of poplyphenolic compounds such as salicylic acid, vanillic acid, ascorbic acid, p-coumaric acid, ferulic acid, caffeic acid, gentisic acid, p-hydroxybenzoic acid, maltol, cinnamic acid, protocatechuic acid, syringic acid, and quercetin, chlorogenic acid, gentisic acid, p- and m-coumaric acid, and rutin etc.
- Plant shows presence of sesquiterpene hydrocarbons such as β-panasinsene, african-2-ene, β-elemene, calarene, (E)-β-farnesene, α-humulene, α-neoclovene, 2-epi-(E)-β-

caryophyllene, β-neoclovene, β-selinene, and bicyclogermacrene, and oxygenated sesquiterpenes like spathulenol, humulene epoxide II, ginsenol, hexadecanoic acid, and falcarino ect.

- Alkaloids such as 1-carbomethoxy-β-carboline, N9-formylharman, harman, norharman, perlolyrine, 4-methyl-5-thiazoleethanol, and spinacine and ginsenine are observed in ginseng.
- Polysaccharides like panasans A–E, and panaxans I–L, M–P, and Q–U are also present in Ginseng roots.

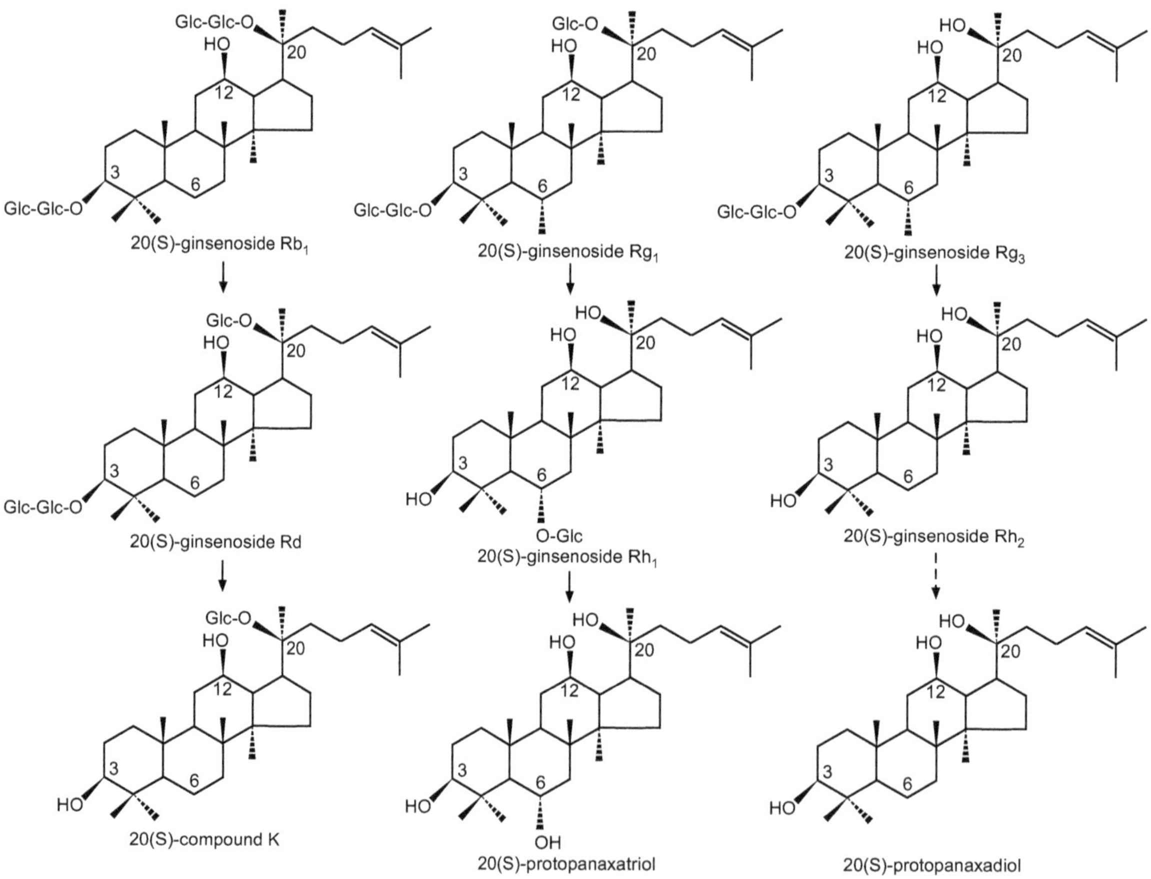

Chemical constituents of Ginseng

Health Benefits of Ginseng:

- Ginseng is used to treat infertility, liver disease, amnesia, colds, menopause, as adaptogen and a restorative tonic, aphrodisiac and erectile dysfunction.
- It can improve stamina, decrease fatigue, antistress agent, and improve concentration.
- Ginseng has various therapeutic activities such as in anaemia, antidiabetic agent, antipyretic, anticancer, antiasthamaytic, antiaging agent.

- It is used in gastritis, neurasthenia, bleeding disorders, loss of appetite, vomiting, colitis, dysentery, insomnia, neuralgia, rheumatism, dizziness, headache, convulsions, disorders of pregnancy, hot flashes due to menopause.
- Ginseng use to treat diabetes. It improves glucose homeostasis, insulin sensitivity, glycated hemoglobin, serum lipid, amino-terminal propeptide concentration, and physical activity.
- Ginseng acts as antimicrobial, antifungal, insecticidal and antifeedant agent.
- It improves sperm count and motility; hence use to treat male infertility.
- Saponins of Ginseng have cytotoxic effects. It inhibits cancer cell proliferation, adhesion and invasion of tumor cells, induces apoptosis and also has anti-angiogenesis activity. Hence, ginseng acts as anticancer agent.
- Panax ginseng acts as antiinflammatory agent by inhibiting cyclooxygenase-2 (COX-2), inducible nitric oxide synthase (iNOS), and nuclear factor kappa B. It also possesses radioprotective effect, antioxidant and immunomodulatory effects.
- It can be used as anti-neurodegenerative agent. It affects neurological functions by interacting with the cholinergic and serotoninergic neurotransmitter systems and improves cognitive performance. Hence, ginseng is used in treatment of Alzheimer's diseases and Parkinson's diseases. By decreasing the levels of apoptotic proteins including p-Akt, Bax, and Bcl-2 it produces beneficiary effects on Parkinson's disease.
- Ginseng is effective against ischemic cerebral damage by promoting clearance of extracellular glutamate, increasing the expression of non-selective cation channels, acid-sensing ion channel, and decreasing the levels of apoptotic proteins such as cytochrome c (CytoC), apoptosis inducing factor (AIF), and caspase-3. It also inhibits synthesis of COX-2 and iNOS.
- Due to antioxidant effects and calcium modulation, ginseng is used to treat various cardiac disorders such as cardiotoxicity, cardiac hypertrophy, myocardial infarction after ischemia and reperfusion, atherosclerosis, angina pectoris and heart failure etc. It inhibits apoptosis in cardiomyocytes by modulating Bcl-2 and caspase-3. It can acts as cardioprotective agent by modulating ion channels and signal transduction, improving lipid profiles, regulating blood pressure, and reducing platelet adhesion.

Side Effects: Long term use and high dose of ginseng may produce side effects such as hypertension, nausea, diarrhoea, headache, mastalgia, insomnia, and skin rash etc. Ginseng should be administered with caution in patients taking medication like phenelzine, coumadin, oral hypoglycemics, insulin and caffeine.

Recommended Dose: For Alzheimer's disease treatment 4.5 to 9 g of ginseng can be administered daily. For mental disorders to 200 to 400 mg daily dose can be given. For COPD treatment 100 mg to 6 g of ginseng can be given three times daily. For treatment of flu 200 mg dose can be given.

(9) ASHVAGANDHA

Synonyms: Asvagandha, Winter cherry, Asgandh, Gandhrapatri.

Biological Name: Dried roots of *Withania somnifera Dunal* belonging to the family Solanaceae.

Geographical Source: In India, Sri Lanka, Afghanistan, Baluchistan, Sind, parts of Africa and in the Mediterranean regions, the Canaries and Cape of Good Hop etc.

Description: Ashvagandha is an evergreen, erect, branching shrub, 30-150 cm in height and has minute star shaped hairs. Plant has simple, ovate, glabrous alternate leaves with sub-acute apex and entire margins. Plant shows axillary, umbellate cymes type Inflorescence. Flowers are greenish or lurid yellow, Monoecious, small about 1 cm long; Fruits (berries) are smooth, orange-red when mature, globose enclosed in the inflated and membranous calyx, and are 5 angled. Seeds are yellow, reniform.

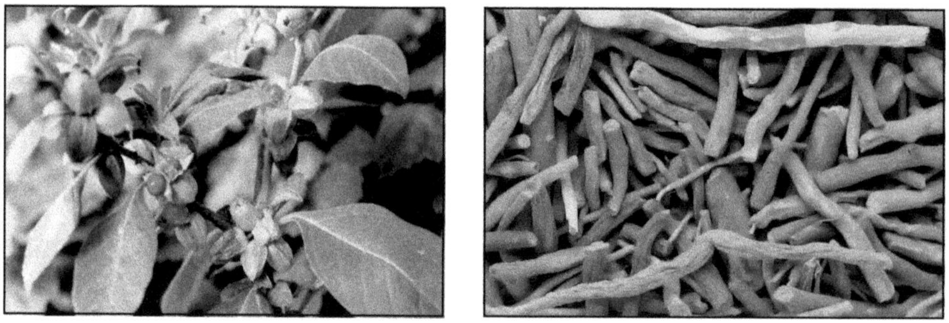

(a) Plant of *Withania somnifera* **(b) Withania roots**

Fig. 4.10

Chemical Constituents:

Plant contains more than 13 alkaloids, 138 withanolides, and several sitoindosides in aerial parts, roots and berries of Withania species. The major chemical constituents are withanolides (0.001 to 0.5% dry weight), Withaferin A, ashwagandhanolide etc. It consists of steroidal compounds including ergostane-type steroidal lactones, withaferin A, withanolides A-Y, withasomniferin A, withasomidienone, withasomniferols A-C, withanone, Plant also contains acylsteryl glucosides, starch, hantreacotane, ducitol, and a variety of amino acids and high amount of iron.

Ashvagandha roots consist of heterogeneous alkaloids such as cuscohygrine, anahygrine, tropine, pseudotropine, anaferine, isopelletierine, withananine, withananinine, pseudo-withanine, somnine, somniferine, somniferinine. Neutral alkaloids like 3-tropyltigloate and others like withanine, withasomnine and visamine. Root also shows presence of free amino acids such as aspartic acid, glycine, tyrosine, alanine, proline, tryptophan, glutamic acid and cystine etc. Total alkaloid content of Indian roots is 0.13 and 0.31%. Apart from alkaloids the root consists of starch, resin, fat, potassium nitrate, phytosterol, reducing sugars, hentriacontane glycosides, dulcitol, withaniol, stearic, palmatic, linoleic, withanic acid, ipuranol and somniro.

Leaves: Leaves showed presence of 12 withanolides, 5 unidentified alkaloids, free amino acids, chlorogenic acid, glycosides, glucose, condensed tannins and flavonoids etc. The leaves from different habitats differ in withanolide content. Leaves and root contains Withaferin A, a steroidal lactone which is therapeutically significant constituent.

Fruits: Green fruits have constituents like a proteolytic enzyme chamase, condensed tannins and flavonoids. Major constituent of fruits are free amino acids such as proline, valine, tyrosine, alanine, glycine, hydroxyproline, aspartic acid, glutamic acid, cystine and cysteine etc.

Shoots: Shoots are rich in crude protein, calcium and phosphorous, and contain scopoletin.

Stem: Stem is rich in condensed tannins and flavonoids.

Bark: It mainly contains free amino acids.

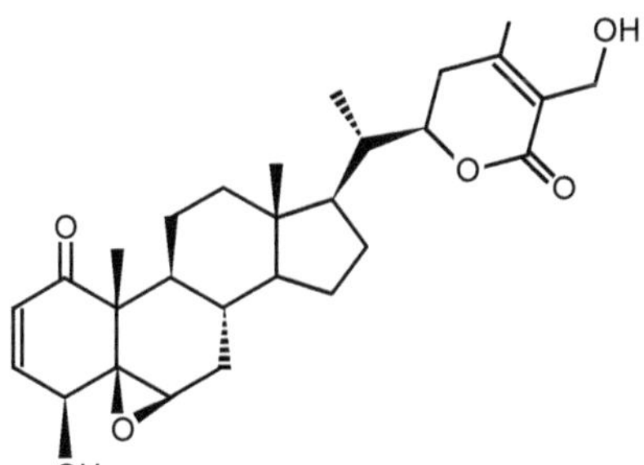

Withaferine A

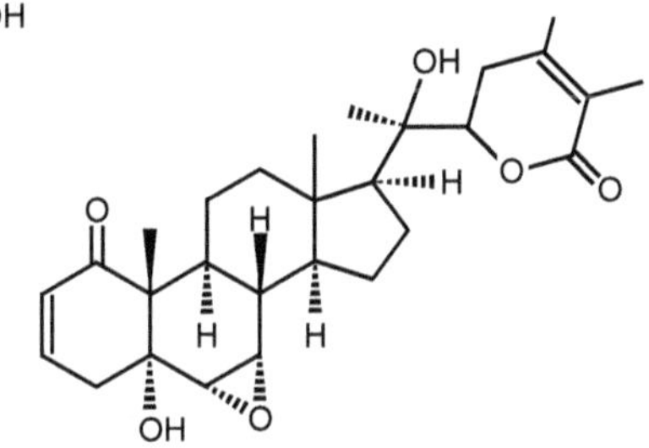

Withanolide A

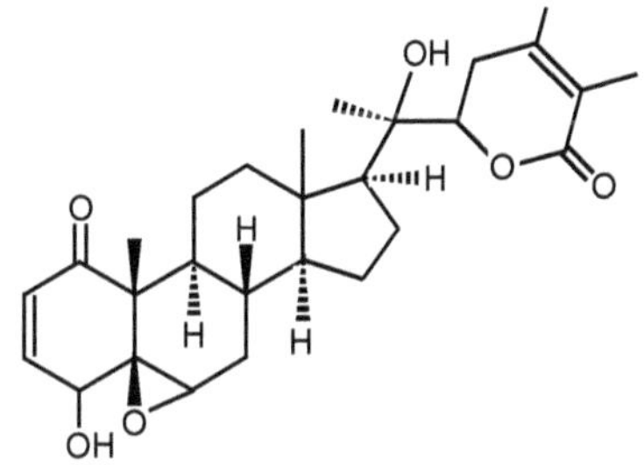

Withanolide D

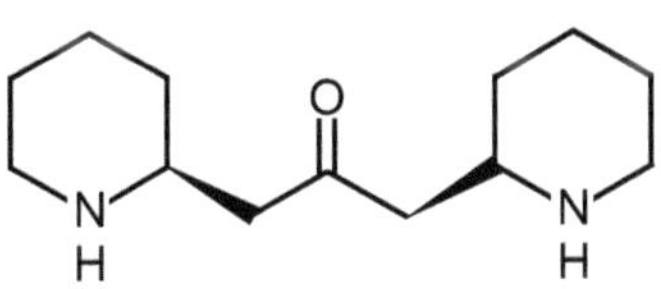

Anaferine

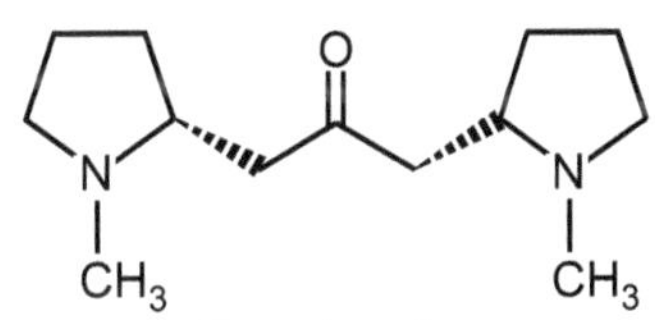

Cusohygrine

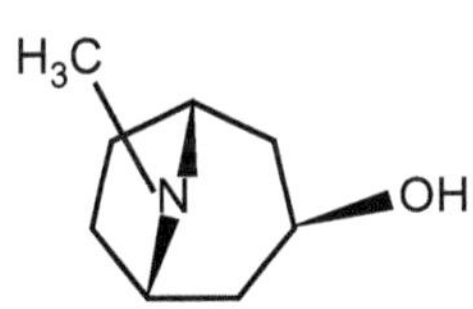

Pseudotropine

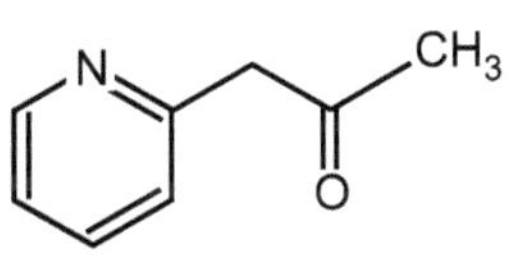

Isopellertierine

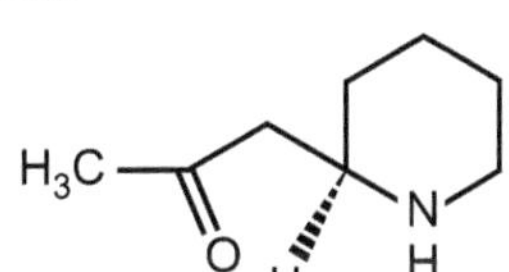

Pellertierine

Chemical constituents of Ashvagandha

Health Benefits of Ashvagandha:

- Due to presence of saponins it act as potent anti-arthritic and anti-inflammatory agent.
- Withaferin A shows antibiotic activity against Gram-positive bacteria, acid-fast and aerobic bacilli, and pathogenic fungi.
- It is potent anticancer and chemoprotective agent.
- Ashvagandha roots acts as hepatoprotictive agent by influencing the levels of lipid peroxidation.
- It has immunosuppressive effect on human B and T lymphocytes. It also has immunomodulatory effects.
- Withania reduces serum cholesterol, triglycerides and lipoprotein levels.
- Ashvagandha improve attention and impulse control in children with ADHD. Effective in patients with bipolar disorder.
- It possesses protective effects against various CNS disorders like epilepsy, anxiety, depression, catalepsy, Alzheimer's disease and sleep disorders.
- It exhibits muscle relaxant and antispasmodic effects on intestinal, uterine, bronchial, tracheal and blood vascular muscles.
- It is used to treat disorders such as osteoarthritis, OCD, parkinson's disease, fibromyalgia and TB etc.
- Active principles of withania increase superoxide dismutase (SOD), catalase (CAT) and glutathione peroxidase (GPX). Thus, due to this, antioxidant property has anti-stress, antiaging and cognition-facilitating effects. Antiaging effects include improvement of Hb, RBC and hair melanin etc.
- Ashvagandha protect oxidative damage to pancreatic islet cells by its free radical scavenging activity. Hence, it can act as antihyperglycaemic agent.
- It activates chemotactic activity of macrophages and enhances production of interleukin-1 (IL-1) and tumour necrosis factor (TNF). Hence, it can regulate immune responses.
- It also exhibits cardioprotective effects.
- Traditionally it is used as sedative, hypnotic, narcotic, galactagouge, blood purifier, general tonic, diuretic aphrodisiac, and uterine tonic. It is implemented in treatment of rheumatoid arthritis, lumbago, painful swellings, leucoderma, asthma, amnesia, anxiety disorders, ulcers, scabies etc.

Side Effects: It is safe by oral route. But in large doses it can produce side effects such as stomach upset, diarrhoea, and vomiting. It should be cautiously administered in patients with diabetes, thyroid dysfunction, ulcers, BP and CNS disorders.

Recommended Dose: It can be decided based on age, health, and several other conditions. It can be given 125 mg to 5 g per day. 250 mg to 3 g per day of ashvagandha can be given in diabetes. For inflammation 250 mg of ashwagandha powder or 12 ml of ashwagandha extract can be given. About 40-50 drops ashwagandha tincture added to 120 ml water can be given 3 times daily. Ashvagandha capsules should be taken 1-2 capsules, twice daily.

(10) SPIRULINA

Synonym: Arthospira, Dihe, Cyanobacteria.

Biologcial Name: These are blue green microalgae of different species like *Spirulina maxima (Arthrospira maxima), Spirulina platensis (Arthrospira platensis),* and *Spirulina fusiformis (Arthrospira fusiformis)* of family Oscillatoriaceae.

Geographical Source: *A. platensis* is distributed in Africa and Asia, while *A. maximum* is observed in Central America.

Description: Spirulina is microscopic blue-green algae or cyanophytes or cyanobacteria). It has cork screw-shaped multicellular filaments. *A. platensis* has cylindrical trichomes that are arranged in a left-handed helix throughout the filament. They are autotrophic. It grows well in high-salt alkaline water.

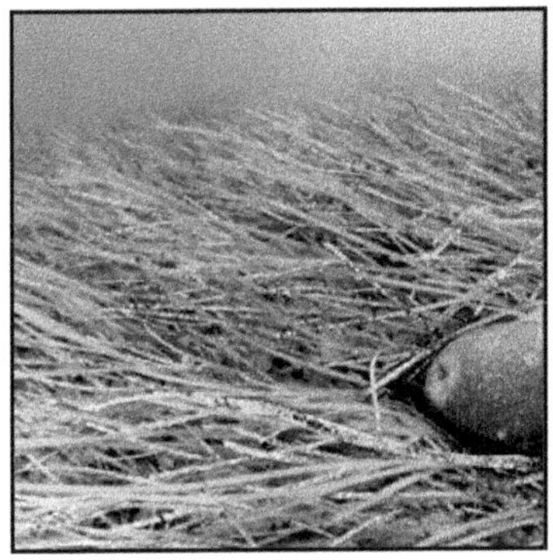

Fig. 4.11: Spirulina microalgae

Chemical Constituents:

Spirulina is rich source of proteins (58%) and also contains carbohydrates (30%), fat (8%), dietary fibres (3%), sugars (3%), vitamins (<1%) etc.

Spirulina shows presence of fatty acids such as α and γ linoleic acid, linolenic acid, docosahexaenoic acid, eicosapentaenoic acid, arachidonic acid, omega 3 and omega 6 polyunsaturated fatty acid and stearidonic acids.

It contains vitamins such as A, C, D, E, vitamin B_{12}, thiamine, nicotinamide, pyridoxine, riboflavin, and folic acid.

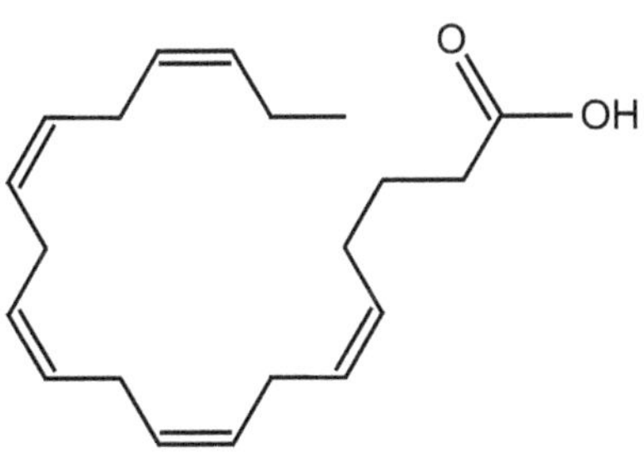

Eicosapentaenoic Acid (EPA)

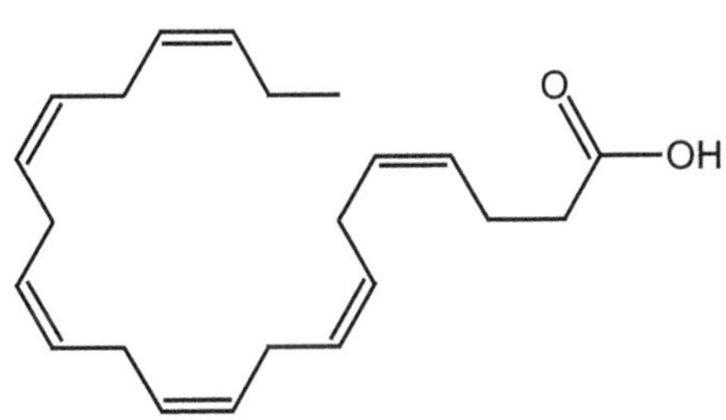

Docosahexaenoic Acid (DHA)

Chemical constituents of Spirulina

Pigments, such as chlorophyll-a, zeaxanthin, diatoxanthin, 3′-hydroxyechinenone, echinenone, β-carotene, xanthophyll, canthaxanthin, c-phycocyanin, β-cryptoxanthin, myxoxanthophyll, oscillaxanthin, phycobiliproteins, and allophycocyanin are present in spirulina. It also contains minerals like calcium, magnesium, manganese, copper, zinc, iron, sodium, potassium, phosphorus, selenium etc.

Health Benefits of Spirulina:

- Spirulina consists of high amount of nutrients hence it is a whole food supplement.
- It is potent antifungal and antibacterial agent. It also possesses antiviral activities against viruses such as Herpes simplex virus type-I, measles virus, HIV-I and influenza virus etc.
- It shows free radical scavenging activity. It improves activity of antioxidant enzymes like GSH, SOD, CAT, GSH PX and also reduces lipid peroxidation. Hence, it has antioxidant effect.
- It exhibit hepatoprotective effects by inhibiting oxidative stress and apoptosis, by reducing lipid peroxidation.
- It maintains proper renal function and histology of cells hence it act as nephroprotective agent.
- It has neuprotective effects. It inhibits brain damage produced by toxic chemicals, enhance locomotor activity and reduce damage to spinal cord.
- It reduces total lipids, cholesterol, triglycerides. It can reduce blood sugar and improve insulin resistance. Hence, it is potential hypoglycemic and hypolipidemic agent. It also protects against various heart diseases.
- Spirulina is potent anticancer agent. It enhances tumour necrosis factor, function of natural killer cells. It prevents expression of proliferating cell nuclear antigen and P_{53}.
- It acts as immunomodulatory agent by enhancing activity of natural killer cells, lysozymes, enhancing phagocytic potential and also increasing production of antibiotics, interferons gamma and cytokinins.
- It acts as anti-inflammatory agent as it inhibits histamine release from mast cells.
- Spirulina also protects reproductive system of poultry animals from oxidative damage.
- Spirulina avoids DNA damage, activates cell nucleus enzymes and DNA repair process. Hence, exhibit anti genotoxic effects.

Side Effects: Spirulina may cause side effects such as headaches, allergic reactions, muscle pain, sweating and insomnia etc. Adverse effects like immunoblistering and rhabdomyolysis are observed. It should not be administered in people with phenyl ketonuria.

Recommended Dose: 1 to 10 g/day.

QUESTIONS

1. What are neutraceuticals? Give their classification.
2. Describe in detail about market, growth, scope of neutraceuticals.
3. Write in brief about neutraceutical products available in market.
4. Explain Health benefits and role of Nutraceuticals Diabetes.
5. Elaborate in detail about role of neutraceuticals in CVS diseases.
6. Describe in detail about management of Cancer with the use of neutraceuticals.
7. What is Irritable bowel syndrome? Discuss the role of neutraceutical in treatment of IBD and various Gastro intestinal diseases.
8. Describe general health benefits and role of neutraceuticals in treatment of various disorders.
9. Explain in detail about Alfalfa and Chicory.
10. Explain the role of Ginger as a neutraceutical in maintaining good human health.
11. Explain Ginseng, as a health food.
12. Explain in detail about role and benefits of Ashvagandha as a neutraceutical.
13. Write short notes on honey and spirulina used as health supplement.
14. Write an elaborative account on role of Garlic as neutraceutical.
15. What is neutraceutical? Explain about Biological source, chemical constituents and role of fenugreek.
16. Explain health benefits of Indian gooseberry.

❖❖❖

Chapter...5

HERBAL-DRUG AND HERB-FOOD INTERACTIONS

Objectives

- To know about definition, classification, types of Herbal-Drug and Herb-Food Interactions.
- To understand mechanisms and effects of interactions.
- To study different drugs and their possible side effects and interactions.

5.1 INTRODUCTION

Herb-Drug Interactions:

The herbal drugs are in great demand throughout the world. But people have very little knowledge about possible herb-drug interactions. The herb-drug interactions may have serious consequences in few cases. Hence, while treating patients with herbal drugs possibility of herb drug interactions should be considered.

Many of the people believe that herbal drugs do not cause any harm. But as herbs can influence body functions, possible herb-drug interactions can occur, when herbs are co-administered with drugs.

Definition:

Drug interaction is defined as 'alteraction in the pharmacological activity of one drug by the concomitant use of another drug or other substance. The concurrent use of herbs may increase, mimic or decrease the effect of other drugs'.

Potential for Herb-Drug Interactions:

There is no chemical reaction between herb and drug. But components of herbs can enhance or diminish the amount of drug present in blood stream.

When herb components bind to drug preventing it from getting into blood stream from gastrointestinal tract or stimulate enzyme degradation activity or help in elimination of drug, there is decrease in drug amount. Hence, drug becomes ineffective.

Herb components can increase amount of drug that may produce toxic effects. The herb can produce similar effect like drug; hence there may be increase in overall drug effect.

Herbal drugs may be toxic intrinsically or when these are taken with combination of other preparations, toxic effects can be observed.

Herbal drugs often contain contaminants such as incorrect species, pollen-grains, insects, allergens, heavy metals (lead, mercury, arsenic) and poisonous drugs etc. These contents may cause toxic reactions.

Few examples of increase or decrease in drug effects due to herbal components are given below:

- Blood thinner warfarin effects may be increased or decreased which leads to bleeding or formation of clots.
- Due to herbal components, the effect of medicines given in the treatment of blood pressure may decrease, which leads to high blood pressure or risks of strokes.
- Herb components can decrease effect of anti-infective agents.
- Effect of antidiabetic drugs may be enhanced leading to dangerously low levels of blood sugar.

About 4th or 6th cause of death in world is due to various drug interactions. The herb–drug or synergy interactions cause various fatal incidences as herbs can increase risk of bleeding causing hepatic failure, renal failure or even death due to adverse reactions.

Significance to Study Herbal-Drug Interactions:

Herb-drug interactions can affects health and the efficiency of treatments. As some herbal therapies might:

- Increase the side effects of drugs, leading to toxicity.
- Leads to treatment failure due to decrease in the therapeutic effect of drugs.
- Unexpected complications may occur due to modification of drug action.
- Enhance the therapeutic effect of drugs.
- Prescription and non-prescription drugs can alter reaction of body to herbal therapies.

Reasons of Herbal-Drug Interactions:

Herbal drug interactions may occur due to some reasons given as follows:

1. Proper information is not available regarding the contents of the herbal product.
2. Product information may be incomplete or inaccurate.
3. Herbal product contains many phytoconstituents and are not characterized properly.
4. Plants are chemically diverse in nature. The chemical makeup of plant depends on part of the plant used, climatic conditions, harvesting and storage conditions, manufacturing conditions and process conditions etc.
5. Lack of adequate knowledge of combinations.

5.2 TYPES OF DRUG INTERACTIONS AS PER AYURVEDA

There are various types of drug interactions according to Ayurveda which are as follows:

1. **Herb-herb interactions:** Examples: Use of *Piper betal* should not be administered with *Garcinia morella*.
2. **Herb-food interaction:** When co-administered some herbs can interact with absorption of food. As per Ayurveda, common food herb interactions are as follows:
   - Milk should not be administered with radish, garlic, mentha or bitter gourd.
   - When *Piper longum* is administered with fish; *Solanum nigrum* with honey or meat; *Semecarpus anacradium* with hot water may cause dreadful side effects or even death.
   - Leaves of asafoetida should not be taken with milk. It may cause loss of strength, complextion, sterility and many other disorders.
   - Combination of lakucha fruits and decoction of masha should be avoided.
   - Sesame seed paste with black cumin can cause diarrhoea.
   - Tea contains anticoagulants called coumarins. When tea is co-administered with garlic, it may cause excessive bleeding.
   - St. John's Wort causes interactions with food containing tyramine such as aged cheeses, sour cream, yogurt, pepperoni, salami, meats, smoked or pickled fish, yeast, red wine, figs, raisins, soy sauce etc. It can cause symptoms like flushing, chills, hypertension, tachycardia, palpitations, restlessness, and insomnia.
3. **Herb and drug of animal origin interactions:** Examples: Meat is contraindicated with *Brassica alba*. Equal quantity of ghee and honey is contraindicated as per Ayurveda.
4. **Interaction related to disease:** Example, Haritaki cannot be administered in pregnancy and anorexia.

5.3 DIFFERENT WAYS OF HERBAL PREPARATIONS TOXICITY

The different ways in which herbal products cause toxicity are:

1. **Toxic ingredients:**

Some herbals may contain toxic ingredients with various potential adverse effects. The examples are as follows:

- Penny royal (*Mentha pulegium*) oil contains a potent abortifacient compound. It can cause liver, kidney damage and death.
- Neuropathy and coma is reported in patients taking herbal laxative to control weight.
- Neurological symptoms are aggrevated due to Podophyllin.
- Noni herbal medicine contains high potassium levels and may cause arrhythmias and even myocardial infarction. The precausion should be taken while using it in patients with renal problems.

- Various herbs such as germander (*Teucrium chamaedrys*), comfrey (*Symphytum* spp) and chapparal (*Larrea tridentata*) can produce hepatoxicity.

2. Unintentional addition of toxic species to herbal medicines:

Few herbal weight reduction formulations use *Aristolochia fangchi* instead of *Stephania tetrandra*. It causes kidney damage and cancer as per animal studies.

3. Intentional addition of drugs:

The intentional addition of drugs is done to potentiate the therapeutic effect of herbals.

Various toxic effects are observed due to such type of admixing.

Many herbal preparations are adulterated with steroids like prednisolone, dexamethasone; pain killer like aminopyrine, acetaminophen; skeletal muscle relaxants like chlorzoxazone; minor tranquilizer like diazepam and glybenclamide etc which can cause serious problems.

Chronical use of traditional medicines containing steroids, poisons and high levels of heavy metals etc. can lead to renal damage.

4. Contamination of the herbs due to environmental factors:

Herbal preparations are not properly evaluated for purity and consistency of active components, and also contain unintentional contaminants as stated above. Various contaminants get mixed from soil, water or from plant's natural habitat which leads to serious toxicity. e.g. various cases of heavy metal poisoning are reported due to use of Chinese herbal preparations.

5. Toxicity due to combination with modern medicines:

The toxicity of herbs with some potential for toxicity can be increased when administered with modern medicines because of their metabolic and physiological effects.

In certain diseases use of herbs should be contraindicated. When used in combination with herbs alterations in the pharmacokinetic and pharmacodynamic properties of drugs are observed.

e.g. herbal-drug interaction may cause decrease or increase in the absorption, distribution, metabolism and excretion of the drug that leads to increase/decrease in the desired pharmacological effects of the drug.

5.4 EFFECTS OF HERB-DRUG INTERACTIONS ON VARIOUS SYSTEMS OF BODY

1. Gastro-intestinal system:

- Horse chestnut acts as irritant to gastro-intestinal tract and can affect efficacy of antiulcer drugs. The activity of laxatives may be enhanced due to use of herbal laxative senna.

2. Cardiovascular system:

- Hawthorn, the cardioactive drug interacts with antiarrhythmic drugs like cardenolide.

- Activity of diuretics may be potentiated due to administration of Dandelion (herbal diuretic).
- Antihypertensive drug therapy can be adversely affected by use of ginseng (lowers blood pressure), broom (increases blood pressure), liquorice (with mineralocorticoid activity), and dandelion etc.
- Alfalfa enhances the effect of hypolipidaemic drugs.
- Parsley develops hypertension when coadministered with sympathomimetic drugs like ephedrine, isoprenaline etc.
- Anticoagulant warfarin shows enhanced activity when used with herb angelica, while activity is reduced when it is used with agrimony. Herb 'willow' when used with warfarin cause increase in risk of bleeding.

3. Central nervous system:

- Sedative herbs like passiflora, valerian react with hypnotic and anxiolytic drugs.
- Evening primrose oil can react with epileptogenic drugs.
- Herbal sedative like hypericum affects activity of antidepressant, analgesic and anti-epileptic drugs.

4. Endocrine system:

- Alfalfa (hypoglycemic activity) and devil's claw (hyper-glycemic activity) can adversely affect antidiabetic drugs.
- Ginseng and red clover (sex hormonal activity) can interfere with activity of sex hormonal treatment and with oral contraceptives.

5.5 PHARMACODYNAMIC AND PHARMACOKINETIC ISSUES OF HERB-DRUG INTERACTIONS

(a) Pharmacodynamics:

Pharmacodynamics is concerned with effect of drug or agent on active sites in human body and its concentrations.

We know that, plant contains primary and secondary metabolites. Primary metabolites are responsible for growth and development of plant which includes enzymes, proteins, lipids, carbohydrates etc. While secondary metabolites are generally excretory products of plant metabolism but are essential for survival of plants in its natural environment.

As per scientific data, secondary metabolites show biological actions in organisms as they share a common ancestry with enzymes and proteins of living organisms. Also there are structural similarities between animal and plant constituents. So following points should be considered while studying pharmacokinetic interactions:

1. The way by which various plant constituents like mucilage, tannins, glycosides, alkaloids, minerals etc. interact with gut and body tissues of organisms.
2. As plant constituents reach the body tissues through digestive tract, it is necessary to understand first pass effect and impact of enterohepatic recycling on them.

3. After digestion what type of constituents will reach systemic circulation.
4. To study change in bioavailability and activity of plant constituents due to change in pharmaceutical preparations.

(b) Pharmacokinetics:

Pharmacokinetics is concerned with what effects the body has with drug and its concentration.

Pharmacokinetics means study of absorption, distribution, metabolism and elimination of phytoconstituents.

Mostly phytoconstituents are administered through oral or topical routes, so it is necessary to study bioavailability of these constituents.

Bioavailability is the degree of absorption of active ingredient into blood after oral administration.

It helps to decide dose of drugs. Phytoconstituents have unusual or poor bioavailability. Also they act at chemical level in the body. Hence, it is necessary to study their pharmacokinetic effects.

Following points should be considered while studying Herbal Pharmacokinetics:

- Information about the traditional and common uses of plants should be collected.
- *In vitro* and *in vivo* research should be well interpreted considering bioavailability of herbal drugs.
- Safety and toxicity of plants should be studied with possibility of herb-drug interaction.
- Synergistic nature of constituents should be supported with evidence.
- Bioavailability and efficacy should be optimized.
- Proper pharmaceutical preparation should be selected.
- The size and solubility of molecule should be considered. More fat soluble molecules have better bioavailability than purely water soluble molecules.
- Transport, metabolism in gut, stability, gastric emptying should be studied.
- First pass metabolism, food-drug interactions are also considered.
- Factors related to patient i.e. pathological factors are also studied.

Herbal pharmacokinetic is a complex study as :

- Plants are chemically complex.
- There are various interactions between constituents and they have different bioavailability.
- Active constituents are not known.
- As phytoconstituents are metabolized in gut, they have unpredictable pharmacokinetic characters.
- Phytoconstituents are large molecules so have poor and unpredictable bioavailability.

5.6 MECHANISMS OF HERB-DRUG INTERACTION

Drug-herb interactions are same as pharmacokinetic and pharmacodynamic drug-drug interactions. Very less is known about these interactions. These are mostly based on assumption or on theoretical interactions rather than evidence-based and mainly observed *in-vitro* studies.

The mechanisms for drug interaction can be classified into two general categories:

A. Pharmacokinetic interactions.

B. Pharmacodynamic interactions.

A. Pharmacokinetic Interactions:

Pharmacokinetic interaction involves absorption, distribution, metabolism and elimination of drug molecules.

Absorption: Herbs and drugs when taken orally are absorbed into blood through the stomach and intestines. The herbs may alter the physical environment of the stomach such as changes in intestinal pH, complexing mechanisms, and intestinal motility which leads to changes in the drug concentration that enters the bloodstream.

For example, common ingredients in herbal weight-loss products are laxative herbs such as aloe leaf, guar gum and senna, which may decrease intestinal transit time and reduce drug absorption.

Gums and mucilages are soluble in water but poorly absorbable. The gum and mucilage containing plants such as psyllium, rhubarb, flaxseed, marshmallow and aloe can bind to other drugs and reduce their action. E.g. the absorption of lithium is inhibited by psyllium. Rhubarb and aloe can cause diarrhoea, which reduces the action of drugs having narrow therapeutic index. It can be avoided by taking drugs one hour before or two hours after consumption of herbal products.

Distribution: Herbs such as Meadowsweet and Black willow can bind to plasma proteins and contain pain-reducing salicylates. These herbs can dislocate highly protein bound drugs such as warfarin and carbamazepine and increases serum drug levels. Thus, the adverse effects of these drugs are enhanced when taken concurrently.

Metabolism: After entering into the bloodstream, drugs are metabolized by the liver either in order to form therapeutically active forms or to remove the drug from the bloodstream. Herbal drugs have the ability to alter liver metabolism by inducing or inhibiting liver enzymes.

Thus, herbs can alter the amount of therapeutically active drugs by two ways:

- By **Enzyme induction activity:** the hebs can stimulate the production and activity of enzymes leading to degradation and elimination of the drug from the body. It decreases the amount of drug. E.g. St. John's Wort induces the activity of the cytochrome P450 enzymes. It may reduce the efficacy of the oral contraceptive pill or concentration of warfarin, digoxin, protease inhibitors, theophylline, carbamazepine etc.

- Herbs may lead to **Enzyme Inhibition.** Herbs inhibit the production of the enzyme required to break down the drug, hence increasing the drug levels. The enzyme induction process may takes several days or weeks while enzyme inhibition can occur within 2-3 days. It leads to rapid development of toxicity. E.g. the metabolism of corticosteroids is reduced due to liquorice leading to adverse and toxic effects. As per *in-vitro* study, herbs like Echinacea and chamomile may inhibit activity of the cytochrome P450 and isoenzyme CYP3A4. When drugs like alprazolam, simvastatin, calcium-channel blockers, and protease inhibitors are used in combination could potentially increase serum drug levels and adverse effects.

Elimination: Few drugs are eliminated through the kidney. The herbs may affect the functioning of the kidney and can influence the level of drug in the blood. The level of drug may increase, if the herb reduces kidney functioning, while it may decrease if the herb increases kidney functioning. The serum drug levels are affected due to changes in excretion. E.g. the chronic use of liquorice may result in hypokalemia and water retention and hence can cause interference with antihypertensive and antiarrhythmic agents.

B. Pharmacodynamic Interactions:

When administered together, herbs and drugs may have synergistic effect (work together) or antagonistic (in opposition) effects. These mutual actions of herbs and drugs inside the body are termed as 'pharmacodynamic interactions'. Pharmacodynamic interactions are difficult to predict and prevent. These interactions are of two types:

(i) Additive interactions: Additive interaction means the herb can produce the similar effect as that of the drug and leads to increase in the drug effect (without increasing the amount of the drug). Hence, concurrent administration of herbal sedatives, anticoagulants, antihypertensives with conventional drugs may increase the effect of such drugs. e.g. valerian increases the hyponotic activity of benzodiazepines. Co-administration of gingko, garlic and ginger increases the anticoagulant action of warfarin. St John's Wort increases effect of serotonergic drugs.

(ii) Antagonistic interactions: It means that, a herb might produce an opposite effect as that of the drug, so reducing the drug effect. e.g. Ephedra and other caffeine-containing herbs like cola nut, guarana, mate, green tea often used in weight loss products, may antagonize the effects of antihypertensive medications.

5.7 TYPES OF HERB-DRUG INTERACTIONS

The herb-drug interactions can occur by following ways:

1. **By modification in intestinal absorption of medicines:** It includes various mechanisms like impairment by hydrocolloidal fiber, selective precipitation of drug by tannins, selective precipitation of drug by iodine and enhancement of drug by pungent herbs.
2. **Potentiation of cardiotonic medicines:** It can occur due to herbal cardiotonics stimulant laxatives, enhancers of urinary potassium excretion, potentiation of sedative or tranquilizers.

3. **Modification of blood sugar in insulin-dependent diabetes:** Due to administration of hypoglycemic and hyperglycemic herbs.
4. **By modification of prothrombopenic anticoagulant effects:** It may be due to potentiation by coumarin-containing plants, potentiation by platelet aggregation inhibitors and antagonism by plants with high vitamin K content.
5. **Incompatibility with medications for gastrointestinal tract:** It is due to use of stimulants for secretion of stomach.

5.8 HERB-DRUG INTERACTIONS OF COMMONLY USED DRUGS

1. ST. JOHN'S WORT (*HYPERICUM*)

Synonyms: Amber, Amber Touch-and-Heal, Demon Chaser, Goat weed, Hardhay Goat-weld.

Biological Source: It consists of dried aerial parts of *Hypericum perforatum* of family Hypericaceae.

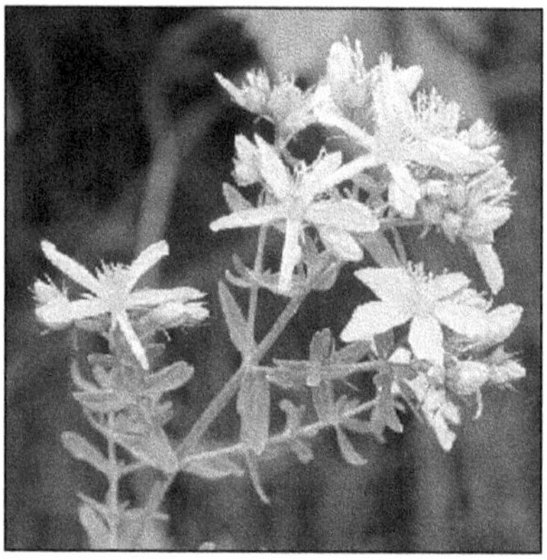

Fig. 5.1: Flowering branch of St. John's Wort

Geographical Source:

The plant is native to Europe and Asia but grows in India in western Himalaya, China, Canada, Africa, Australia and United States.

Description:

St John's Wort is herbaceous perennial plant with extensive, creeping root system. The plant has erect branched stems and it can grow to 1 m high. The leaves are opposite, sessile, narrow, glabrous with entire margin, oblong about 1–2 cm long, and are yellow-green in colour with translucent dots of glandular tissue. The plant has bright yellow coloured, star shaped flowers with conspicuous black dots. The flowering occurs between late spring and early to mid summer.

Chemical Constituents:

The main constituents are Hyperborean and adhyperforin (Prenylated Phloroglucinol derivatives). The plant also contains constituents like:

- **Flavonoids:** Plant contains rutin,Epigallocatechin,hyperoside, isoquercetin, quercitrin, quercetin, amentoflavone, biapigenin, astilbin, myricetin, kaempferol, luteolin.
- **Naphthodianthrones:** Hypericin, pseudohypericin, protohypericin, protopseudo-hypericin.
- **Phenolic acids:** Chlorogenic acid, caffeic acid, p-coumaric acid, ferulic acid, p-hydroxybenzoic acid, vanillic acid.
- Tannins, volatile oils, saturated fatty acids (isovaleric acid, myristic acid, palmitic acid, stearic acid).
- **Alkaloids:** Vitamins, pectin, β-sitosterol, hexadecane, caffeine, vitamin C, carotenoids, triacontane, kielcorin, norathyriol etc.

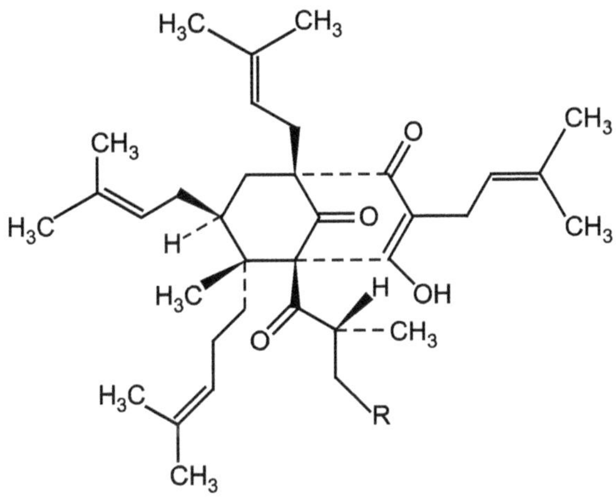

Hyperforin R = H
Adhyperforin R = CH_3

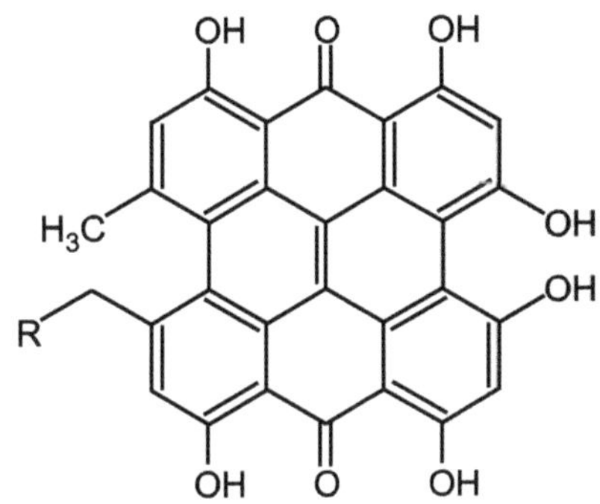

Hypericin R = H
Pseudohypericin R = OH

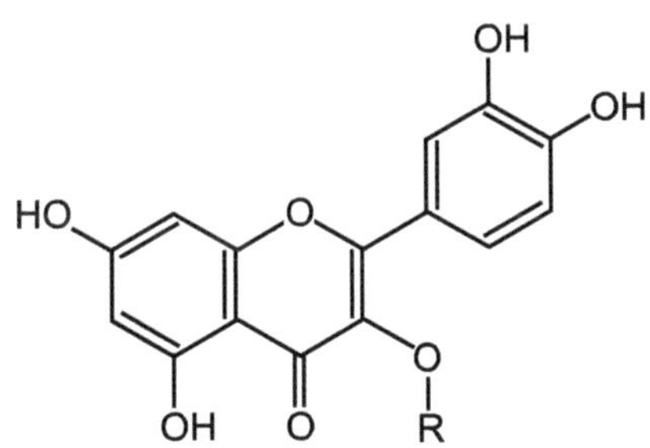

Quercitrin R = Rha *p*
Hyperoside R = Gal *p*
Isoquercitrin R = Glc *f*

Gal *p* =

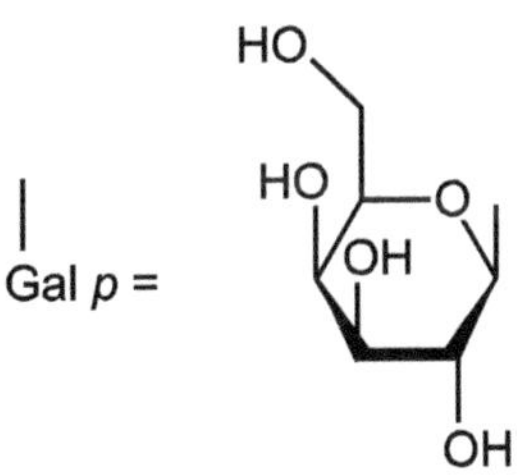

B-D-Galactopyranosyl

Glc *f* =

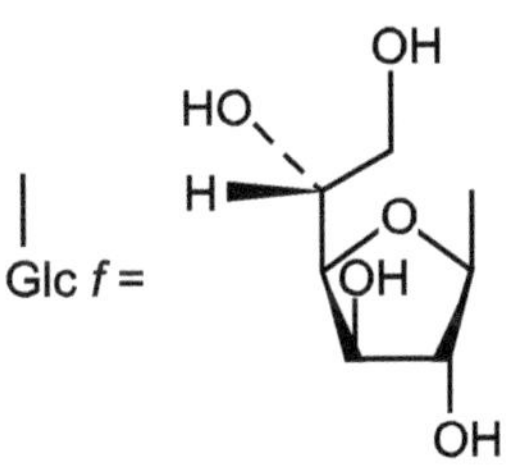

B-D-Glucofuranosyl

Rha *p* =

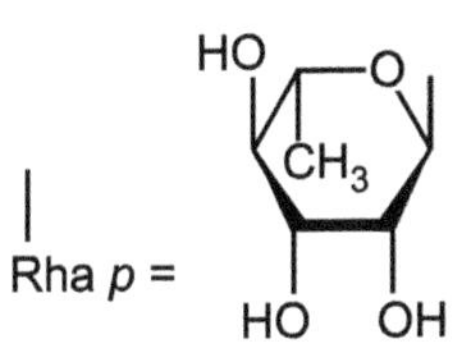

6-Deoxy-a-L-mannopyranosyl

Chemical Constituents of St. John's Wort

Uses:

It is used in treatment of depression, heart palpitations, moodiness and symptoms of menopause, mental disorders, premenstrual syndrome (PMS), attention deficit-hyperactivity disorder (ADHD), obsessive-compulsive disorder (OCD), social phobia, and seasonal affective disorder (SAD). It can be used to treat fibromyalgia, chronic fatigue syndrome (CFS), burning feelings in the mouth, migraine and other types of headaches, pain, irritable bowel syndrome, cancer, HIV/AIDS, hepatitis C, herpes simplex, weight loss, and skin diseases.

Herb-Drug Interactions:

- It can cause multiple drug interactions due to induction of the cytochrome P450 enzymes CYP3A4 and CYP1A2.
- St. John's wort can increase metabolism of anti-anxiety drug alprazolam, hence decrease its effectiveness.
- St. John's wort also decreases the efficacy of birth control pills by enhancing its breakdown by induction of CYP3A4.
- St. John's wort might decrease the effects of cardiotonic drug digoxin (Lanoxin) by reducing its absorption.
- Fenfluramine (Pondimin) increases serotonin level in brain. Its co-administration with St. John's wort further increases serotonin causing serious side effects such as heart problems, shivering, nausea, headache and anxiety.
- It decreases effectiveness of various drugs such as Imatinib, Irinotecan, Ketamine, mitriptyline, carisoprodol, citalopram, diazepam, lansoprazole, omeprazole, phenytoin, warfarin, and many others by enhancing their metabolism by liver.
- It also decreases effects of anti HIV/AIDS drugs like amprenavir, nelfinavir, ritonavir, and saquinavir by Induction of CYP 3A4.
- Methadone is a narcotic pain reliever. St. John's wort decreases its effectiveness by induction of CYP 3A4, 2C8 and CYP 2D6.
- Phenytoin effectiveness may decrease due to St. John's wort increasing the possibility of seizures.
- When administered with warfarin it might increase the risk of blood clotting.
- St. John's wort increases effects and side effects of fexofenadine by reducing its break down by liver.
- When St. John's wort is administered with antidepressant drugs like fluoxetine, paroxetine, sertraline clomipramine, imipramine etc. increases serotonin levels and cause serious side effects including heart problems, shivering and anxiety.
- It also causes serious side effects with medications for migraine such as frovatriptan, naratriptan, rizatriptan, sumatriptan etc.
- If St. John's wort is taken with medications that increase sensitivity to sunlight, it may also increase the chances of sunburn, blistering or rashes on areas of skin exposed to

sunlight. Such type of medications are amitriptyline, ciprofloxacin, norfloxacin, ofloxacin), levofloxacin, tetracycline, methoxsalen etc.

- Cyclosporine when taken with St. John's wort leads to decrease in drug concentration and rejection of transplanted organ by Induction of CYP3A4 and P–g P.

Possible Side Effects:

St. John's wort when taken orally upto 12 weeks, it is considered to be safe. Its possible side effects includes trouble sleeping, vivid dreams, restlessness, anxiety, irritability, stomach upset, fatigue, dry mouth, dizziness, headache, skin rash, and diarrhoea. In persons taking antidepressant drugs it can cause agitation, hallucinations, fever, fast heart rate, overactive reflexes, nausea, vomiting, diarrhoea, loss of co-ordination, fainting etc.

2. KAVA KAVA:

Synonyms: Ava Pepper, Ava Root, Awa

Biological Source:

It consists of dried roots of plant *Piper methysticum* belonging to family Piperaceae.

Geographical Source:

The plant is found in Melanesia, Micronesia and Polynesia. It grows well in shade and moist areas.

Description:

It is shrub and has heart-shaped leaves and woody stems. The stems are green with swollen nodes. The male flowers are approximately six inches long solitary, auxiliary, with greenish white spikes. The female flowers are rare. The fruits are berries with one seed.

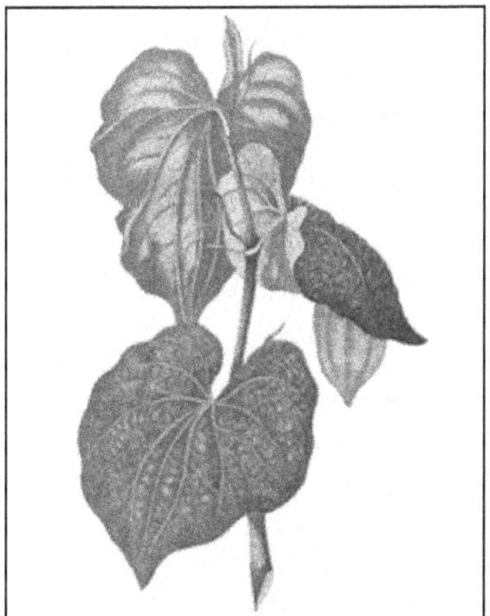

Fig. 5.2: *Piper methysticum* plant

Chemical Constituents:

Dried kava root consists of 12% water, 43% starch, and 20% fibers, protein, sugars and minerals. The main phytoconstituents found in kava roots are kavalactones, chalcones and other flavanones. kawain, 7,8-dihydrokawain, methysticin, 7,8- dihydromethysticin, yangonin, and demethoxy yangonin are main kavalactones present in plants. Minor constituents found in kava are three chalcones, flavokavain A, flavokavain B, and flavokavain C, and toxic alkaloid pipermethystine.

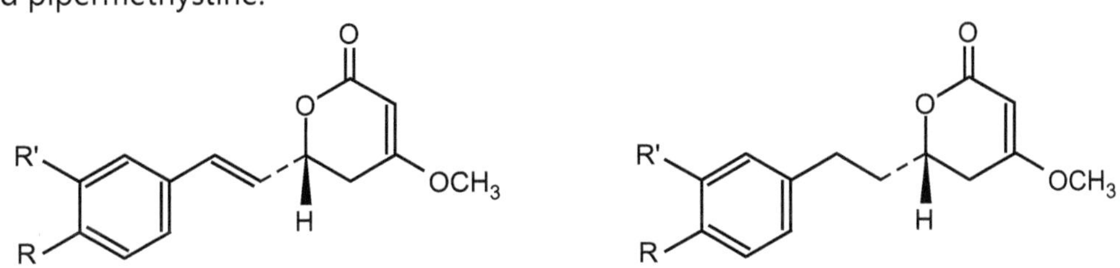

Kawain **Dihydrokawain**

Chemical Constituents of Kava Kava

Uses:

Kava kava may decrease anxiety, stress, insomnia and menopausal symptoms. It may used in treatment of cancer, attention deficit-hyperactivity disorder (ADHD), epilepsy, psychosis, depression, chronic fatigue syndrome (CFS) and headaches. It is also used in treatment of common cold, respiratory tract infections, Tuberculosis, muscle pain, urinary tract infections, skin diseases and wounds etc. Other uses include urinary infections, vaginitis, fatigue, asthma, rheumatism and pain.

Herb Drug Interactions:

- Kava when taken together with alprazolam may cause drowsiness.
- Kava also interacts with CNS depressant medications such as clonazepam, lorazepam, Phenobarbital, zolpidemetc and cause drowsiness.
- By decreasing dopamine, secretion kava decreases the effectiveness of levodopa.
- Kava may cause side effects by decreasing liver metabolism of drugs such as clozapine, cyclobenzaprine, fluvoxamine, haloperidol, imipramine, omeprazole, lansoprazole, phenytoin, phenobarbital, diclofenac, ibuprofen, warfarin, ondansetron and tramadol etc.
- Kava enhances the absorption of medications such as etoposide, paclitaxel, vinblastine, vincristine, vindesine, ketoconazole, itraconazole, amprenavir, indinavir, nelfinavir, saquinavir, cimetidine, ranitidine, diltiazem, verapamil, corticosteroids causing serious side effects.
- Kava when administered with medicines such as acetaminophen, amiodarone, carbamazepine, isoniazid, methotrexate, methyldopa, fluconazole, itraconazole, and erythromycin etc. can cause hepatotoxicity.

Possible Side Effects:

When taken orally, it may cause liver damage. Kava aggravates the symptoms of depression and Parkinson's disease. It is not safe during pregnancy and lactation. It may cause adverse effects like visual disturbances, urinary retention, GI discomfort and rhabdomyolysis etc.

3. GINKGO BILOBA

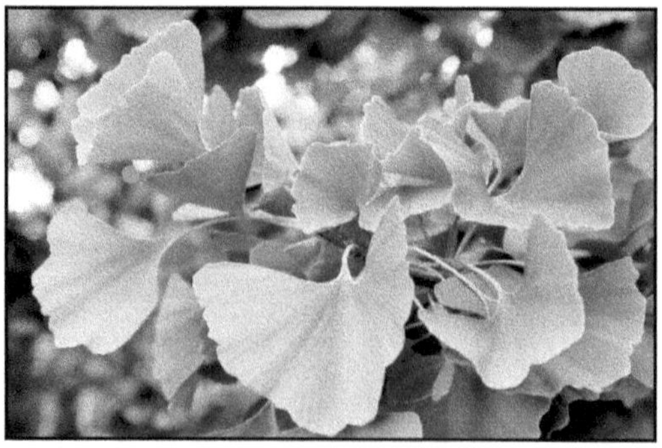

Fig. 5.3: Leaves of *Ginkgo biloba* plant

Synonym: Ginkgo, gingko, maidenhair tree.

Bioilogical Source:

It consists of dried leaves of *Ginkgo biloba L* belonging to family Ginkgoaceae.

Geographical Source:

The plant is widely distributed in China, Korea and Japan.

Description:

Gingko biloba is deciduous tree with tough branches having elongated and spur shoots. The leaves are fan-shaped, alternate, leathery, with parallel venation; and occur in clusters. The leaves turn bright yellow, and then fall within 15 days during autumn. The male and female plants occur in 1:1 ratio. Seeds are yellow in colour, drupe like with long peduncle; outer coat is fleshy and inner coat stony.

Chemical Constituents:

The leaves of the plant mainly consist of flavonoid glycosides (24%), proanthocyanidins (7%) and terpenoids. The major phytoconstituents are Quercetin-3-β-D glucoside, Quercitrin, Rutin. The minor constituents include Quercetin, Kaempferol, and Isorhamnetin etc. Terpene lactones present in plant are Ginkgolide A, Gingkolide B, Ginkgolide C, Bilobalide and Ginkgotoxin. It contains diterpenes like ginkgolides A, B, C and J and the sesquiterpene, bilobalide.

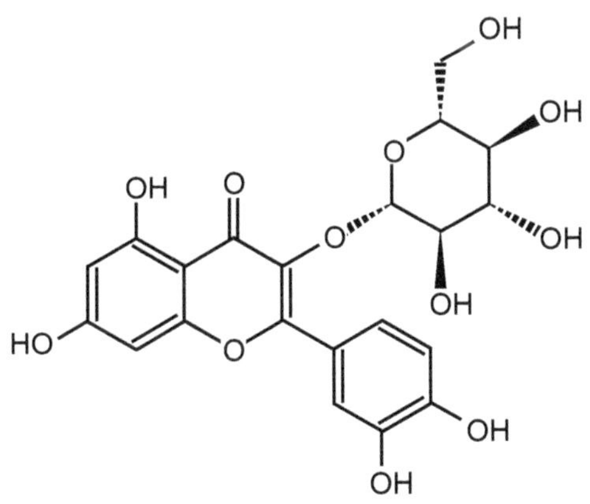

Quercetin-3-β-D glucoside

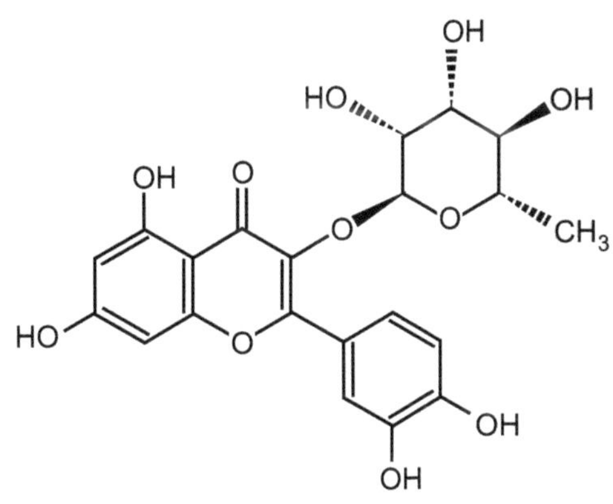

Quercitrin

Chemical Constituents of *Ginkgo biloba*

Uses:

Ginkgo biloba acts as anti-inflammatory and hepatoprotective agent. The plant has antilipidemic, antidiabetic and antioxidant activity. It reduces anxiety and treats dementia related to Alzheimer's disease. The plant also acts as anti-allergic, anti-inflammatory, anti-viral, anti-proliferative, anti-tumorigenic, and anti-carcinogenic agent.

Herb Drug Interactions:

- When ginkgo is administered with ibuprofen, it can increase the chances of bruising and bleeding due to slow blood clotting. Ginkgo should not be given with medications such as aspirin, clopidogrel, diclofenac, naproxen, dalteparin, heparin which slow down blood clotting.
- Ginkgo can decrease the effect of alprazolam.
- When ginkgo is administered with buspirone, it may cause over excitation of central nervous system.
- Ginkgo decreases the effect of anti HIV drug, efavirenz.
- Ginkgo and St. John's wort when administered with fluoxetine may cause hypomania.
- Ginkgo may slow down the liver metabolism of certain drugs such as clozapine, cyclobenzaprine, fluvoxamine, haloperidol, imipramine, mexiletine, olanzapine, pentazocine, propranolol, tacrine and theophylline etc. Hence, it may cause side effects.
- Gingko may decrease the effects of drugs such as amitriptyline, carisoprodol, citalopram, diazepam, lansoprazole, omeprazole, phenytoin and warfarin etc. Ginkgo may increase rate of liver metabolism of these drugs.
- Gingko may cause side effects when taken with drugs such as lovastatin, clarithromycin, cyclosporine, diltiazem, estrogens, indinavir and triazolam, due to alteration in liver metabolism of these drugs.
- When Gingko is administered along with antidiabetic drugs such as glimepiride, glyburide, insulin, pioglitazone, rosiglitazone, chlorpropamide, glipizide and tolbutamide etc. decreases their effects.
- Gingko when taken along medications such as anesthetic, antiarrhythmics, antibiotics, antidepressants, antihistamines, immunosuppressants, narcotics and stimulants etc. it may increase the chances of getting seizures in few patients.
- Gingko decreases the effects of anticonvulsant drugs such as phenobarbital, primidone, valproic acid, gabapentin, carbamazepine and phenytoin etc.
- Trazodone when taken with Gingko may cause serious side effects.
- Hydrochlorothiazide when administered with gingko cause increase in blood pressure.

Possible Side Effects: Gingko can cause possible side effects such as stomach upset, headache, dizziness, constipation, increase in force of heartbeat, and allergic skin reactions etc. High dose of leaf extract may increase the risk of liver and thyroid cancers. It may increase the risk of bruising and bleeding. Gingko seeds may cause seizures and death. In patients with G6PD enzyme deficiency gingko may cause severe anemia. It is not safe in pregnancy and lactation.

4. GINSENG:

Synonyms: Panax ginseng, Red berry, Renshen, Hong shen, Shang, Shi yang seng.

Biological Source:

It consists of dried roots of Panax ginseng of family Araliaceae.

Geographical Source:

Ginseng is native of Manchuria, Chinese tartary and other parts of eastern Asia, and is largely cultivated in Korea and Japan.

Description:

It is a smooth perennial herb, and has large, fleshy, spindle-shaped, annulated very slow-growing root. It is pale yellow to a brownish in colour, odourless with mucilaginous taste with slight bitterness. The stem is simple and erect, with five finely-toothed leaflets. It has a single, terminal umbel, with a few small, yellowish flowers. The fruit consists of cluster of bright red berries.

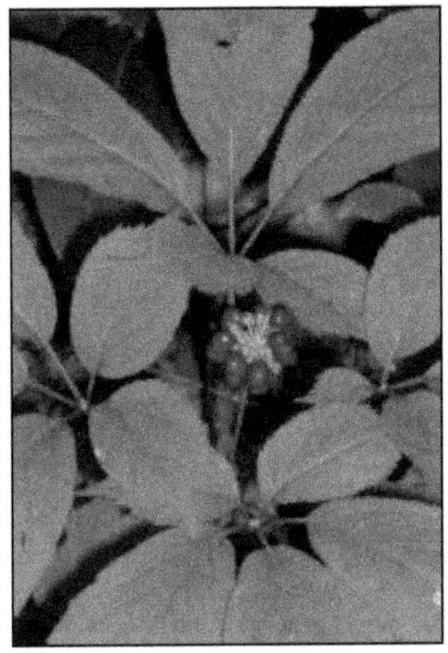

Fig. 5.4: Ginseng herb

Chemical Constituents:

Ginseng contains active components called 'Ginsenosides', which are steroid-like saponins. About 100 ginsenosides are known among them. Ginsenosides Rb1, Rb2, Rc, Rd, Re and Rg1 etc. comprise over 90% of the total ginsenosides. Other constituents include Ginsenoside Rg2, Re, Rd, Panaxadione, 3-keto-20(S)-protopanaxatriol, Dencichine, α,β-N-oxalyl-L-α,β-diaminopropionic acid (β-ODAP), Saringosteryl and its glycoside, Daucosterol and 5a, 6b-dihydroxydaucosterol.

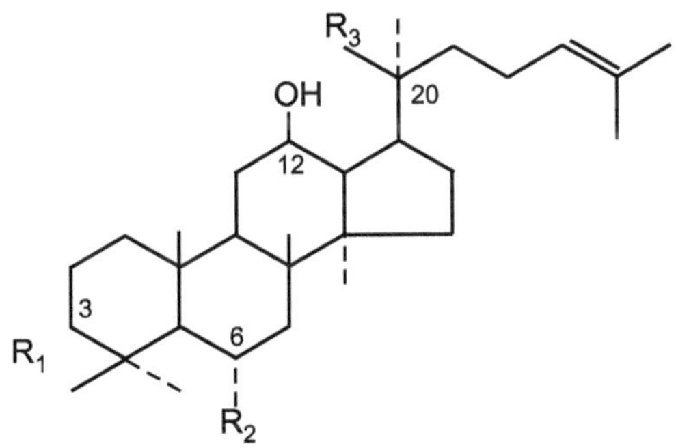

Ginsenosides	R_1	R_2	R_3
Ginsenoside-Rb_1	–O–Glc^2-Glc	–H	–O–Glc^6-Glc
Ginsenoside-Rc	–O–Glc^2-Glc	–H	–O–Glc^6-Ara (pyr)
Ginsenoside-Re	–OH	–O–Glc^2-Rha	–O–Glc
Ginsenoside-Rf	–OH	–O–Glc^2-Glc	–OH
Ginsenoside-Rg_1	–OH	–O–Glc	–O–Glc

Chemical Constituents of Ginseng

Uses:

Ginseng is used to treat depression, anxiety, general fatigue, chronic fatigue syndrome (CFS), multiple sclerosis, anemia, chronic bronchitis, swine flu, pre-diabetes and diabetes, inflammation of the stomach lining (gastritis) and fever, chronic obstructive pulmonary disease (COPD), HIV/AIDS, fertility problems, for boosting the immune system. It has wide applications in treating bleeding disorders, loss of appetite, vomiting, intestinal problems, gallstones, bad breath, fibromyalgia, sleeping problems (insomnia), nerve pain, joint pain, dizziness, headache, hearing loss, convulsions, disorders of pregnancy and childbirth, hot flashes due to menopause, common cold and flu, heart failure, high blood pressure, wrinkled skin, and as antiaging agent.

Herb-Drug Interactions:

- When taken with caffeine, Panax ginseng might cause serious problems such as increased heart rate and high blood pressure as both are CNS stimulants.
- Panax ginseng decreases effects of estrogen pills.
- Panax ginseng can decrease effect of furosemide.
- Panax ginseng slows down the metabolism of imatinib, hence increasing its effects and side effects.
- The blood sugar level should be closely monitored when ginseng is taken along with insulin, as ginseng may also decrease in blood sugar level.
- Medications like amitriptyline, clozapine, codeine, desipramine, donepezil, fentanyl, flecainide, fluoxetine, meperidine, methadone, metoprolol, olanzapine, ondansetron, tramadol are metabolized by liver. Panax ginseng decreases break down of these medications thereby increasing their side effects.
- Panax ginseng may stimulate the body. When ginseng is introduced with anti-depressant medications like phenelzine, tranylcypromine can cause side effects such as anxiousness, headache, restlessness and insomnia.
- Panax ginseng when administered with medications that affect the heartbeat such as amiodarone, disopyramide, dofetilide, ibutilide, procainamide, quinidine, sotalol, and thioridazine can cause heart rhythm problems.
- Panax ginseng might decrease the effectiveness of immunosuppressant drugs such as azathioprine, basiliximab, cyclosporine, daclizumab, muromonab-CD3, orthoclone, mycophenolate, tacrolimus and sirolimus etc.
- Panax ginseng slows down blood clotting. Hence, when it is used with anticoagulant or antiplatelet drugs such as aspirin, cilostazol, clopidogrel, diclofenac, cataflam, ibuprofen, naproxen, enoxaparin, heparin, ticlopidine and warfarin etc. might increase the chances of bruising and bleeding.
- Panax ginseng can decrease the effects of midazolam, nifedipine.

- Ginseng when used along with anti HIV drug like Raltegravir, can increase the chances of liver toxicity.
- Ginseng when administered with CNS stimulant drugs such as diethylpropion, epinephrine, phentermine, pseudoephedrine etc. can cause serious side effects. It may increase heart rate and blood pressure.

Possible Side Effects:

Common side effects of ginseng include skin reaction, diarrhoea, insomnia, headache, rapid heartbeat, increased or decreased blood pressure, loss of appetite, itching, rash, breast tenderness and vaginal bleeding.

5. GARLIC:

Synonyms: Allium, Lasun

Biological Source:

It consists of dried bulbs of *Allium sativum L* of family Liliaceae.

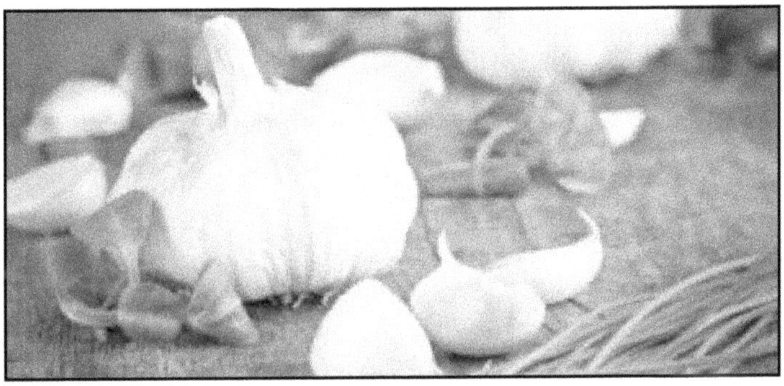

Fig. 5.5: Garlic bulbs

Geographical Source:

The plant is native to central Asia, and also grows at Africa, United States, India and Europe.

Description:

It is a bulbous perennial plant with about 4 ft in height. It consists of several cloves covered with white or pink membrane. It has hermaphrodite flowers. It is pollinated by bees and other insects.

Chemical Constituents:

Garlic contains about 1.0% volatile oil.

Oil contains allicin responsible for particular odour. It contains alliin, allixin, allylpolysulfides, diallylsulphide (DAS), diallyldisulphide, diallyltrisulphide (DATS), N-acetylcysteine (NAC), N-acetyl-S-allylcysteine (NASC), S-allylcysteine (SAC), S-allylmerca, 2-vinyldithiin (1,2-DT) and thiacremonone, amino acids etc.

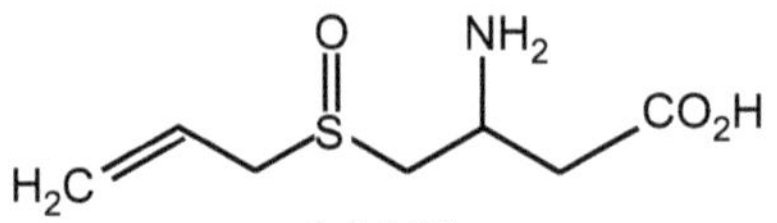

(a) Alliin

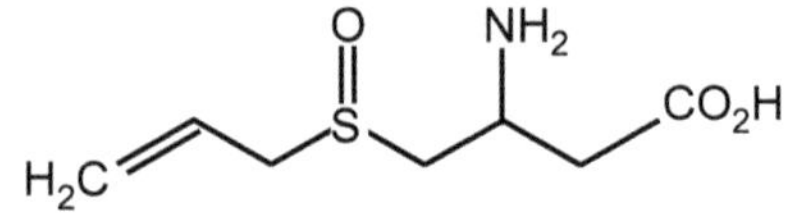

(b) Allicin (Diallyl thiosulphinate)

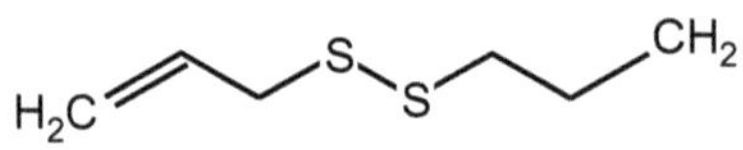

(c) Diallyl disulphide

Chemical Constituents of Garlic

Uses:

It acts as aphrodiasiac, carminative, expectorant, stimulant. It is used to treat fever, hyperlipidemia, bronchial asthma, tuberculosis, GIT disorders, diabetes, and infections and to prevent arteriosclerosis.

Herb-Drug Interactions:

- Garlic may increase bleeding times with anticoagulants.
- Garlic may induce hepatic CYP3A4 metabolism of protease inhibitors like ritonavir, indinavir etc. It decreases blood levels of protease inhibitors and leads to toxicity.
- During and after surgery, garlic causes spontaneous bleeding.
- *In-vitro* and *in-vivo* studies demonstrated inhibition of platelet aggregation by bio-organic constituents of garlic.
- Saquinavir levels are decreased due to possible induction of p-glycoproteins by garlic. Hence, patients taking saquinavir should be advised to minimize their consumption of garlic or garlic supplements.
- When co-administered with chlorpropamide, produces antihyperglycemic effect.
- Major reaction is observed with isoniazide. Garlic reduces absorption of isoniazid and hence its effects.
- Minor interactions include changes in paracetamol pharmacokinetics and hypoglycaemia when combined with the antidiabetic drug chlorpropamide.
- Garlic decreases effects of anti HIV medications such as nevirapine, delavirdine and efavirenz by increasing their break down.
- Garlic decreases effectiveness of calcium channel blockers (diltiazem, nicardipine, verapamil), cancer drugs (etoposide, paclitaxel, vinblastine, vincristine, vindesine), fungus-fighting drugs (ketoconazole, itraconazole), glucocorticoids, alfentanil, cisapride, fentanyl, lidocaine, losartan, midazolam etc. This occurs due to increase in the liver break down of such medications because of garlic.
- Garlic decreases blood pressure when administered with medications used for lowering high blood pressure such as nifedipine, verapamil, diltiazem, isradipine, amlodipine etc.

Possible Side Effects:

Allergic reactions such as difficulty in breathing, swelling of your face, lips, tongue or throat etc. can occur due to garlic consumption. Various side effects such as redness, swelling, or blistering, easy bruising or bleeding, unpleasant breath or body odour, heartburn, burning in mouth or throat, nausea, vomiting, gas or diarrhoea etc. are observed.

6. PEPPER:

Synonyms: Black pepper, Kali miri, Pippali

Biological Source:

It consists of dried ripe fruits of the plant *Piper nigrum* of family Piperaceae.

Geographical Sources:

The plant grows well in Brazil, Indonesia and India.

Description:

The plant grows well in shade and need support. The leaves are heart shaped, alternate with palmate veins. The male and female flowers are small, monoecious and separate. The fruits are drup with single seed and red in colour when mature. The single stem shows 20-30 spikes of fruits. The fruits are globular brownish to black in colour, with uneven surface, seeds are almost brown or black, with aromatic odour and pungent taste.

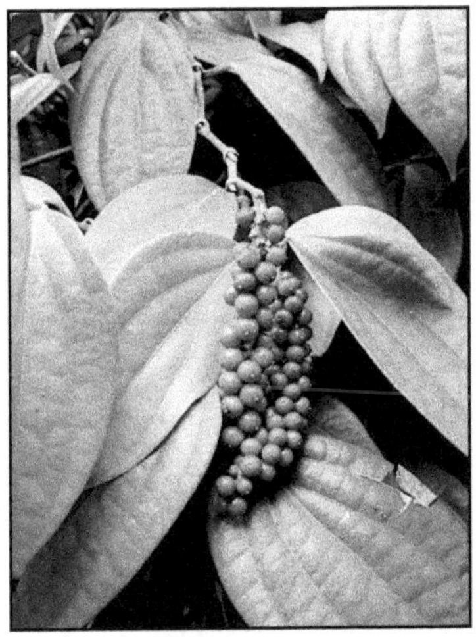

Fig. 5.6: Fruits and leaves of plant *Piper nigrum*

Chemical Constituents:

Fruits contain 1.0 – 2.5 per cent volatile oil. The main pharmacologically active principle is pungent alkaloid piperine which occurs in four isomers such as Piperine, Isopiperine, Chavicine and Isochavicine. The plant also shows presence of phytoconstituents such as Brachyamide B, Dihydro-pipericide, (2E, 4E)-N-Eicosadienoyl-pereridine, N-trans-Feruloyltryamine, N-Formylpiperidine, Guineensine, pentadienoyl as piperidine, (2E, 4E)-Nisobutyl-ldecadienamid, isobutyl-eicosadienamide, Tricholein, Trichostachine, isobutyl-eicosatrienamide, Isobutyl-octadienamide, Piperamide, Piperamine, Piperettine, Pipericide, Piperine, Piperolein B, Sarmentine, Sarmentosine, Retrofractamide A. The volatile oil consists of phytoconstituents such as Sabinene, Limonene Camphene, α-Pinene, α-Phellandrene, α-Terpinolene, β-Pinene Caryophyllene oxide, α-Cis-Bergamotene, Cinnamic acid, Benzaldehyde and Eugenol.

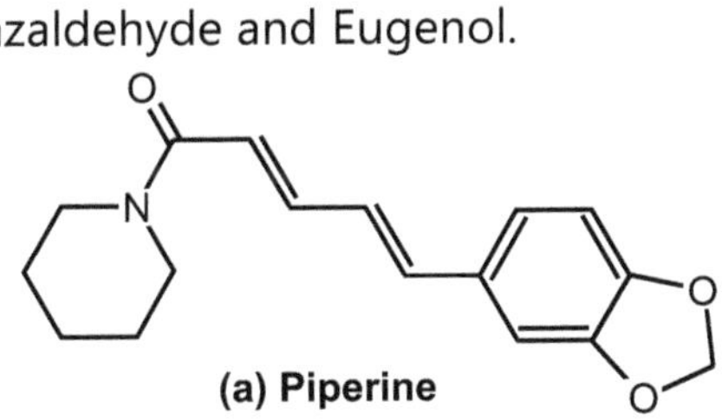

(a) Piperine

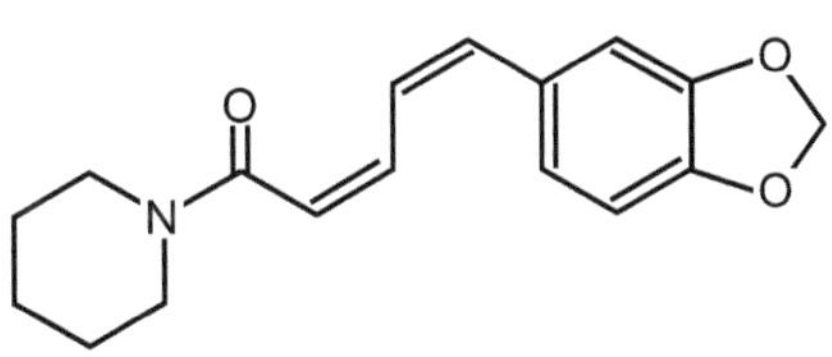

(b) Chavicine

Chemical Constituents of Black Pepper

Uses:

Black pepper shows wide array of therapeutic activities such as antihypertensive, antiplatelet, antioxidant, anticancer, antiasthmatics, analgesic, anti-inflammatory, antidiarrhoeal, antispasmodic, antidepressants, immunomodulatory, anticonvulsant, anti-thyroids, antibacterial, antifungal, hepatoprotective, insecticidal and larvicidal activities etc. It acts as bioenhancers and increases absorption of many drugs and nutrients.

Herb Drug Interactions:

- As black pepper has diuretic effects, it decreases clearance of lithium and increases the concentration of lithium in body hence cause serious side effects.
- Black and white pepper increases the side effects of various drugs such as lovastatin, ketoconazole, itraconazole, fexofenadine and triazolam by altering their liver metabolism.
- Black pepper enhances absorption of various drugs such as etoposide, paclitaxel, vinblastine, vincristine, vindesine, ketoconazole, itraconazole, amprenavir, indinavir, nelfinavir, saquinavir, cimetidine, ranitidine, diltiazem, verapamil, digoxin, corticosteroids, erythromycin, cisapride, fexofenadine and cyclosporine etc. by deactivating various pumps in the body. Hence, can cause serious side effects.
- Black pepper enhances the effects and side effects of phenytoin.
- Propranolol, rifampin, theophylline, amoxicillin absorption in the body increases when they are taken with black pepper.
- Carbamazepine absorption increases and metabolism decreases when administered with black pepper. It increases its effects and side effects.
- By inhibiting P-glycoprotein (PGP), piperine increases bioavailability of fexofenadine.
- Piperine may decrease blood sugar level hence should be administered with caution with antidiabetic drugs like glimepiride, glyburide, insulin, pioglitazone etc.
- Piperine slows down blood clotting. Hence, when it is administered with anticoagulant medications such as aspirin, clopidogrel, dalteparin, enoxaparin, heparin, ticlopidine and warfarin, it may increase the chances of bruising and bleeding.
- Piperine may increase the sedative side effects of pentobarbital.

Possible Side Effects:

It is generally safe when given orally in small doses. It it get into eyes may cause redness and burning. In case of children if pepper accidentally gets into the lungs, it may cause death. In small doses it is safe during pregnancy and lactation but in large doses it may cause miscarriage.

7. EPHEDRA:

Synonyms: Ma-Huang, Mahuang, Yellow horse, Yellow astringent, Pinellia.

Biological Source:

It consists of dried young stem of *Ephedra gerardiana* (India), *Ephedra nebrodensis* (India), *Ephedra sinica* (*China*), *Ephedra equisetina* of family Ephedraceae.

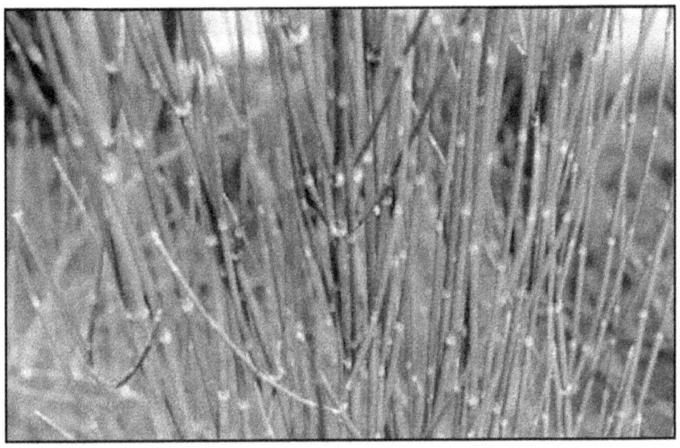

Fig. 5.7: Ephedra stems

Geographical Source:

Ephedra is native to northern China and Inner part of Mongolia. It also grows in southern Europe, North Africa to Asia as well as in the mountains of North and South America. Ephedra plants typically grow in dry and desert regions.

Description:

Ephedra is an evergreen shrub 2 to 3 feet hight and has no leaves. Stems are green, jointed, smooth, woody, branching. During flowering, it shows small yellow-green buds. It has scale like leaves, cone-like reproductive structures and bright red or orange berry-like fruits.

Chemical Constituents:

Ephedra consists of 1.0 percent of amino alkaloids such as ephedrine, pseudoephedrine (isoephedrine), norpseudoephedrine (cathine), norephedrine, methylephedrine, methylpseudoephedrine, including quinoline and 6-hydroxykynurenic acid and tannins.

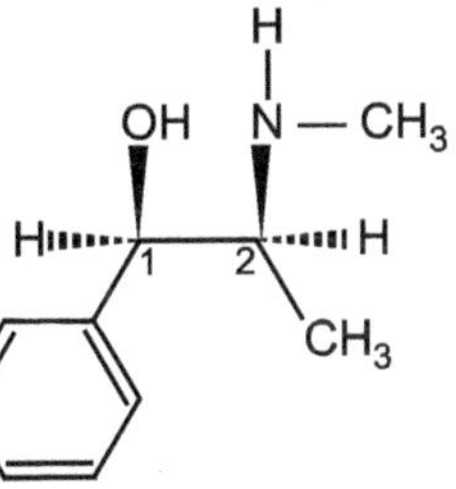

(1R, 2S)-(–)-Ephedrine

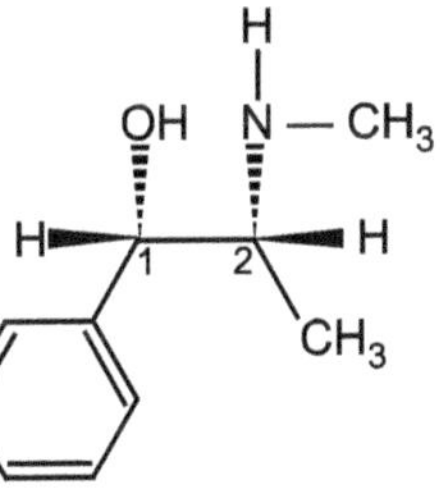

(1S, 2R)-(+)-Ephedrine

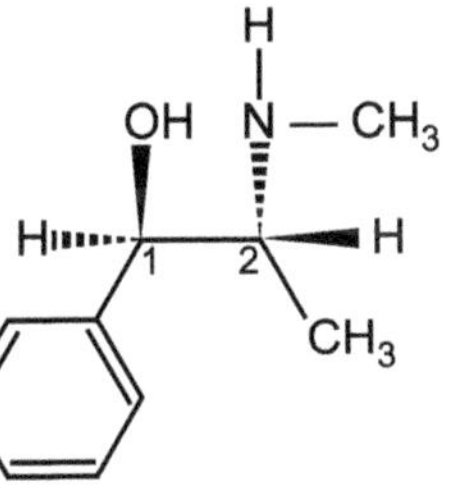

(1R, 2R)-(–)-Pseudoephedrine

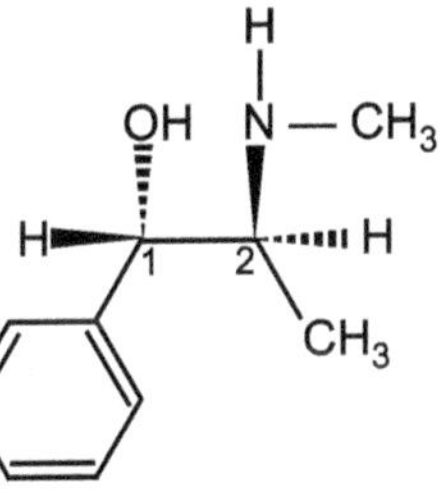

(1S, 2R)-(+)-Pseudoephedrine

Chemical Constituents of Ephedra

Uses:

It is used in asthma, bronchitis, bronchospasm, allergies, nasal congestion, colds, flu, fever and other breathing problems.

Herb-Drug Interactions:

- Ephedra when administered with medications like amiodarone, disopyramide, dofetilide, ibutilide, procainamide, quinidine, sotalol, thioridazine etc. can cause serious side effects like heart attack.
- Ephedra when taken with methylxanthines (aminophylline, caffeine, and theophylline) might cause side effects such as nervousness, fast heartbeats, high blood pressure and anxiety as both can stimulate body.
- When ephedra is administered with CNS stimulants it may cause serious problems like increased heart rate and high blood pressure.
- Effectiveness of dexamethasone may decrease due to ephedra. This is due to enhanced break down of dexamethasone by ephedra.
- Ephedra and Ergot derivatives can increase blood pressure. Hence, when ephedra is taken with ergot derivatives might drastically increase blood pressure.
- The serious side effects such as fast heartbeat, high blood pressure, seizures, nervousness can caused when ephedra is taken with antidepressant drugs,
- Ephedra decreases efficacy of antidiabetic drugs.
- Ephedra can decrease the efficacy of anticonvulsant drugs such as Phenobarbital, primidone, valproic acid, gabapentin, carbamazepine, phenytoin.

Possible Side Effects:

It may cause side effects such as dizziness, restlessness, anxiety, irritability, headache, loss of appetite, nausea, vomiting etc. It also causes arrhythmia and sudden death, myocardial infarction, stroke, psychiatric symptoms, autonomic hyperactivity, seizures, ischemic colitis and gastric mucosal injury etc.

QUESTIONS

1. What are drug interactions? Give reasons of interaction and its significance to study herb-drug interactions.
2. Classify drug interactions.
3. How herbal preparations can produce toxicity?
4. Write a short note on effects of herb drug interactions on body.
5. Write in brief about pharmacokinetic and pharmacodynamic considerations of herb-drug interactions.
6. How does herb-drug interaction occur?
7. Write in brief about mechanisms of herb-drug interaction.

8. Write an elaborative note on Hypercium.
9. Discuss in brief about kava-kava, its possible side effects and interactions.
10. Discuss in detail about herb-drug interaction of *Gingko biloba*.
11. Write an exhaustive note on Ginseng.
12. Write about Garlic, its possible side effects and interactions.
13. How Pepper & Ephedra does interact with other drugs?

❖❖❖

UNIT-III

Chapter...6

HERBAL COSMETICS

Objectives

- To know about definition, advantages and classification of herbal cosmetics.
- To learn about raw materials used in skin care products.
- To study about excipients used in hair care products.
- To learn about raw materials used in oral care products.

6.1 INTRODUCTION

Since ancient age human beings are using cosmetics to improve their external appearance, to improve chances of social success and to highlight their self esteem. The word cosmetic was derived from the Greek word 'kosm tikos' which means something having the power, arrange, skill in decorating. Human beings are using products derived from plants, animals, minerals and other organic products as cosmetics. **Herbal cosmetics** are the products which contain various cosmetics as a base in permissible limit and one or more herbal ingredients having defined cosmetic benefits. The demand for herbal cosmetics is increasing at faster rate as they contain nature friendly ingredients and lack side effects. Currently worldwide turnover of herbal industry is more than US$10 billion dollars and which is expanding at a rate of three to four percent annually. Herbs do not provide instant cure but they help the body to tune with the nature.

Raymond Reed, founder member of U.S Society of Cosmetics Chemist, coined the term Cosmeceuticals in 1961. This term was further tailored by Dr Albert Kligman in the year 1984, which means substances having therapeutic and cosmetic applications. Cosmeceutical is a combination of two words cosmetic and pharmaceuticals which are intended to enhance health and beauty of human body.

Definition:

As per the **consumer products (Safety) Regulations 1989;** a cosmetic product is defined as 'any substance or preparation intended for external application of the human body (epidermis, hair system, nails, lips and external genital organs), or to the teeth or buccal mucosa wholly or mainly for the purpose of cleaning, perfuming or protecting them, or keeping them in good condition or changing their appearance or combating body odour or perspiration except where such activities are for the purpose of treating or preventing disease'.

As per the **Drugs and Cosmetic Act 1940 of India** Cosmetic is defined as "Any article intended to be rubbed, poured, sprinkled or sprayed on or introduced into or applied to any part of the human body for cleansing, beautifying, promoting attractiveness or altering the appearance and includes any article intended for use as a component of cosmetic".

Herbal cosmetics are defined as, "the beauty products which contain herbal ingredients and have skin healing, smoothening, appearance enhancing and conditioning properties".

Advantages of Herbal Cosmetics over Synthetic Cosmetics:

The following are few advantages of herbal cosmetics over synthetic cosmetics:

- Herbal cosmetics are made up from natural products free from all the harmful synthetic chemicals. Herbal cosmetics utilize plant parts, plant extracts or nutrients which are easily available in nature such as aloe vera gel, neem, coconut oil, vitamin E.
- Natural cosmetics are safe to utilize as proved and tested by dermatologists. As they contain natural ingredients there are less chances of getting skin rashes, skin itchiness or allergies.
- Herbal cosmetics are compatible with all skin types as they contain natural ingredients and avoid skin degradation.
- Wide varieties of herbal cosmetics are now available.
- They are available at affordable prices.
- Herbal cosmetics are tested in laboratories using state of the art equipment and there is no need of their animal testing.
- They are mostly free from side effects.
- Herbal cosmetics have long history of use and better patient acceptance.
- Herbal ingredients are widely available at cheaper rates.

Classification of Herbal Cosmetics:

Herbal cosmetics are classified by main two ways:

1. Based on dosage form
2. Based on application on body parts.

1. Based on dosage form: The categories of cosmetics based on dosage forms are

- Emulsion: e.g. Cold cream, Vanishing cream, Liquid cream.
- Powders: e.g. Face powder, Talcum powder, Tooth powder.
- Cakes: e.g. Rouge compacts, Make-up cake.

- Oils : e.g. Hair oils.
- Paste : e.g. Tooth paste, Deodorant paste.
- Soaps : e.g. Shaving soap, Toilet soap.
- Solutions : e.g. After shave lotions, Hair set solutions.

2. **Based on application on body parts:** Different types are as follows:

- Cosmetics for skin care: e.g. Creams, Lotions, Sunscreen products, Deodorants, Bath products.
- Cosmetics for hair care: Oils, Shampoos, Dyes, Tonics, Hair removal products, Shaving products.
- Cosmetics for nail care: Nail polishes, Manicure products.
- Cosmetics for dental and oral care: Toothpastes, Dentifrices, Mouth washes.

6.2 RAW MATERIALS USED IN SKIN CARE COSMETICS

Skin is largest organ of the human body. It protects against external environment, microbes, sunlight and chemicals and regulates temperature and fluid balance. Skin consists of epidermis, dermis and subcutaneous layers. The dermis is made up of connective tissue consisting of elastin and collagen fibers, abundance of blood vessels and specialized nerve endings. Epidermis has two layers mainly the stratum germinativum and the stratum corneum, (the outermost horny layer). Herbal cosmetics are formulated with the purpose to protect the skin against endogenous and exogenous harmful agents and maintain homeostasis. Herbal cosmetics are formulated with the composition closely related to human sebum. It has high amount of phospholipids. These phospholipids maintain skin hydration; act as antioxidant, anti-inflammatory agent and have natural sun-blocking effects. They also contains polysaccharides, complex sugars and starch derivatives which acts as emollient. Various seed oils or fixed oils used in herbal cosmetics are rich in fatty acids and triglycerides. Fixed oils maintain skin hydration, has antiaging, anti-inflammatory, antimicrobial and antifungal properties. Tannins present in plant provide astringent effect and maintain skin tone.

Basic Requirements of Skin Care Products are:

- **Cleansing agent:** These agents should remove the dust, dead cells and dirt that blocks skin pores. E.g. Vegetable oils like coconut, sesame and palm oil.
- **Toners:** They help to tighten the skin and avoid the contact with toxins present in air or other environmental pollutants. E.g. hazel, geranium, sage, lemon, ivy burdock and essential oils.
- **Moisturizing agents:** Moisturizers keep the skin soft and supple, maintains healthy glow and have antiaging effects. E.g. Vegetable glycerin, sorbitol, rose water, jojoba oil, aloe vera etc.

6.2.1 Fixed Oils Used for Dry Skin Treatment

1. **Coconut oil:** It is also called as copra oil. It is edible oil obtained from fruit or seed of the coconut palm tree *Cocos nucifera*, family Arecaceae. Coconut oil is extracted by dry pressing of dried copra or by wet processing from coconut milk. It can be used in both liquid and solid forms as its melting point is 24 to 25°C. Coconut oil contains 99% of saturated fat. Coconut oil mainly consists of lauric acid (41.8%), myristic acid (16.7%), palmitic acid (8.6 %), and caprylic acid (6.8 %). It contains 6% Monounsaturated fats, 2% polyunsaturated fats and phytosterols. It is potent skin moisturizer and softener. It helps to prevent protein loss from the wet combing of hair.
2. **Sunflower Oil:** It is the fixed oil expressed from sunflower seeds of plant *Helianthus annuus*, family Asteraceae. The largest producers of sunflower oil are Ukraine and Russia as. Sunflower oil is extracted using chemical solvents like hexane, or by crushing seeds or by cold-pressing, means crushing the seeds under low-temperature conditions. It is light amber color with a mild flavour. Sunflower oil consists of Palmitic acid (5%), Stearic acid (6%), Oleic acid (30%), Linoleic acid (59%), polyunsaturated fat, monounsaturated fat, lecithin, tocopherols, carotenoids and waxes. It has soothing properties. It is widely used in face and body care products.
3. **Jojoba oil:** Jojoba oil is extracted from the seeds of shrub *Simmondsia chinenesis*, family Simmondsiaceae. The plant is native to southern Arizona, southern California, and northwestern Mexico. At room temperature unrefined jojoba oil is clear golden liquid with a slightly nutty odour while refined jojoba oil is colourless and odourless. The melting point of jojoba oil is about 10 °C. It consists of fatty acids such as stearic acid, palmitic acid, palmitoleic acid, oleic acid, linoleic acid, linolenic acid, Behenic acid, Erucic acid, Nervonic acid, Lignoceric acid, 11-Eicosenoic acid and arachidonic acid, and triglycerides. It is used in cosmetics as a moisturizer and as solvent for exotic fragrances. It functions like Human sebum. Jojoba oil acts as humecant, create a protective film over the skin, thus it protects and moisturizes the skin and hair, replenishes skin and hair loss and restores their natural pH balance. Jojoba oil is used in lotions, moisturizers, hair shampoos and conditioners. The pure oil can be directly applied on skin, hair, or cuticles. It also has analgesic, antipyretic, antiinflammatory, antioxidant, antibacterial and antiparasitic properties.
4. **Olive oil:** Olive oil is a fixed oil extracted from the fruits of *Olea europaea*, family Oleaceae. Olive plant mainly grows in Mediterranean basin. Spain, Italy and Greece are largest producers of olive oil. Olive oil contains oleic acid (up to 83%), linoleic acid (up to 21%) and palmitic acid (up to 20%). It also contains Myristic acid, heptadecanoic acid and eicosanoic acid in traces. It also consists of phyconstituents such as triolein, tripalmitin, trilinolein, tristearate, monosterate, triarachidin, squalene, β-sitosterol and tocopherol etc. It is good skin and hair conditioner and antioxidant. It is used to treat

various skin problems such as contact dermatitis, atopic dermatitis, xerosis, eczema, rosacea, seborrhoea, psoriasis, thermal and radiation burns, skin inflammation and aging etc. It is also used in treatment of UVB-induced skin tumours. Along with beeswax, it acts as cleanser, moisturizer and antibacterial agent. It is also popular for massaging infants and toddler.

5. **Castor oil:** This is obtained from the Castor seeds *Ricinus communis* of family Euphorbiaceae. Castor plant is commonly observed in southeastern Mediterranean Basin, Eastern Africa and India. Castor oil is viscous, colourless to very pale yellow liquid with a distinct taste and odour with boiling point 313 °C. The main chemical constituent is ricinoleic acid. Other constituents include oleic acid, palmitic acid, stearic acid, Linoleic acid; α-Linolenic acid, Dihydroxystearic acid. Water-soluble toxin ricin is also present in oil. The oil protects skin from against harsh climate, and has skin soothing effect. It is moisturizer and use to treat rough skin and acne. Hydrogenated castor oil or its esters, act as vehicles or carriers, emollients or solvent for toiletry, cosmetic, hair and skin care formulations. It is potent skin cleanser and conditioner.

6. **Cocoa butter:** It is also known as theobroma oil which is yellow coloured fat obtained from *Theobroma cacao* of family Sterculiceae. It is extracted from dried; fermented and roasted seeds separated from their hulls. The cocoa nibs are ground to form chocolate liquor. Then to separate the cocoa butter chocolate liquor is pressed. It melts at temperature 34–38 °C. It is rich in saturated fats and monounsaturated oleic acid (34.5%). Other constituents are Arachidic acid 1.0%, Linoleic acid 3.2%, Palmitic acid 26.0%, Palmitoleic acid 0.3%, Stearic acid 34.5%, and Other Fatty Acids 0.5%. It has soothing effect on windburn or sunburn. It acts as vehicle in suppositories and pessaries. Cocoa butter consists of oleic, stearic and palmitic acids. It is good emollient and a natural antioxidant.

7. **Mango kernels:** It is obtained from fruit stone of *Mangifera indica* of family Anacardiaceae. The plant is native to the Indian subcontinent. It is also called as mango kernel fat or, mango butter. The oil is semi-solid at room temperatures, but can melts easily on contact with warm skin. It is soft yellow colour oil with a melting point of 32–42 °C. Mango kernel oil consists of Palmitic acid (5.5 %), Stearic acid (40-45%), Oleic Acid (40-46 %), Linoleic Acid (3-4 %) and Arachidic acid (2-2.5 %). It is used in ointment base and is used in cosmetics. It is suitable ingredient for baby creams, suncare balms, hair products, and other moisturizing products. It is useful in treatment of skin eruptions, sores, boils and infections.

6.2.2 Skin Protecting Agents and Anti-Aging Treatment

Ultraviolet radiations are of 3 types UVA (320-400 nm), UVB (280-320 nm) and UVC (200-280 nm). These radiations are responsible for skin cancer, immunosupression and melanoma. Natural skin protective agents are sunscreen agents which can block UV-induced sunburns. Sunscreens protect the skin from damaging effects of sun by improving body's defense mechanism. The reactive oxygen species ROS and reactive nitrogen species (RNS) are generated when skin is exposed to UV radiation. Various naturally occurring antioxidants, flavonoids, carotenoids and phenolic acids fight against these free radicals and protect the skin from damage.

1. **Aloe:** It is obtained from leaves of *Aloe vera, Aloe barbadensis* Miller family Liliaceae. Plant is fleshy, spiny-toothed leaves with red or yellow flowers. The mucilage obtained from inner part of leaf act as potent moisturizer, skin softener, antioxidant and use to heal cuts, wounds and burns. Aloe contains various constituents such as amino acids like leucine, isoleucine, saponin 12 anthraquinone glycosides, proteins, carbohydrates, minerals, vitamins A,C,E,B, choline, B12 and folic acid which can soothe, heal, moisturize and regenerate the skin. Aloe gel consists of 99% water, glucomannans, amino acids, lipids, sterols and vitamins etc. Aloe gel is useful to treat burns, sunburn and mild abrasion, and inflammation of skin. It can act as antibacterial, antifungal, antiviral, antioxidant and antihistaminic agent. Aloe gel also act as a cleanser, anaesthetic, antiseptic, antipyretic, antipruritic, nutrient and moisturizer and promote cell proliferation. Aloe sticks the epidermal cells together and softens the skin. It stimulates collagen and elastin fibres synthesis hence exhibit antiageing properties. Aloe possesses wound healing effect by keeping the wound moist and allowing oxygen to penetrate the wound, leading to regeneration of skin. Mucopolysacharides present in aloe causes remodeling of the wound. Aloe also protects the skin against harmful effects of UV rays.

2. **Oats:** It is obtained from *Avena sativa* L of family Graminae. Main producers of oats are European union, Russia Canada, Poland, Australia and Finland. Oats are rich in protein, and other constituents include minerals, lipids, β-glucan, polysaccharide, fibers, avenanthramides, an indole alkaloid-gramine, flavonoids, flavonolignans, triterpenoid saponins, sterols and tocols etc. Oats protect and repair the skin and hair from damaging effects of UVA or UVB irradiation, pollution, smoke, bacteria, chemicals and free radicals etc. It is used in treatment of geriatric dermatosis, eczema and sunburn, irritation and inflammation of the skin. Because of its soothing, moisturizing and an anti-irritating properties it is used in preparation of facial masks, facial scrubs and soap-free skin cleansers. Hydrolysed oat protein form protective film on skin and is used in formulation of baby cleansing products. Its constituent Polysaccharide β-glucan reduces signs of aging, protect skin against UV damage, stimulate metabolic activity, collagen synthesis, and improve the tensile strength of hair. Oat protein and β-glucan moisturizes, soothe the skin and reduce redness due to abrasion.

3. **Golden Root:** It is plant *Rhodiola rosea* of family Crassulaceae. It grows in cold regions of the world. It is also called as roseroot, Aaron's rod, arctic root, king's crown etc. The roots of plant consists of phenols, rosavin, rosin, rosarin, organic acids, terpenoids,

phenolic acids and their derivatives, flavonoids, anthraquinones, alkaloids, tyrosol, and salidroside. It also contains polyphenols such as proanthocyanidins, quercetin, gallic acid, chlorogenic acid and kaempferol. It reduces fine lines and wrinkles hence acts as antiaging agent. It protects the skin from environmental stress caused by extreme changes in temperature and oxidative stress caused by sun exposure. Golden root stimulates the skin for oxygen consumption, boost vitality and respiration in the cells. It possess wide therapeutic activities such as it increase physical endurance, work productivity, longevity, resistance to high altitude sickness, and also used to treat fatigue, depression, anemia, impotence, gastrointestinal ailments, infections, and nervous system disorders etc. It acts as antioxidant and has antistress properties.

4. **Carrot:** It is obtained from the plant *Daucus carota* belonging to family Apiaceae. It is rich source of β-carotene, Vitamin A, B, C, E and K, and lesser amount of α-carotene, γ-carotene, lutein, and zeaxanthin. Polyacetylenes such as Falcarinol and falcarindiol are observed in carrot. Other constituents such as pyrrolidine, 6-hydroxymellein, 6-methoxymellein, eugenin, 2,4,5-trimethoxybenzaldehyde (gazarin) or falcarindiol 3-acetate are also present in carrot. Carrot seed oil possesses anti-aging, revitalizing, rejuvenating properties and is natural toner. Carrot keeps the skin healthy, removes scars and blemishes, prevents wrinkles, and protects the skin against sun rays. As carrot is rich in potassium, it keeps the skin hydrated. It helps to treat pimples, acne, rashes, dermatitis and other skin problem. It can be applied on wounds, cuts, and inflammation for quick healing.

5. **Ginkgo:** It is obtained from *Ginkgo biloba* belonging to family Ginkgoaceae. It consists of phenolic acids, proanthocyanidins, flavonoid glycosides, such as myricetin, kaempferol, isorhamnetin and quercetin, and the terpene trilactones, ginkgolides and bilobalides, ginkgo biflavones, alkylphenols and polypenols. It is rich in antioxidants so helps to reduce wrinkles and other signs of skin aging. It can acts as natural sunscreen. It has anti-inflammatory and skin cleansing properties. As Gingko is rich in vitamin E, it helps to combat skin problems like scars, stretch marks, acne, patchiness and pimples. It keeps the skin healthy and fresh. It is used in various ailments such as poor blood circulation, hypertension, and poor memory, and depression, male impotence. It is potent antioxidant and anti-inflammatory agent. It is also used to reduce sunburns.

6. **Turmeric:** It is obtained from the underground stems of herb *Curcuma longa* of the family Zingiberaceae. Turmeric contains curcumin, demethoxycurcumin, bisdemethoxy curcumin, zingiberene, curcumol, curcumenol, eugenol, tetrahydrocurcumin, triethylcurcumin, turmerin, turmerones and turmeronols. It is used as antiseptic, analgesic, anti-inflammatory, antioxidant, antimalarial, insect-repellant, natural colourant etc. It inhibits activity of phosphorylase kinase, hence is used for prevention, treatment or control of psoriasis, acne, wounds, burns, ulcers, eczema, sun damage to the skin and premature aging.

7. **Ginseng:** It consists of roots of various species of Ginseng such as *Panax ginseng* (Korean ginseng), *P. notoginseng* (South China ginseng) and *P. quinquefolius* (American ginseng) of family Araliaceae. Phytoconstituents present in Ginseng are saponins, ginseng oils and phytosterol, carbohydrates and sugars, organic acids, nitrogenous substances, amino acids and peptides, vitamins and minerals, and enzymes. It has 13 saponins called asginsenosides or panaxosides. Ginseng activates the skin's metabolism, reduces keratinization and wrinkles and enhances skin fairness. It moisturizes skin; enhance skin nutrition, increases blood circulation and cell proliferation. It has skin lightening and brightening property. It also possesses free radical scavenging activity, keeps the skin firm and inhibits lipoperoxidation. Hence, it acts as anti-ageing agent.

8. **Vitamin C:** Vitamin C stimulates collagen repair and stimulates collagen gene expression. Proline and lysine hydroxylases stabilizes the collagen molecule tertiary structure. Vitamin C acts as cofactor for these enzymes. Vitamin C protects the skin from environmental pollutants and ultraviolet radiations. It avoids photo-aging effects on skin. It decreases melanogenesis hence avoids conditions such as melisma or age spots. Vitamin C enhances the production of lipid barrier, formation of stratum corneum, induces differentiation of keratinocytes thereby avoids water loss. It is helpful in inflammatory skin conditions.

9. **Vitamin E:** Vitamin E is fat soluble vitamin mainly present in nuts, spinach, whole grains, olive oil and sunflower oil etc. There are eight types of vitamin E mainly α-, β-, γ- and σ-tocopherols and related corresponding tocotrienols. It scavenges lipid peroxyl radicals, arrests chain propagation and lipid peroxidation, hence protecting the cell membrane from destruction. It protects the skin from UVB radiations and also decreases melanin production.

6.2.3 Volatile Oils Used in Skin Care Products

1. **Calendula:** It is obtained from *Calendula officinalis* of family *Asteraceae*. The plant is mainly obtained from southwestern Asia, Western Europe, Macaronesia, and the Mediterranean region. The Calendula essential oil consists of constituents such as α-thujene, α-pinene, 1, 8-Cineole, dihydrotagetone and T-muurolol. It acts as antioxidant, anti- inflammatory and wound healing agent.

2. **Rose oil:** It is obtained from four species of roses mainly *Rosa damascena* Mill., R. *gallica* L., R. *moschata* Herrm. And R. *centifolia* L. belonging to family Rosaceae. It is used to treat depression, grief, nervous stress and tension. It also helps to heal wound and maintain good skin health. It contains constituents such as citronellol, geraniol, nerol, linalool, phenyl ethyl alcohol, farnesol, stearoptene, α-pinene, β-pinene, α-terpinene, limonene, p-cymene, camphene, β-caryophyllene, neral, citronellyl acetate, geranyl acetate, neryl acetate, eugenol, methyl eugenol, rose oxide, α-damascenone, β-damascenone, benzaldehyde, benzyl alcohol, rhodinyl acetate and phenyl ethyl formate etc.

3. **Eucalyptus oil:** It is obtained by steam distillation from the leaves of various *Eucalyptus* species mainly *E. cinerea F. Muell., E. baueriana F. Muell., E. smithii R. T. Baker, E. bridgesiana R. T. Baker, E. microtheca F. Muell., E. foecunda Schau., E. pulverulenta Sims, E. propinqua Deane and Maiden, E. erythrocorys F. Muell.* of family Myrtaceae. They are widely used in the preparation of liniments, inhalants, cough syrups, ointments, toothpaste and also as pharmaceutical flavours. It consists of 1,8-cineole (eucalyptol; not less than 70%), limonene (4-12%), α-pinene (2-8%), α-phellandrene (less than 1.5%), β-pinene (less than 0.5%), camphor (less than 0.1%). The essential oil has soothing, cooling properties hence useful for massage. It is anti-inflammatory and analgesic agent.

4. **Chamomile:** It is obtained from German chamomile *Matricaria recutita L.* and Roman chamomile *Anthemis nobilis* Linn belonging to family Compositae. Chamomile oil is used to treat inflammation of skin and mucous membranes, eczema and other skin disorders. It helps to reduce itching and improve damaged skin. It possesses skin repairing, regenerating, and strengthening properties. Roman chamomile oils consist of α-pinene, camphene, β-pinene, sabinene, myrcene, 1,8-cineole, γ-terpinene, caryophyllene, and propyl angelate and butyl angelate. While German chamomile oil contains chamazulene, α-bisabolol, bisabolol oxide A, bisabolol oxide B and bisabolone oxide A. α-bisabolol (levomenol) and chamazulene present in chamomile inhibit leukotriene synthesis and thus act as anti-inflammatory and analgesic agent. It is also helpful in treatment of age spots, boil, minor wound, burn, or an insect bite, dry skin, windburn, sunburn, and chronic skin conditions such as acne and psoriasis.

5. **Citrus oil:** It is essential oil extracted from rinds of *Citrus sinensis* [L.] Pers and other citrus species belonging to family Rutaceae. Citrus oil is mixture of acids, alcohol, aldehydes, esters, ketones and hydrocarbons. It is composed of limonene, sabinene, α-pinene, β-pinene, myrcene, octanal, linalool, decanal etc. It is strong antioxidant, antibacterial, immunomodulator, flavouring agent, anti-stress agent, cleanser and helps to get rid of skin problems such as warts, bunions, corns or calluses etc.

6. **Geranium oil:** It is obtained from water and steam distillation of shoots of plant *Pelargonium graveolens* (L.) L Her. ex Ait of family Geraniaceae. Oil consists of α-pinene, myrcene, limonene, menthone, linalool, geranyl acetate, citronellol, geraniol and geranyl butyrate. Geranium oil is acts as cleansing, toning and sharpening agent. It is helpful in treatment of greasy, over-oily skin, acne, congested skin and eczema. It helps in skin tightening and has antiageing effects. It helps to avoid scars and after marks of fat-cracks, surgeries, boils, acne or pox. It has wide applications in fragrance industry and in aromatherapy. It helps to balance hormones, acts as tonic antiaxiety, anti-inflammatory, antihypertensive, anthelmintic agent. It eliminates problems of menopause, improve circulation and dental health and boost kidney health etc.

7. **Lavender oil:** It is obtained from plants *Lavendula angustifolia, L. latifolia, L. stoechas* and *L. x intermedia* of family Lamiaceae. The essential oil consists of linalool, α and γ-terpeniol, borneol, perillyl alcohol, linalyl acetate, geranyl acetate, neryl aceatae, α-pinene, β-pinene, camphor, limonene, tannins, triterpenes, coumarins, β-caryophyllene and cineole. It stimulates cell growth and used widely in skin disorders like bites, stings, boils, burns, stretch marks, rashes, spots, cold sores and sunburns etc. It is antibacterial agent hence helps to avoid acne. It is used in treatment of psoriasis and eczema. It helps to avoid wrinkles and hyperpigmentation.

8. **Tea tree oil:** It is obtained from distillation of leaves of plant Melaleuca alternifolia Cheel of family Myrtaceae. The oil consists of terpinen-4-ol, γ-terpinene and α-terpinene ρ-cymene, terpinolene, α-terpineol, sabinene and α-pinene. It is ingredient of choice in various cosmetics like personal care products, hair preparations and skin creams. It has antibacterial, antifungal, antiviral properties. It is useful to treat sores, blisters, spots, rashes, psoriasis, warts, burns and acne etc.

6.2.4 Protection Agents Against Acne, Spots and Pimples

The skin condition which affects sweat glands and hair follicles, causing inflammation, black heads, white heads and pustules is termed as acne. They can leave scars and pitting.

1. **Artemisia:** It is obtained from *Artemisia vulgaris, Artemisia absinthum, A. campestris* of family Compositae. The plant is mainly found at Europe, Asia, northern Africa, Alaska and North America. The volatile oil mainly contain camphor, camphene, 5-thujone, germacrene D, 1,8-cineole, and C-caryophyllene etc. The plant decoction is used to treat skin diseases like eczema, herpes and prurulent scabies, ulcerative sores and wounds.

2. **Tulsi:** It is obtained from *Ocimum sanctum* of family Lamiaceae. Tulsi consists of oleanolic acid, ursolic acid, rosmarinic acid, eugenol, carvacrol, linalool, β-caryophyllene. Tulsi acts as anti-inflammatory agent by inhibiting both the cyclo-oxygenase and lipoxygenase pathways of arachidonate metabolism. It also has antiseptic properties. It has anti acne, skin brightening, tightening properties. It helps to remove the scars and spots from the face.

3. **Pumpkin:** It is obtained from *Cucurbita pepo* of family Cucurbitaceae. Pumpkin seed oil has linoleic, oleic, palmitic, stearic acid, vitamin A, vitamin C, β-carotene, carbohydrates, fats and proteins. It acts as anti-inflammatory agent. It is used in treatment of herpes lesions, venereal sores, acne, pimples, blackheads, chronic leg ulcers, as a poultice on sprains and pulled ligaments etc. It is suitable for all skin types. It avoids skin damage, soothes and moisturizes skin.

4. **Onion:** It is obtained from red onion, *Allium cepa* of family Liliaceae. It consists of constituents such as quercetin, quercetin-3-glucoside, isorhamnetin-4-glucoside, xylose, galactose, glucose, mannose, fructose, organosulfur compounds, allylsulfides, flavonoids,

flavenols, S-alkyl cysteine sulfoxides, cycloalliin, selenium, thiosulfinates, sulfur and seleno compounds, vitamins, minerals, proteins etc. It is used to treat acne, boils, abscesses and blackheads. It has antiageing and skin brightening properties. It helps to avoid hyperpigmentation and moles. Due to presence of flavonoids it acts as antiallergic, antifungal, antibacterial and anti-inflammatory agent.

6.2.5 Antioxidants used in Skin Care Products

Most of the plants contain polyphenolic compounds hence they have free radicals scavenging effect. Various antioxidants used in skin care products are as follows:

1. **Tea:** It is obtained from *Camellia sinensis* of family Theaceae. It has black and green variety. Black tea is prepared by fermentation process, while green tea is produced by steaming the leaves immediately after harvesting. Tea consists of tannins, flavonoids, amino acids, vitamins, caffeine and polysaccharides. It has antiinflammatory, antioxidant, antiallergic, antibacterial and antiviral effects. Green tea mainly contains Catechins, flavandiols, and flavonols to repair UV photo-damage and phototoxicity. Green tea stimulates the formation of ceramides and sphingolipids in the skin and thus stimulates the lipid barrier. Black tea also acts as antioxidant and has skin protective properties.
2. **Grape seed:** The seeds are obtained from *Vitis vinifera L.* of family Vitaceae. Procyanidins present in grape seed are potent antioxidants. They inhibit lipid peroxidation, collagen and elastin degradation, acts as tyrosinase inhibitor and enhance wound healing process. Hence, it is applied in various skin disorders.
3. **Red clover:** It is obtained from *Trifolium pretense* L. of family Fabaceae. It is rich in isoflavones. It is useful in treatment of various skin disorders such as psoriasis, eczema, acne and rash. It also acts as anti-inflammatory agent and sunburn protective agent.
4. **Fenugreek:** It consists of herb of *Trigonella foenum-graeceum* L. of family Fabaceae. Diosgenin, coumarin, hydroxy-isoluceine, luceine, tyrosine, protein, B-Complex Vitamins, vitamin C and β-carotene are the constituents of fenugreek. Its seeds have antioxidant potential and mucilage has emollient properties. Fenugreek is used to treat severe skin inflammations, chapped lips and mouth ulcers.

Tabel 6.1: Various Antioxidants as Skin Protective Agents

Sr. No.	Chemical constituent	Source	Mechanism
1.	Anthocyanins	Strawberry, banana, radish, potato	Antioxidant, neutralize enzymes that destroy connective tissue, repair protein damage

Contd....

2.	Proanthocyanidin	Grapes, oak, white chestnut, pine, apples, berries, barley, chocolate	Inhibit DNA mutation, antioxidant, inhibit elastase
3.	Resveratrol	grapes, wine, cranberries, peanuts, and peanut products, *Polygonum cuspidatum, Veratrum grandiflorum*	Antioxidant, antimutagen; anti-inflammatory effects
4.	Quercetin	Evening primrose, tea, sunflower, may apple, cranberry, neem, onion.	Anti-inflammatory, antioxidant effects, immunomodulator
5.	Apigenin	Marigold, artemisia, cumin, arnica, carrot, citrus, peppermint	Prevention of UVA/UVB-induced carcinogenesis, anti-inflammatory agent
6.	Silymarin	Milk Thistle	Reduced UV-induced sunburn cell formation and apoptosis, antitumour, prevents UVB-induced immune suppression and oxidative stress
7.	Curcumin	Turmeric	Anti-inflammatory, antitumoral, and antioxidant, prevent UV irradiation-induced apoptotic changes
8.	Carotenoids	Fruits and vegetables	Decreased UV-induced erythema, lipid peroxidation, and sunburn cell formation
9.	Polyphenolics	Fruits, vegetables, tea, grains, wine	Antioxidants, anti-inflammatory, immunomodulator
10.	Glycyrrhetinic acid	Liquorice	Antioxidant property, Sunprotection

6.2.6 Natural Colourants in Skin Care Products

1. **Annatto:** It is an orange-red coloured compound obtained from seeds of the achiote tree *Bixa orellana* of family Bixaceae. It mainly contains coloured compounds carotenoids bixin and norbixin. Bixin is lipophilic constituent while norbixin is hydrophilic, thus annatto colour has duel solubility property. Bixin gives orange shade while norbixin gives yellow colour.

2. **Avocado:** The oil is obtained from *Persea gratissima* of family Lauraceae. Plant contains constituents such as carotenoids and chlorophylls mainly lutein, α-carotene, β-carotene, neoxanthin, violaxanthin, zeaxanthin, antheraxanthin, chlorophylls a and b, and pheophytins a and b. Lutein is main colourant responsible for producing green or yellow colour and is lipophilic in nature.

3. **Beet root:** It is obtained from *Beta vulgaris* belonging to family Amaranthaceae. It contains natural colourant betanin. It is hydrophilic compound but degrades when subjected to light, heat and oxygen. It produces red or pink coloured shades.

4. **Butterfly Pea:** It is obtained from flowers of *Clitoria ternatea* of family Fabaceae. The flower shows presence of anthocyanins, p-coumaric acid and ferulic acid. Flowers are used to produce purple or blue coloured shades. It is due to presence of hydrophilic constituent Delphinidin.

5. **Calendula:** It is obtained from flowers of plant *Calendula officinalis* of family Asteraceae. Flower extract produces yellow, orange to red coloured shades because of presence of carotenoids. Flavoxanthin is the main colourant present in calendula. Flavoxanthin is water soluble colourant. It also shows presence of lycopene, lutein and about nineteen different carotenoids.

6. **Carrot:** It is obtained from roots of *Daucus carotasativa* belonging to family Apiaceae. It contains lipophilic colourant β-carotene and produces orange coloured shades. It also shows presence of α-carotene, γ-carotene, lutein and zeaxanthin.

7. **Chamomile:** It is obtained from essential oil of *Matricaria recutita*, family Asteraceae. The oil consists of Lipophilic pigment Chamazulene responsible for giving blur colour.

8. **Henna:** It is obtained from leaves of plant *Lawsonia inermis* of family Lythraceae. Leaves contain hydrophobic compound called Lawsone (2-hydroxy-1,4-naphthoquinone) or hennotannic acid. It yields red-orange coloured shades. Lawsone is also present in flower of water hyacinth *Eichhornia crassipes.*

9. **Hibiscus:** It is obtained from flowers of plant *Hibiscus rosa-sinensis* belonging to family Malvaceae. It consists of red hydrophilic pigments Cyanidin-3-sophoroside.

10. **Indigo:** It is obtained from leaves of *Indigofera tinctoria* of family Leguminosae. Indigo dye is a derivative of indican, a glucoside and this is converted to blue indigotin by an enzyme process. It produces blue to mauve coloured shades. The dye is obtained from fermented leaves of plant which is processed into cakes. Then cake is finely powdered. When powder is exposed to air, blue colour develops. The dye shows good fastness property.

11. **Iris:** It is obtained from roots of plant Iris germanica of family Iridaceae. It consists of main constituents Mangiferin, Delphinid which produces Purple or Blue or Green coloured shades.

Table 6.2: List of Plants Used as Natural Colourants

Sr. No.	Common Name	Botanical Name	Constituents and Nature	Colour
1.	Saffron	*Crocus sativus* Iridaceae	Crocin, Crocetin, Picrocrocin, Riboflavin Hydrophilic	Yellow
2.	Turmeric	*Curcuma longa* Zingiberaceae	Curcumin Hydrophobic	Yellow / Orange
3.	Madder	*Rubia tinctorum* Rubiaceae	Alizarin and Purpurin Mildly hydrophilic	Red to purple
4.	Monascus	*Monascus purpureus* Elaphomycetaceae	Rubropunctamine Hydrophilic	Red to purple
5.	Nettle	*Urtica dioica* Urticaceae	Chlorophyll Lipophilic	Green
6.	Paprika extract	*Capsicum anuum* Solanaceae	Capsanthin, Capsorubin Lipophilic	Red / Purple
7.	Pomegranate	*Punica granatum* Punicaceae	Punicalagin Hydrophilic	Red or Purple
8.	Red cabbage	*Brassica oleracea* Brassicaceae	Cyanidin-3-glucoside and Delphinidin-3-glucoside Hydrophilic	Pink or Purple
9.	Red clover	*Trifolium pretense* Fabaceae	Formononetin Hydrophilic	Golden yellow
10.	Red sandalwood	*Pterocarpus santalinum* Fabaceae	Santalin Hydrophobic	Red
11.	Rosehip fruit	*Rosa canina,* Rosaceae	Lycopene, β-carotene Lipophilic	Red
12.	Safflower	*Carthamus tinctorius* Asteraceae	Lipophilic: Carthamin Hydrophilic: Carthamidin	Yellow or Red

Contd...

13.	Sea buckthorn	*Hippophae Rhamnoides* Elaeagnaceae	β-carotene, Zeaxanthin, Lycopene Lipophilic	Orange
14.	Spinach	*Spinacia Oleracea* Amaranthaceae	Chlorophyll Lipophilic	Green / Yellow
15.	Spirulina	*Spirulina platensis* Oscillatoriaceae	Phycocyanin and Phycoerthyrin Hydrophilic	Blue or Green
16.	St. John's Wort	*Hypericum perforatum* Hypericaceae	Hypericin Lipophilic and Hydrophilic	Red
17.	Tomato	*Solanum lycopersicum* Solanaceae	Lycopene Lipophilic	Red / Orange
18.	Walnut	*Juglans nigra* Juglandaceae	Juglone, Lipophilic	Orange / Brown
19.	Woad	*Isatis tinctoria* Brassicaceae	Indigotin, Hydrophilic	Blue / Indigo
20.	Yarrow	*Achillea millefolium* Asteraceae	Chamazulene Lipophilic	Blue

Table 6.3: Different Plants Used for Skin Care

Sr. No.	Name of Plant	Chemical Constituents	Uses
1.	Mango *Mangifera indica*, Anacardiaceae	Mangiferin, isomangiferin, tannins, gallic acid protocatechic acid, catechin, mangiferin, alanine, glycine, γ-aminobutyric acid, kinic acid, shikimic acid.	anti-oxidant
2.	Akashbel , *Cuscuta reflexa*, Convolvulaceae	7'-(4'-hydroxy,3'-methoxyphenyl)-N-[(4-butylphenyl)ethyl]propenamide, 6,7-dimethoxy-2H-1-benzopyran-2-one, 3-(3,4-dihydroxyphenyl)-2-propen-1-ethanoate, 2-(3-hydroxy-4-methoxyphenyl)-3	Control dermatitis, itching and ringworm infection
3.	Amla, *Phyllanthus emblica*,	Ellagitannins, emblicanin A, emblicanin B, punigluconin, pedunculagin, punicafolin	Anti-oxidant

	Euphorbiaceae	phyllanemblinin A, phyllanemblin, ellagic acid, gallic acid	
4.	Aswagandha, *Withania somnifera*, Solanaceae	Withanolides, (-)-sominolide, withanolide-R, corydaldine, Oxyhydrastine, fumaritine, protopine, fumariline, juziphine, etrahydropalmatine, N-feruloyltyramine, (+)-bicuclline, (-)corlumine	Skin cleansing and antioxidant
5.	German chamomile *Matricaria chamomilla,* Asteraceae	Herniarin, umbelliferone, chlorogenic acid, caffeic acid, apigeni, luteolin, luteolin-7-O-glucoside, quercetin, rutin, naringenin	Leaves have anti-acne property
6.	Almond, *Prunus amygdalus* Rosaceae	3-O-methylquercetin 3-O-β-d-glucopyranoside, naringenin 7-O-β-d-glucopyranoside, catechin, protocatechuic acid, vanillic acid, p-hydroxybenzoic acid	Kernel : for fair skin and beautification , sunscreen
7.	Chameli, *Jasminum grandiflorum*, Oleaceae	Secoiridoid glucosides, 2''-epifraxamoside, demethyl-2''-epifraxamoside, secoiridoid, jasminanhydride	Essential oil : skin diseases, protection from sunburn
8.	Sandal *Santalum album*, Santalaceae	α- and β-santalol, cedrol, esters, aldehydes, phytosterols, squalene	Essential oil: Skin soothing, cooling, antioxidant, perfume
9.	Cucumber, *Cucumis sativus* Cucurbitaceae	vitamins, minerals, amino acids, phytosterols, phenolic acids, fatty acids, and cucurbitacins, pectins, starch, sugars, vitamin C, and curcurbitacin	skin cooling, toning and skin tightening properties
10.	Palas, *Butea frondosa* Fabaceae	6, 8 di-C-rhamnosyl apigenin, luteolin, Chrysoeriol 7-O-β-D-4C1-glucuronic acid.	Leaves : for pimples Seed : anti fungal infection and bruises.

Contd...

11.	Gophaa, *Leucas aspera*, Lamiaceae	Triterpenoids, oleanolic acid, ursolic acid, β-sitosterol, nicotine, sterols, glucoside, diterpenes	Leaves : for scabies, skin psoriasis, chronic skin eruption and eczema
12.	Maca *Lepidium meyenii* Brassicaceae	Vitamins (B_1, B_2, C, E), minerals and trace elements	Radiant complexion, healthy, firm, smooth skin, antiaging
13.	Lemon, *Citrus limon* Rutaceae	Limonene, β-myrcene and decanal	Source of vitamin C : to treat skin itching and skin nourishment, health skin.
14.	Takla, *Cassia tora*, Caesalpiniaceae	Anthraquinone, naphthopyrone glucoside cinnamaldehyde, gum, tannins, mannitol, coumarins and essential oils	Leaves and seed : skin infection, ringworm, skin eruption
15.	Papaya, *Carica papaya* Caricaceae	Papain, chymopapain, carpain, carpasemine, benzyl isothiocyanate	Milky juice : soft and healthy skin; remove blemishes
16.	Haraddodi, *Plukenetia volubilis*, Euphorbiaceae	Omega 3 fatty acids, Omega 6 fatty acids and Vitamin A	Protect the skin balances skin's oiliness and moisturizer. For soft and younger skin
17.	Sea buckthrons, *Genus Hippophae*, Elaeagnaceae	Vitamins, pro-vitamins, antioxidants,	Skin emollient, nourishment, Main ingredient in many hair and skin care products.
18.	Sunflower, *Genus Helianthus*, Asteraceae	Vitamin E, K and polyphenols	Healthy skin and hairs
19.	Water lettuce, *Pistia stratiotes*, Araceae	Palmitic acids, anthocyanin-cynidin-3-glucoside, luteolin-7-glycosid, vitexin, orientin	Leaves: treat chronic skin disorders
20.	Vasaka, *Adhatoda vasica*, Acanthaceae	Vasicine, vasicine acetate, 2-acetyl benzyl amine, vasicinone, quinazoline	Treat skin infections

6.3 RAW MATERIALS USED IN HAIR CARE PRODUCTS

6.3.1 Medicinal Plants Used as Hair Tonic in Hair Care Products

- **Amla:** It consists of fresh or dried fruits of *Emblica officinalis* of family Euphorbiaceae. It is commonly observed in India and cultivated at commercial level in Uttar Pradesh, Gujarat, Rajasthan and Maharashtra. Active principle of amla is 6% of tannins such as gallic acid, ellagic acid, phyllembelin, vitamin C, and minerals such as phosphorus, iron and calcium. It is commonly used as oil or aqueous extract in the hair care formulations like hair oil or shampoo. It acts as hair tonic, stimulates hair growth and prevents premature graying of hairs.
- **Brahmi:** It consists of herb of *Centella asiatica* belonging to family Umbelliferae. It grows well in wet damp and marshy places of north India. Brahmi shows presence of essential oils, sterols, flavonol, glycoside, triterpenoid, saponins etc. Brahmi is used as oil and extract in hair care formulations. It is rasayana drug hence maintain proper body health. It avoids premature graying of hairs and helps to relieve mental fatigue and stress.
- **Bhringraj:** It is obtained from plant *Eclipta alba* Linn of Family Asteraceae. It is an annual or perennial plant grows in moist places throughout India. Plant shows presence of coumestans like wedelolactone and dimethyl wedelolactone; ecliptine alkaloid; β-amyrin glycosides, triterpenic acid and ecalbasaponins steroids etc. Brahmi oil is very good hair tonic and used for getting healthy, black and long hairs.
- **Henna:** It is natural colourant obtained from leaves of *Lawsonia inermis* of Family Lythraceae. Henna leaves are used as natural colour dye in hair formulations. It contains lawsone which give dark intense orange color at basic pH.
- **Neem:** It consists of dried or fresh leaves of plant *Azadirachta indica* belonging to family Melliaceae. The plant is indigenous to all plains in Indian subcontinent. Neem leaves shows constituents such as flavonoids, steroids, terpenoids, sterols and nimbolide. Neem seed and seed oil consists of nimbin, nimbibin, salanin etc. It is used in treatment of ticks, fleas and lice. Neem oil is used in herbal hair oils, hair tonics, shampoos and conditioners.
- **Hibiscus:** It consists of flowers of *Hibiscus rosa sinensis* of family Malvaceae. Hibiscus has constituents such as taraxeryl acetate, β-sitosterol, campesterol, stigmasterol, cholesterol, erogosterol, flavonoids and flavonoid, glycosides, lipids, citric and oxalic acids. It acts as hair tonic, stimulates hair growth and prevents premature graying, hair loss and scalp disorders. It is used as hair conditioner and in hair washes.
- **Jatamansi:** It consists of rhizomes of plant *Nardostachys jatamansi* belonging to family Valerianaceae. It is found in north India to east India. It shows presence of 1 to 2 % of pale yellow volatile oil, jatamansic acid, jatamansone, nardostachone, resin, sugar oil Jatamansi oil is hair tonic, promote hair growth and used as hair dye.

- **Fenugreek:** It consists of herb of *Trigonella foenum graecum* of family Leguminoseae. In India it is cultivated in Rajasthan, Gujarat, Uttar Pradesh, Maharashtra and Tamilnadu. Seeds are used in hair care formulations. Fenugreek seed contain alkaloids like Neurin, Trigonelline, Choline, Gentianine; amino acids like Isoleucine, 4-Hydroxyisoleucine, Histidine, Leucine, Lysine; Saponins like Graecunins, fenugrin B, fenugreekine, trigofoenosides A-G, lipids, vitamins and fibers. Fresh fenugreek leaves are hair growth promoter, preserves natural color, keeps hair silky and used in dandruff treatment.
- **Shikakai:** It consists of pods of plant *Acacia concinna* of family Mimosacea. It is observed in plains of central and south India. Shikekai consists of lupeol, spinasterol, acacic acid, lactone, natural sugars, hexacosanol, spinasterone, oxalic acid, tartaric acid, citric acid, succinic acid, ascorbic acid, alkaloids calyctomine and nicotine. Shikakai acts as natural hair cleanser, astringent and detangle hairs. It is used to make hair formulations like soaps and shampoos for hair wash. It promotes hair growth; strengthen hairs and acts as antidandruff agent.
- **Ginko:** It consists of dried leaves of plant *Ginko biloba* belonging to family Ginkgoaceae. It is mainly found in North India. It consists of terpenes, ginkolides, flavanol glycosides and kaemferol. Leaf extract is used in formulations like shampoos and hair lotions.
- **Arnica:** It is obtained from dried roots and flowers of *Arnica Montana* belonging to family Apiaceae. It consists of phytoconstituents such as arnicin, volatile oil, tannin and phulin. Arnica is hair tonic and anti-dandruff agent.
- **Senna:** It consists of dried leaves of *Cassia angustifolia* or *Cassia acutifolia* of *family* Leguminoceae. It grows well in south India and some part of north part of India. It shows presence of sennosides, rhein, chrysophanol, emodin, aloe emodin, mono and diglucosides, kaemferol, palmidin, myricyl alcohol and mucilage. It acts as black hair dye.

6.3.2 Volatile Oil and Fixed Oils Used in Hair Care Products

- **Coconut oil:** It consists of fixed oil obtained from kernels of plant *Cocos nucifera Linn*, of family Palmae. Phytoconstituents of coconut oil are lauric, caproic, caprylic, capric, myristic, palmitic, and stearic acid. It has good saponification value hence it is used in shampoos and hair oil.
- **Eucalyptus oil:** It consists of volatile oil obtained from leaves of *Eucalyptus globules* of family Myrtaceae. The volatile oil is composed of cineole, aldehyde, terpenes, alcohol and phenol. It is colourless or pale yellow liquid with characteristic aromatic odour and a pungent, spicy and cooling taste. It acts as anti-dandruff agent.
- **Rose oil:** It is volatile oil obtained from petals of *Rosa damascena* and *Rosa centifolia* of family Rosaceae. The steam-distilled product is called as rose otto while the solvent extracted product is rose absolute. β-damascenone, β-damascone, β-ionone and oxide are main constituents of Rose oil. It is used as perfume.

- **Basil Oil (Tulsi oil):** It is essential oil obtained by steam distillation of leaves and flowering tops of *Ocimum Sanctum* belonging to family Labiatae. The basil oil consists of 1, 8 cineol, linalool, citral, methyl chavicol (estragole), eugenol and methyl cinnamate etc. It is good hair growth promoter.
- **Lemon oil:** It is essential oil obtained from cold expression of peels (fruit) of *Citrus limonum* belonging to family Rutaceae. It is cultivated in north-west region of India. The constituents of lemon oil are α-pinene, camphene, β-pinene, sabinene, myrcene, α-terpinene, linalool, β-bisabolene, limonene, trans-α-bergamotene, nerol and neral. It is potent hair cleaning agent.
- **Rosemary oil:** It is obtained from plant *Rosmarinus officinale* Linn of family Labiatae. It consists of volatile oil, resin, ursolic acid, α-pinene, borneol, β-pinene, camphor, bornyl acetate, camphene, 1,8-cineole and limonene etc. It is good hair growth promoter and used in hair lotions and gels.
- **Cedar wood oil:** It is essential oil extracted from the wood of *Juniperus virginiana* of family Pinaceae. The oil contains α-cedrene, β-cedrene, cedrol, widdrol, thujopsene etc. It helps to treat dry hairs, hair loss and dandruff.
- **Sandal wood oil:** It is essential oil obtained from steam distillation of heartwood of *Santalum album*, of family Santalaceae. It grows well in South India, western ghat. The the main constituents of sandalwood oil are 90-97% of sesquiterpenes alcohol (Santalol), hydrocarbons, acids, aldehydes and ketones. It is used as perfume in hair care products.
- **Sage oil:** It is essential oil obtained by steam distillation of dried leaves of *Salvia officinalis Linn* of family Labiatae. The sage oil is composed of α-pinene, cineole, linalyl acetate, thujone, borneol, bornyl acetate, farnesol, and camphor. It is potent anti-dandruff agent.
- **Jojoba oil:** It is fixed oil obtained from cold expression of seeds of *Simmondsia chinensis* of family Simmondiaceae. In India it is cultivated in Rajasthan, Gujarat, Maharashtra, and Tamilnadu. It consists of eicosenoic acid, docosenoic acid and oleic acid. It is potent hair revitalizing agent.
- **Almond oil:** It is fixed oil obtained from cold expression of ripe seeds of plant *Prunus dulcis* of family Rosaceae. It has nourishing, softening, cleansing and hair strengthening property. It contains 40-55% fixed oil, 20% proteins, mucilage etc. The fixed oil composed of oleic acid, linoleic acid, and palmitic acid. It is used in formulations like hair lotion and hair tonic.
- **Arachis Oil:** It is fixed oil obtained from the seeds of the *Arachis hypogea* belonging to the family Leguminoseae. Arachis oil is pale yellow with a faint nutty odour. It is cultivated at Brazil, Southern United States, China, Africa and India. Arachis oil consists of oleic acid, linoleic acid, palmitic acid, stearic acid, arachidic acid, behenic acid, lignoceric acid and other fatty acids. It is used in hair oils.

- **Sesame oil:** It is fixed oil expressed from ripe seeds of *Sesamum indicum* of family Pedaliaceae. It is cultivated in Gujarat, West Bengal, Rajasthan, Tamilnadu, Orissa, Madhya Pradesh, Andhra Pradesh, Maharashtra, Uttar Pradesh, Punjab and Karnataka. Sesame oil contains palmitic acid, oleic acid, linoleic acid, linolenic acid, stearic acid, arachidic acid, behenic acid and gandoleic acid as major phytoconstituents. It is potent hair tonic and avoids premature graying of hairs.
- **Olive oil:** It is a fixed oil extracted from the fruits of *olea europaea* belonging to family Oleaceae. It is mainly produced at Spain, Italy and Greece. Olive oil contains phytoconstituents like triolein, tripalmitin, trilinolein, tristearate, monosterate, triarachidin, squalene, β-sitosterol and tocopherol. It is skin and hair conditioner and fatty acid penetration enhancer.
- **Neem oil:** It is fixed oil expressed from seeds, kernels or leaves of *Azadirachta indica* belonging to family Meliaceae. It is native of India. Neem oil contains linoleic acid, palmitic acid, stearic acid and oleic acid. It acts as hair tonic and anti-dandruff agent.
- **Castor oil:** It is obtained from seeds of *Ricinus communis* belonging to the family Euphorbiaceae. It consists of ricinoleic acid, stearic acid, oleic acid, palmitic acid, linoleic acid and α-Linolenic acid. It acts as emollient. It is used in formulation of lipstick, hair oils, creams and lotions.

6.3.3 Natural Colourants Used in Hair Care Products

- **Henna:** Henna leaves consist of active principle lawsone which is responsible for red–orange colour. It is used as non-oxidizing hair dye. Tannins and flavonoids present in henna acts as mordant. Carbohydrates present in Henna helps to bind it on hairs. It also balances pH of hairs hence avoids graying of hairs and avoid hair fall.
- **Madder:** It consists of roots of Rubia tinctorum belonging to family Rubiaceae. It is red coloured dye. The colouring property is due to presence of anthraquinones such as alizarin and purpurin. Madder has anticancer, antimicrobial, antifungal, hypotensive, analgesic, antiseptic, blood purifier and antirheumatic properties.
- **Chamomile:** These are obtained from leaves and flowers of *Matricaria recutita* (German chamomile) and *Chamaemelum nobile* (Roman chamomile) of family Asteraceae. It is responsible for producing yellow coloured shades. Chamomile flower contains active principle apigenin (1,3,4- trihydroxyflavone). The plant is used as softening agent, moisturizing agent and has skin soothing properties. It is also used for indigestion, diarrhea, sleeplessness and sciatica etc.
- **Walnut:** It is obtained from fruits of *Juglans regia* of family Juglandaceae. Leaves and hull of walnut fruits is used for hair dyeing and responsible for producing brown coloured shades. The active principle of walnut is Juglone, and other constituents are oleic acid, macadamia, linoleic acid, linolenic acid, methionine, cysteine, tryptophan,

threonine. Walnut is used in semipermanent hair formulations. It is used to treat eczema, loss of hair, scalp itching, peeling, dandruff and sun burns etc.

- **Onion skin:** It is responsible for producing yellow colour. The main constituents in onion skin are quercetin aglycone and quercetin-4'-glucoside.
- **Bringraj:** It consists of herb of *Eclipta Alba* of family Asteraceae. It can acts as hair dye because of presence of various constituents like alkaloids, flavonoids, polyacetylenes, triterpenes and their glycosides. It contains flavonesapigenin, luteolin, wedelolactone and demethylwedelo lactone etc. It is hair growth promoter and has anti-graying activity.

6.3.4 Fats and Waxes Used in Hair Care Products

- **Light and heavy liquid paraffin:** It is colourless or odourless oily liquid consisting of a mixture of hydrocarbons. Due to good spreadibility it is used to formulate bath oils, hair oils, lotions and creams etc.
- **Waxes:** They are the esters formed from condensation of high molecular straight chain fatty acids and high molecular straight chain monohydric alcohol. Waxes forms base of cosmetics. The different waxes used in cosmetics are:
  1. **Beeswax:** It is most commonly used purified wax obtained from the honeycomb of bees, *Apis mellifera* of family Apidae. Beeswax contains 70% ester myricyl palmitate. It is solid in nature, yellowish brown in colour, sweet in taste and has characteristic odour. Its melting point is 60 to 65°C.
  2. **Carnauba wax:** It is obtained from leaves of plant *Copernica cerifera* belonging to family Palmae. It is light brown to pale yellow in colour, occurs as coarse powder or flakes with characteristic odour and taste. Its melting range is 81-86°C.
  3. **Paraffin wax:** It is distillation product of petroleum. It mainly consists of paraffins and their isomers. It is white, transluscent wax, colourless, odourless and greasy to touch. Its melting range is 50 to 57°C.
  4. **Spermaceti:** It is wax obtained from *Physester colodon* belonging to family Physeteridae. Spermaceti contains cetyl palmitate and cetyl myristate. It is transluscent, crystalline, pearly white with characteristic odour and taste.

Table 6.4: Different Plants Used for Hair Care Products

Sr. No.	Name of Plant	Chemical Constituents	Uses
1.	Walnut, *Juglans regia*, Juglandaceae	Oleic acid, macadamia, linoleic acid, linolenic acid, methionine, cysteine, tryptophan, threonine	Leaves and hull: hair dyeing

Contd...

2.	Arnica, *Arnica Montana,* Asteraceae	Helenalin, 11α, 13-dihydrohelenalin	Flowers: Hair tonic , stimulates the hair follicles
3.	Bringraj, *Eclipta alba* Asteraceae	Alkaloid ecliptine, wedelolactone, wedelic acid, apigenin, luteolin, Beta -amyrin	Hair growth promoter
4.	Umber, *Ficus racemosa* Moraceae	Beta-sitosterol, p-amyrinj, lupiol acetate	Aerial root : Hair fall resistant
5.	Behera, *Terminalia bellirica,* Combretaceae	Tryptophan, threonine, phenylalanine, tyrosine, termilignan, thannilignan, flavan, anolignan B	Fruit and oil: Hair dye
6.	Birch, *Betula pendula* Betulaceae	Carotenoid, rubisco, uronic acids, lignin	Leaves: Antidandruff
7.	Kushtha, *Saussurea lappa* C.B. Asteraceae	P-hydroxybenzaldehyde, ethyl 2-pyrrolidinone-5(s)-carboxylate, 5- hydroxymethyl-furaldehyde, palmitic acid, succinic acid, glucose, daucosterol, β-sitosterol	Hair dye
8.	Lavender, *Lavandula augustifolia,* Lamiaceae	α-pinene, limonene, 1,8-cineol, linalool, perillyl alcohol, linalyl acetate, camphor, limonene, tannins, triterpenes, coumarins, cineole, and flavonoids	Improves blood circulation, tonic, controls oil production from scalp
9.	Ritha, *Sapindus mukorossi,* Sapindaceae	Saponins, sugars and mucilages	Hair cleanser
10.	Safflower, *Carthamus tinctorius,* Asteracea	Benzyl-O-β-D-glucopyranoside, syringarenol, lirioresinol-A, β-sitosterol, stigmasterol	Hair tonic

6.4 RAW MATERIALS USED IN ORAL HYGIENE PRODUCTS

Oral hygiene is important part of human health but it is neglected. Oral health problems like dental carries and periodontal diseases are increasing day by day. Dental treatments are usually expensive and utilize mainly analgesics and antimicrobial agents. These agents have several side effects such as alteration in oral microflora, diarrhoea, vomiting, burning sensation and tooth staining etc. It is well documented that many of the phytochemicals have anti-microbial activity and are safe, effective and economic option to treat oral diseases. Herbs used for oral hygiene are classified as:

- **Antimicrobial agents:** e.g. Aloe, black pepper, eucalyptus, garlic, turmeric etc.
- **Antioxidant agents:** e.g. Spinach, pepper, black tea, broccoli, green tea, carrot, potato tomato, blackberry, grape etc.
- **Analgesic agents:** e.g. Capsicum, clove, ginger, peppermint etc.
- **Anti-inflammatory agents:** e.g. Aloe, garlic, ginger, onions, neem, periwinkle, turmeric etc.

6.4.1 Herbs Used in Oral Hygiene Products

- **Aloe:** It is obtained from mucilage of *Aloe vera* or *Aloe barbadensis Miller* of family Liliaceae. Aloe vera consists of Anthraquinones aloin, barbaloin and emodin, mono and poly saccharides, Prostaglandins, amino acids, vitamins, Cholesterol, triglycerides, steroids, uric acid, lignins, β-sitosterol, gibberellin, salicylic acid. It contains enzymes such as acid phosphates, alkaline phosphatase, amylase, lactic dehydrogenase and lipase. Vitamins like B_1, B_2, B_6, C, niacin amide and choline are also present. It consists of minerals such as barium, aluminium, calcium, iron, boron, magnesium, phosphorous, silicon etc.

  It acts as moisturizing, analgesic, antibacterial, antiviral, antifungal, antioxidant, immune modulatory, anti-inflammatory agent, wound healing. It is used to treat burns, skin irritation, psoriasis etc.

  Aloe can be widely used to treat various oral problems. Aloe can be directly applied in periodontal surgery. It can be applied on traumatized or injured gum tissues. Chronic dental problems such as gum problems associated with tongue, and burning mouth syndrome can be improved. Aloe vera gel is useful for sore gums and teeth with denture maladaption. It is used to treat inflammation around dental implants. Aloe vera is used to treat chemical burns, aphthous ulcers, gum abscesses, dry socket, lichen planus, benign pemphigus and gingival problems associated with AIDS, leukemia, migratory glossitis etc. It can be utilized in disorders such as candidiasis, desquamative gingivitis, vesiculobullous diseases, acute monocytic leukemia, xerostomia etc.

- **Turmeric:** It consists of rhizomes of *Curcuma longa Linn.* of family Zingiberaceae. It possesses wide range of therapeutic activities such as analgesic, antibacterial, anti-inflammatory, anti-tumor, anti-allergic, antioxidant, antiseptic, antispasmodic, appetizer, astringent, cardiovascular, carminative, cholagogue, digestive and diuretic etc.

  Turmeric consists of 6% volatile oil composed of a number of monoterpenes and sesquiterpenes, including zingiberene, curcumin, α- and β-turmerone etc. The main colouring principles are curcuminoids, 50-60% containing main constituents such as curcumin, mono des methoxy curcumin and bis des methoxy curcumin.

  It is used in dental caries, oral lichen planus and halitosis. It also acts as colorant in pit, fissure sealant and used in dental-plaque detection system. Turmeric can be utilized in the treatment of premalignant lesions in oral cavity. Roasted, turmeric may eliminate pain and swelling of teeth. Turmeric water boiled with clove and guava leaves gives instant relief from dental problems. Burnt turmeric powder along with bishops seed powder not only cleanses teeth but also make them strong.

- **Neem:** It consists of leaflets of *Azadirachta indica* of family Meliaceae. Neem contains chemical constituents such as genin, sodium nimbinate, salannin, nimbin, azadirachtin, nimbidiol, quercetin, nimbidin, fiber, carbohydrates, amino acid, proteins, calcium, carotenoids etc.

  It acts as antiviral, antifungal, antimicrobial, antibacterial, antipyretic, anti-inflammatory, antitumor, analgesic, antihelminthic, anticariogenic, antioxidant agent. Neem is used in dental problems such as dental caries, gingivitis and periodontitis. It has anti-plaque activity by removing bacteria from teeth surface, inhibiting bacterial growth, adhesing to hydroxyapatite on tooth surfaces, and producing insoluble glucan. It avoids sore and bleeding gums. Neem oil is used to treat mouth ulcers.

- **Miswak:** It is dried stem bark of *Salvadora persica* of family Salvadoraceae. It contains salvadorin, trimethylamine, tannins, flavonoids, saponins, silica, chloride, and high amount of fluoride, sulphur, vitamin C. Miswak keeps the gum healthy and prevents inflammation. Calcium salts and fluorides prevent dental decay. Trimethylamine decreases plaque formation. Tannins and sulphated compound, benzylisothiocyanate has antimicrobial effect.

- **Kantkari:** It is obtained from seeds of *Solanum xanthocarpum* of family Solanaceae. It consists of chemical constituents such as solanocarpine, carpesterol, solanocarpidine, potassium nitrate, fatty acid, diosgenin, sitosterol, isochlorogenic acid, neochronogenic acid, chronogenic acid, caffeic acid, solasodine, solasonine, solamargine, quercetin, apigenin, histamine, acetylcholine etc. It acts as anti-caries agent.

- **Tulsi:** It consists of herb of *Ocimum sanctum* of family Lamiaceae. It contains 0.7% volatile oil containing about 71% eugenol and 20% methyl eugenol. It acts as expectorant, analgesic, anticancer, antiasthmatic, antiemetic, diaphoretic, anti-diabetic, antifertility, hepatoprotective, hypotensive, hypolipidimic, antipyretic, antimicrobial, immunomodulator and antistress agents. Tulsi is effective against oral infections. It is used to treat gingivitis and periodontitis.

- **Pomegranate:** It consists of fruits of *Punica granatum* of family Punicaceae. Pomegranate consists of constituents such as ellagic acid, ellagitannins, punicalagins, punicic acid, flavonoids, anthocyanidins, anthocyanins, flavonols and flavones etc. It is used in treatment of diabetes, cardiovascular diseases, cancer, stress, throat infections, coughs and fever etc. It reduces oxidative stress in the oral cavity, acts as antioxidant, anti-inflammatory, antibacterial agent, removes plaque, hence used to treat gingivitis. Pomegranates also act by lowering saliva activities of α-glucosidase enzyme and increasing activities of an antioxidant enzyme ceruloplasmin.

6.4.2 Volatile Oils Used in Oral Care Products

Volatile oils are antibacterial, antifungal and antioxidant in nature. In dentistry, volatile oils has following applications:

- Volatile oils inhibit plaque hence acts as oral hygiene adjunct.
- They reduce anxiety in dental patients and reduce needle insertion pain.
- They possesses wound healing activity after dental procedures
- Volatile oils have antibiofilm activity hence used in dental implant.
- They also act as preservatives.

1. **Clove oil:** It is volatile oil obtained from *Syzygium aromaticum* of family Myrtaceae. Clove oil contains eugenol, eugenol acetate and β-caryophyllene. It has analgesic, antibacterial, antiviral, anti-inflammatory, antioxidant property. It acts as mild anesthetic and an anti-bacterial agent. Clove oil is used in root canal therapy, in temporary fillings, and to relieve dental and gum pain.
2. **Eucalyptus oil:** It is volatile oil obtained from leaves of *Eucalyptus globules* of family Myrtaceae. The eucalyptus oil mainly consists of 1,8-cineole, cryptone, α-pinene, p-cymene, α-terpineol, trans-pinocarveol, phellandral, cuminal, globulol, limonene, aromadendrene, spathulenol and terpinene-4-ol. It exhibits antimicrobial property against gram-positive and gram-negative bacteria. Eucalyptus oil significantly affects plague accumulation, gingival index, bleeding on probing, periodontal depth probing. It reduces gingivitis and gingival bleeding.
3. **Lavender oil:** It is volatile oil obtained by steam distillation from the flowers of *Lavandula angustifolia* of family Lamiaceae. The main chemical constituents in Lavender oil are linalyl acetate, linalool, lavandulol, 1,8-cineole, lavandulyl acetate, and camphor etc. The oil has good antimicrobial activities against most of the bacteria, fungi, and yeast. It helps to reduce stress, anxiety and improve mood of patients.

4. **Tea Tree oil:** It is volatile oil obtained from distillation of leaves of plant *Melaleuca alternifolia* Cheel of family Myrtaceae. It is antiseptic, immunomodulator, an antifungal agent, non-irritant and a mild solvent. The major constituent is terpinen-4-ol (30%–40%). When used orally, it may cause serious side effects such as confusion, loss of muscle control or coma. In dentistry, tea tree oil is used as antimicrobial agent in the mouth before dental surgery, it removes smear layer when used in root canal and to alleviate mouth soreness.

5. **Rosemary:** It consists of volatile oil obtained from *Rosmarinus officinalis* of family Lamiaceae. Rosemary consists of volatile oil, carnosol, ursolic, linalyl acetate (25-46%), linalool (20-45%), lavendulyl acetate (>1.0%), 1,8-cineole, eucalyptol (<2.5%), 3-octanone (<2.5%), camphor (<1.2%), limonene (<1.0%), and α-terpineol (<2.0%) etc. It is used as antibacterial, antifungal, antioxidant, anti-inflammatory property. It helps to relieve toothache and disinfects GP cones.

6. **Sage:** It is obtained from volatile oil of *Salvia officinalis* belonging to family Lamiaceae. The main constituents of volatile oil are α- and β-thujone, camphor, cineole, rosmarinic acid, tannins and flavonoids etc. Because of its antibacterial, antifungal, and antiviral activity, it is used in treatment of sore throat, mouth inflammations and gingivitis. It should not be used in pregnant women, children. It may cause adverse effects such as increased heart rate, mental confusion and convulsions in high dose.

7. **Thyme:** It consists of volatile oil obtained from plant *Thymus vulgaris* belonging to family Lamiaceae. It mainly contains phenols, thymol and carvacrol. Thyme is used to treat chronic candidiasis and halitosis. It can cause side effects such as dizziness, vomiting, and difficulty in breathing.

8. **Propolis:** It is complex mixture of plant-derived and bee released compounds. Propolis is composed of 50% resins, 30% waxes, 10% essential oils, 5% pollen and 5% of various organic compounds. It shows presence of constituents such as caffeic acid phenanthryl ester, polyisoprenylated benzophenone, galangal, pino banksin and pino cembrin, amino acids, phenolic acids, phenolic acid esters, flavonoids, cinnamic acid, terpenes etc. It is used as anesthetic, antibacterial, antifungal, antiviral, antioxidant, anticarcinogenic, antithrombotic agent and immunomodulatory agent.

   It is used to prevent dental caries, gingivitis, stomatitis, halitosis, lichen planus, candidal infections, angular cheilitis, xerostomia, traumatic ulcers and periodontal pocket/abscess. It is used as storage medium, intracanal medicament, relieve denture ulceration. It avoids dentinal hypersensitivity. Propolis acts as mouth freshener, pulp capping, used for temporary restorations and dressings, covering tooth preparations etc.

- **Gum Acacia:** It is dried gummy exudations obtained from *Acacia catechu Wild* of family Fabaceae. Acacia consists of phytoconstituents such as catechin, catechutannic acid, epicatechin, catechin tetramer, dicatechin, gallocatechin, kaempferol, taxifolin, isorhamnetin, afzelechinn, L-arabinose, D-galactose, D-rhamnose and aldobiuronic acid. Acacia acts as antipyretic, antiinflammatory, anti-diarrhoeal, hypoglycaemic, hepatoprotective, antioxidant and antimicrobial agent. It can be used to treat bleeding, piles, uterine haemorrhages, leucorrhoea, tonic, dyspepsia, chronic bronchitis, cough and cold etc. It is effective remedy for gingivitis, stomatitis and other oral problems. It removes tarter, plaque, stain and helps in cleansing and polishing tooth surface.

- **Gum Myrrh:** It is gummy exudation obtained from plant Commiphara molmol of family Burseraceae. It contains volatile oil (2–8%), resin (23–40%), gum (40–60%) and bitter principles (10–25%). Myrrh has antiseptic properties and used to treat stomach and lung disorders. It helps to cure pyorrhoea and gum diseases. It also acts as cytotoxic, analgesic, anti-inflammatory, anticancer, antiparasitic and hypolipidemic agent.

Table 6.5: Different Plants Used in Oral Hygiene Products

Sr. No.	Name of Plant	Chemical Constituents	Use
1.	Cayenne pepper *Capsium annum. l.* Solanaceae	Pungent principle, capsaicinoids including capsaicin, 6,7-dihydrocapsaicin, nordihydrocapsaicin, homodihydrocapsaicin, and homocapsaicin; capsanthin, capsorubin, α- and β-carotene, steroid glycosides, capsicosides, vitamins A and C; trace of volatile oil	Antiseptic and tooth ache.
2.	Chickweed (*Stellaria sps*) Caryophyllaceae	Borneol, menthol, linalool, 1,8-cineole, ascorbic-acid, β-carotene, Calcium, Coumarins, Genistein, γ-linolenic-acid, flavonoids, minerals.	Oral cancer and mouth sores.
3.	Comfrey *Symphsytum asperum* Boraginaceae	Allantoin abundant mucilage; rosmarinic acid, chlorogenic acid, caffeic acid (0.004%) and α-hydroxy caffeic acid phosphorus, potassium, starch, tannins, and vitamins A, C and E.	Treat pain of jaw and tooth fractures or adjustments to braces.

Contd...

4.	Dandelion *Taraxacum officinale*, Asteraceae	Biotin, calcium, choline, fats, iron, magnesium, niacin, PABA, phosphorus, proteins, sulfur, zinc, and a variety of vitamins.	Abscesses in oral cavity and blood purifier.
5.	Ginseng *Panax Ginseng*, Araliaceae	Ginsenosides, calcium, camphor, iron, starch, and vitamins A, B_{12}, and E.	Improves blood circulation and treat gum disorders.
6.	Kelp *Macrocystis pyrifera* Laminariaceae	Biotin, bromine, calcium, choline, copper, iodine, PABA, potassium, a variety of B vitamins, vitamins C and E.	Healthy gums and bones.
7.	Licorice root *Glycyrrhiza glabra* Fabaceae	Triterpenoid saponins glycyrrhizin and glycyrrhetinic acid, liquiritin, chalcones and isoflavones.	Inhibits plaque growth, antiulcer, flavouring agent.
8.	Green Tea *Camellia sinensis* Theaceae	Catechin (C), epicatechin (EC), gallocatechin (GC), epigallocatechin (EGC) epicatechingallate (ECG), and epigallocatechingallate	Anti-inflammatory, antibacterial, antiviral, To treat periodontal disease.
9.	Marigold , *Calenelula officinalis*, Asteraceae	Cadinol, carotenoids, isorhamnetin, saponins, triterpenes, sesquiterpenoids, scopoletin, flavonoids, quercetin, kaempferol.	Treat ulcers, wounds, or inflamed areas. Relieve tension in the jaw joint and pressure from braces.
10.	Red clover, *Trifolium pratense* Fabaceae	Daidzein, Genestein, Biochannin-A, Formonentin, apigenin, luteolin, phenolic acids, minerals, and saponins.	Antiseptic, treat abscessed gums or inflamed gums from root canal therapy.
11.	Grape seed extract *Vitis vinifera*, *Vitaceae*	Proanthocyanidins	For non-invasive root caries therapy.

Contd...

12.	Chamomile *Matricaria recutita* Asteraceae	1-2% volatile oils, chamazulene (1-15%)., α-bisabolol, flavonoids apigenin, luteolin, and quercetin	Gingivitis, periodontal disease and mouth ulcers.
13.	Bloodroot *Sanguinaria canadensis,* Papaveraceae	Sanguinarine	Gingivitis, periodontal disease, remineralization of enamel lesions and acute sore throat.
14.	Cranberry *Vaccinium macrocarpon* Ericaceae	Coumaroyl iridoid glycosides, flavonoids substituted cinnamic acids, stilbenes, triterpenoids alpha-linolenic acid, omega 3 and 6 fatty acids.	Dental caries, periodontal disease, oral squamous cell carcinoma.
15.	Garlic, *Allium sativum* Amaryllidaceae	Alliin, ajoene, diallyl sulfide, dithiin, S-acetylcysteine, and enzymes, B vitamins, proteins, minerals.	Dental caries and periodontitis.

QUESTIONS

1. What are herbal cosmetics? Give their advantages and classification.
2. Write an elaborative note on raw material used for skin care cosmetics.
3. Write a note on antioxidants used in skin care products.
4. Explain in brief about herbal protective agents used in skin care products.
5. Discuss about various volatile oils and fixed oils used as raw material in skin care products.
6. Explain in detail about natural colourants used in cosmetics.
7. Explain various volatile oils and fixed oils used in hair care products.
8. Write an elaborative note on medicinal plants used as hair tonic.
9. Describe various raw materials used in oral hygiene products
10. Discuss in detail about various volatile oils used as raw material in oral care products.

❖❖❖

Chapter...7

HERBAL EXCIPIENTS

Objectives

- To understand the concept of natural excipients. Their functions, classification, advantages and disadvantages.
- To know about significance of natural colourants, sweeteners, flavours and perfumes.
- To understand the concept, natural products used as binders, diluents, viscosity builders and disintegrants.

7.1 INTRODUCTION

Drugs are formulated in suitable dosage forms with the help of excipients. The word 'excipient' is derived from Latin word. It means to receive, to gather and to take out. Excipients may acts as binding, lubricating, gelling, coating, stabilizing suspending, flavouring, sweetening, surfactant, preservative and bulking agents. Excipients play important role to determine performance, safety, efficacy and stability of active pharmaceutical ingredients. Now-a-day's herbal excipients are in great demand as they are economic, easily available and less toxic.

Definition:

According to the International Pharmaceutical Excipients Council, The excipients are defined as, "substance, other than the active drug substances of finished dosage form, which have been appropriately evaluated for safety and are included in a drug delivery system to either aid the processing of the drug delivery system during its manufacture; protect, support or enhance stability, bioavailability, or patient acceptability; assist in product identification; or enhance any other attributes of the overall safety and effectiveness of the drug delivery system during storage or use.

According to WHO excipient is defined as, "the substance other than active ingredients which have been appropriately evaluated for safety and or included in a drug delivery system to

- Aid in processing of drug delivery system during its manufacture.
- Protect, support and enhance stability, bioavailability or patient acceptability.
- Assist in product identification.
- Enhance any other attribute of the overall safety and effectiveness of the drug during storage or use.

In simple words, Pharmaceutical excipients may be defined as in-active substance added to medicinally active compounds to formulate dosage forms.

Natural excipients used to make formulations that are obtained from various natural sources like Plants, Animals, Minerals, Microbes.

Functions of Excipients:

- Add bulk to the formulation.
- During manufacturing it helps to handle API.
- Assist in drug administration.
- Enhance patient compliance.
- Enhance drug solubility and bioavailability of APIs.
- Avoid drug degradation.
- Give robust and reproducible result of formulation.
- Modify the pH and osmolarity of the liquid dosage forms.
- Prevents drug aggregation and helps in drug particles dispersion.
- Helps to mask unpleasant taste, colour and odour.
- Helps to maintain stability.

Advantages of Herbal Excipients

- Natural excipients are natural gums and mucilage which are:
- Biocompatible,
- Economic,
- Easily available,
- Less toxic,
- Have soothing action and have non-irritant action.
- Safe and biodegradable
- Can be chemically modified

Disadvantages of Herbal Excipients:

- Natural excipients are mainly carbohydrates and during manufacturing they come in contact with external environment and hence are prone to microbial contamination.
- Natural excipients are obtained from natural resources which are varying in environmental conditions, regions and climates. Hence, yield and chemical composition of natural excipients vary in different conditions.
- The process of manufacturing the natural excipients depends on various cultivation, collection, processing and storage factors.
- There are possibilities of heavy metal contamination.

Ideal Properties of Excipients:

- They can be used practically.
- They should be non-toxic and non-irritant in nature.
- They should be non-volatile in nature.
- They should not be affected by temperature, light and hydrolysis.
- They should be easily available and cheap.
- They should not have specific colour, odour and taste.
- They should possess good water and lipid solubility.
- They should be compatible with the active ingredient in the preparation and should not affect its function.
- They should be pharmacologically inert.

7.2 CLASSIFICATION OF EXCIPIENTS

The excipients are classified based on various parameters as follows:

1. **Based on regulatory aspects there are three main categories:**
   - **Approved excipients:** This category includes excipients from food industry or pharmaceutical industry. They are safe and are in use for very long time.
   - **Intermediate category Essentially new excipients:** This category includes structurally modification compounds which are in use as excipients.
   - **New compounds:** These are are not used in the pharmaceutical industry and are new compounds
2. **Classification based on sources of excipients:**
   - Products from animal source: e.g. Beeswax, Cochineal, Gelatine, Honey, Spermaceti, Lanolin etc.
   - Products from vegetable source: e.g. Kokum butter, Pectin, Starch, Peppermint oil, Cardamon, Vanilla etc.
   - Products from mineral source: e.g. Bentonite, Kieselghur, Kaolin, Paraffins, Talc, Fuller's earth etc.
   - Products from marine source: e.g. Agar, chitin, chitosans, Carrageenans, Alginates.
   - Synthetic products: PEGs, Polysorbates, Povidone.
3. **Classification based on chemical nature:**

Table 7.1: Classification based on Chemical Nature

Sr. No.	Chemical nature	Role	Examples
1.	Alcohols	For patient compliance.	Volatile oils, lanolin, polyphenolic compounds.

Contd...

2.	Esters, Ethers, Aldehydes Carboxylic acids	For dose precision and accuracy.	Fixed oil, citric acid, vanillin.
3.	Glycerides and waxes	To enhance stability.	Bees wax, lanolin.
4.	Carbohydrates (mono-, di- and polysaccharides)	Assist in manufacturing process.	Gums and mucilages.
5.	Hydrocarbons and halogen derivatives	Drug tolerance.	Paraffins, polyphenolic compounds.
6.	Polymers (natural and synthetic)	To avoid drug disaggregation.	Cellulose, pectin.
7.	Minerals	Help in drug dDissolution	Bentonite, talc, calamine.
8.	Protein	To prepare controlled release formulations.	Gelatin, soyabean.
9.	Preservatives, dyes, sweeteners, surfactants	To enhance absorption, to preserve, to make bitter taste and colour.	Stevia, Honey, Henna, Cochineal, Antioxidants, Polysorbates, Emulsifying waxes.

4. Classification according to application of excipients:

Table 7.2: Classification of Excipients According to their Application

Sr. No.	Category	Examples
1.	Fillers	Plant cellulose, Gelatin, Lactose, Sucrose, Glucose.
2.	Binders	Acacia, Alginic acid, Corn starch.
3.	Disintegrating agents	Silicone, Guar gum, Agar.
4.	Coating agents	Gelatin, Shellac, Natural polymers.
5.	Lubricants	Castor oil, Mineral oil, Paraffin oil.
6.	Antioxidants	Ascorbic acid, Potassium metabisulphite, Sodium metabisulphite, Gallic acid.
7.	Colouring agents	Annatto, Carotene, Chlorophyll, Cochineal, Curcumin.
8.	Flavouring agents	Strawberry, Raspberry, Lemon, Orange, Peppermint.
9.	Solvent	Purified water, Oils.
10.	Chelating agents	Onions, Garlic, Chlorella, Brazil nuts.
11.	Buffering agents	Lemon
12.	Surface active agents	Waxes, Saponins.
13.	Viscosity builder or emulsifiers	Gelatin, mucilage of Aloe, Gums.

7.3 DIFFERENT TYPES OF NATURAL EXCIPIENTS

7.3.1 Natural Colourants

Natural colourants are highly coloured compound capable to impart colour to fabric, paper, leather, drugs, cosmetics and plastic. Dye is compound which gets absorbed by the material and gives permanent colour. While pigment is coloured compound only applied to the surface. Natural colourants should have intense colour, should be highly water soluble. It should possess reactivity and substantivity. The colourant should have fastness property. The colourant have chromophore and auxochrome properties. Chromophore imparts colour to compound while auxochrome makes the dye water soluble and helps to bind it to substrate. The main function of colouring agent is to impart attractive colours to dosage forms, with patient compliance and for easy identification of dosage forms.

Advantages/Significance of Natural Colourants:

- Natural colourants are soft, lustrous and soothing.
- Wide ranges of colours are available.
- Natural dyes are usually renewable so no disposal problem.
- Ecofriendly and stable.
- Non-hazardous to human health.
- Show some medicinal properties.

Disadvantages of Synthetic Colourants:

- Can produce allergies.
- May be carcinogenic in nature.
- Can produce toxic effects and teratogenic effects.
- As per WHO report, synthetic colourants can cause problem like immune system problems, ADHD, low temperature to frustration, impulsivity etc.

Some of the natural colourants are discussed below:

1. HENNA:

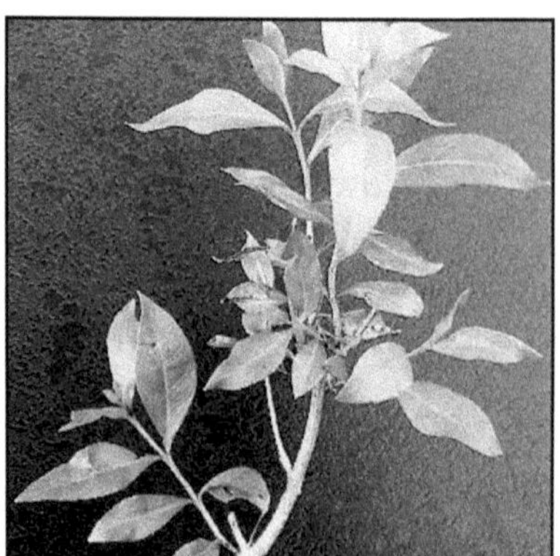

Fig. 7.1: Plant of *Lawsonia inermis* herb

Synonyms: Egyptian private, Mignonnette, Mehendi.

Biological Source: It consists of dried leaves of *Lawsonia inermis (L. alba)* belonging to Family Lythraceae.

Geographical Source: North Africa, India, Srilanka.

Constituents: It contains colouring principle Lawsone (2,5-dihydroxy-1,4-naphthoquinone). Other constituents are phenolic glycosides, coumarins, xanthene, flavonoids, fats, resin and tannin etc.

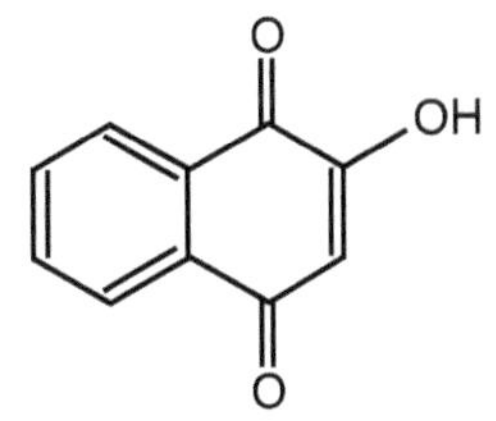

Lawsone

Colourant can be extracted from the leaves by sodium bicarbonate. It imparts yellow to orange coloured shades. Its colour vanishes at acidic pH.

Chemical Tests: On addition of acid in decoction of henna, the orange red colour vanishes. On addition of alkali, colour darkens.

Applications: It is used as hair dye. It is used as colourant in hair care products and other cosmetics.

2. TURMERIC:

Synonyms: Haldi, Indian saffron.

Biological Source: It consists of dried, as well as fresh rhizomes of the plant *Curcuma longa Linn* belonging to family Zingiberaceae.

Geographical Source: It mainly grows in India and also in China, Malaysia, Italy and Australia.

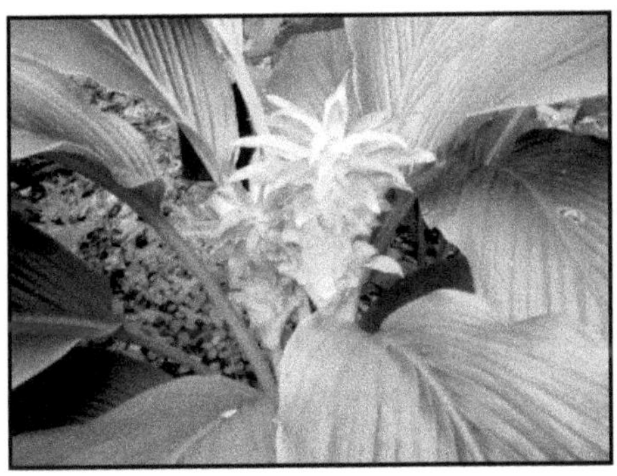
Fig. 7.2: Turmeric plant, flowering

Description: It occurs as yellow coloured powder with aromatic odour and warm and slight bitter taste. It is insoluble in ether, water and soluble in alcohol.

Constituents: It contains 5% of volatile oil, resin and diaryl heptanoid yellow colouring substances known as curcuminoids. Curcumin is the main component of curcuminoids. It is responsible for producing yellow coloured shades. Other phytoconstituents are atlantone, bisdemethoxycurcumin, demethoxycurcumin, diaryl heptanoids, tumerone, sugars, resins, proteins, vitamins and minerals etc.

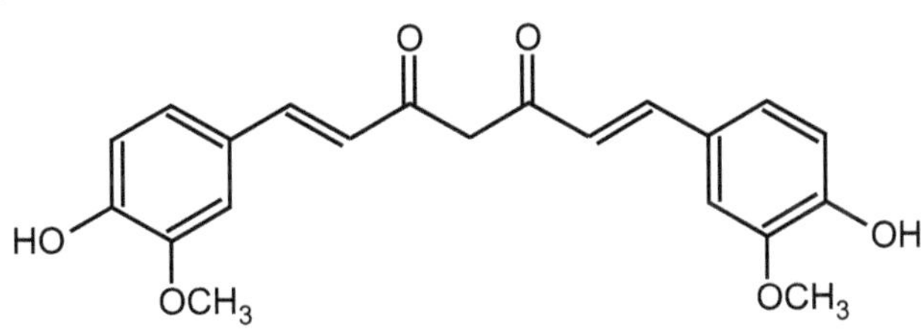

Curcumin

Chemical tests: Curcumin gives crismson red colour with sulphuric acid.

On addition of boric acid to turmeric extract, reddish brown colour develops which on alkali treatment changes to greenish blue.

Incompatibilities: With alkali and with direct sunlight colour of turmeric fades away.

Applications: It is used as colourants in various pharmaceutical dosage forms, cosmetics and food products.

3. ANNATTO:

Synonyms: Chiote tree; Lipstick tree; Annotta.

Biological Source: It consists of dried seeds of *Bixa orellana* belonging to family Bixaceae.

Geographical Source: It is indigenous to central and South America and grown in India also.

Description: Bixin occurs as orange yellow crystals or Dark red-brown to red-purple powder. It produces yellow coloured shades. It is stable at neutral and alkaline pH but forms precipitate at acidic pH. It is soluble in alcohol, ether and oils but insoluble in water. Bixin occur in the cis-form, but converted to trans-bixin, during extraction process. Dye is stable at pH 8 and stability decreases between pH 4 to 8.

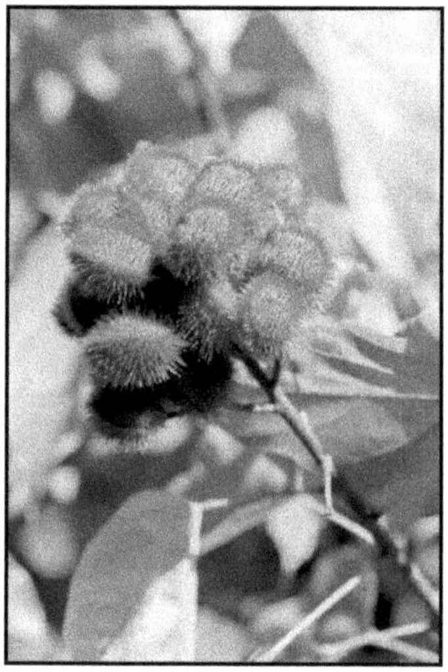

Fig. 7.3: Annatto herb

Constituents: It consists of major colourant bixin. It consists of minor constituents like trans-bixin and cis-norbixin. The seeds contain 4.5-5.5% pigment, which consists of 70-80% bixin.

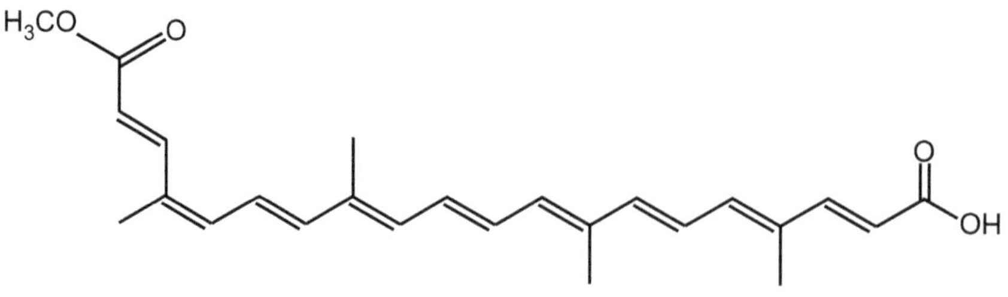

Bixin

Identification: The annatto dissolved in acetone shows absorbance maxima at about 425, 457 and 487 nm.

Uses: It acts as colouring and coating agent for solid and liquid pharmaceutical dosage forms. It is used as colouring agent in food and dairy products. It is also used in the manufacture of wood stains and varnishes and for silk dyeing.

4. INDIGO:

Synonyms: Neel, Indigo.

Biological Source: It is obtained from *Indigo tinctoria, Indigo suffruticosa,* belonging to family Leguminosae.

Geographical Source: India, America, Europe, Africa

Description: Indigo dye is obtained from leaves. Leaves are soaked in water and fermented. It converts the glycoside indican present in the plant to the blue dye indigotin.

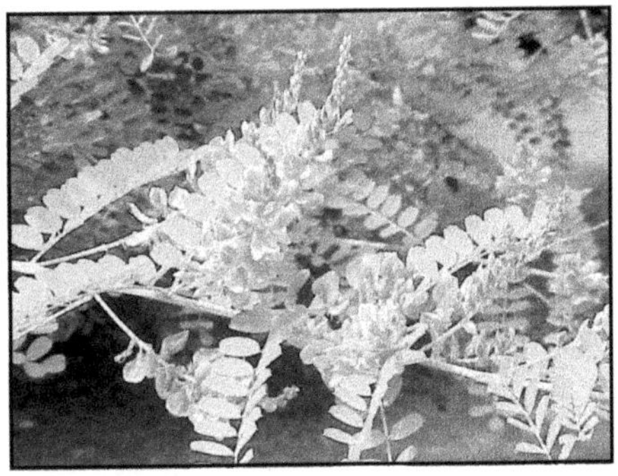

Fig. 7.4: Plant of *Indigo tinctoria*

Indigo dye occurs as dark blue crystalline powder. It get sublimes at 390–392 °C. Indigo dye is insoluble in water, alcohol, or ether, but soluble in DMSO, chloroform, nitrobenzene, and concentrated sulfuric acid. Its λ_{max} is 613 nm.

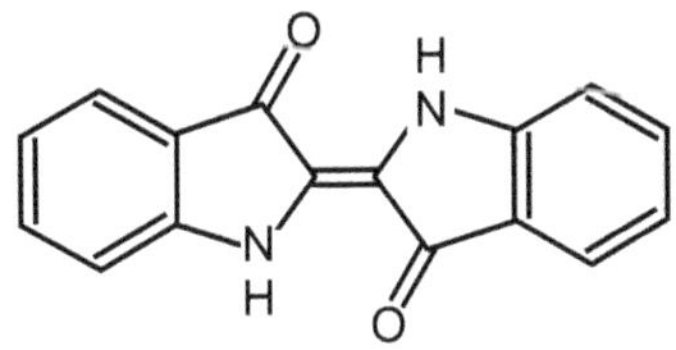

Indigo

Chemical Constituents: The plant contains main constituent glycoside indican which produces colour dye. Other constituents are rotenoids deguelin, dehydrodeguelin, rotenol, rotenone, tephrosin and sumatrol etc.

Applications: It is used as colourant in pharmaceutical and food industry. It is used in dyeing of jeans. It is a textile dye.

7.3.2 Natural Sweeteners

Sweetening agents are the substances which are added to drug formulation to mask its bitter taste and can be used by diabetic patients also. These are of two types nutritive and non-nutritive sweetners. Nutritive sweeteners are mainly sugar or sugar alcohols which contain calories. E.g. sorbitol, mannitol, xylitol, lactitol. Non-nutritive sweeteners are artificial sweeteners without any calories or carbohydrates. E.g. Aspartame, Saccharin, Cyclamate, Acesulfane-k etc. Natural sweetners are saccharide and non-saccharide type. Non-saccharide sweeteners are of various types such as terpenoids, dihydrochalcones, dihydrocoumarins, sweet proteins and steroidal saponins.

Advantages/Significance of Natural Sweeteners:

- They are non-calorific in nature.
- Have less possible side-effects.
- The Quality and quantity can be improved by modern technologies.
- Economic.
- No rise in blood sugar level.
- Avoid decay of teeth.

Some of the Natural Sweeteners are discussed below:

1. STEVIA:

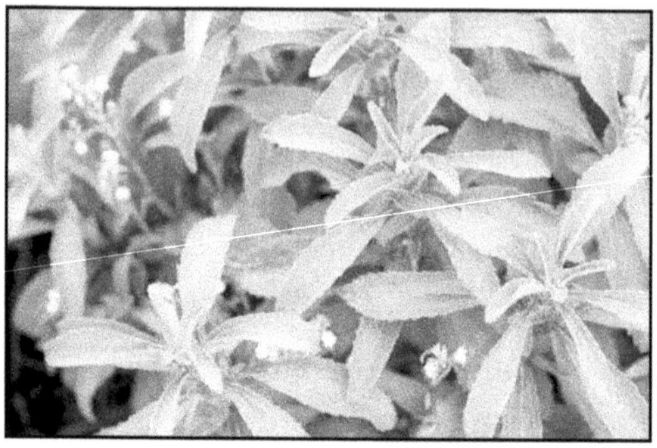

Fig. 7.5: *Stevia rebaudiana herb*

Synonyms: Honey leaf, Sugar leaf.

Biological Source: It is natural sweetener extracted from plant *Stevia rebaudiana* belonging to family Compositae.

Geographical Source: Paraguay, South Brazil and cultivated in Japan, Southeast Asia, USA etc.

Description: Stevioside is 200-250 times sweeter than sucrose but it has bitter and undesirable after taste. Rebaudioside is 200-300 times sweeter than sucrose. It is sweeter than Stevioside and has no significant undesirable taste characteristics. But it is unstable and gets easily decomposed due to light. Stevioside is poorly water soluble but highly soluble in alcohol. Its stability is not affected by pH and at high temperature. Stevioside occurs as white powder or light yellow crystalline powder.

Constituents: Stevioside is diterpene glycoside and is the major component with sweet tasting compound present in leaf. Other principles having sweet taste are steviosides A and B, Steviobioside, Rebaudioside A, B, C, D, E and Dulcoside A etc. To isolate stevioside, leaves of the plant are treated with water or water-ethyl alcohol mixture and purified by treatment with calcium or magnesium hydroxide or magnesium carbonate.

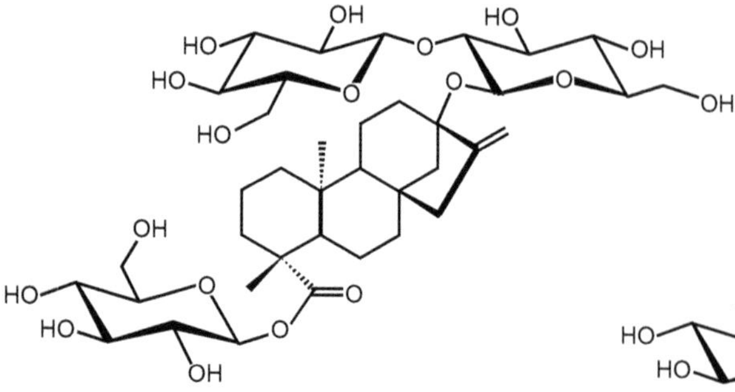

Stevioside

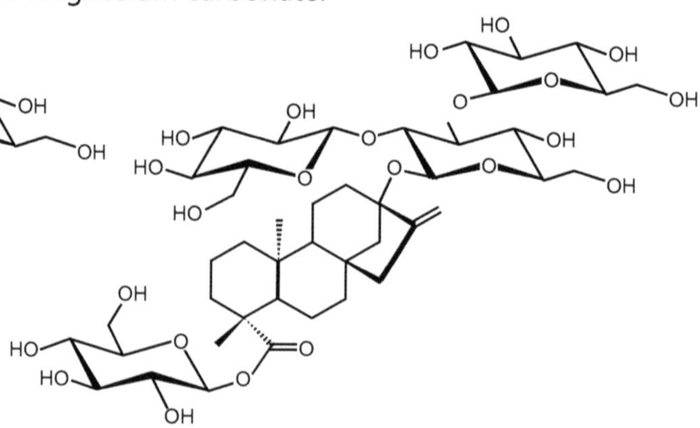

Rebaudioside A

Uses: Stevia is used as natural calorie free sweetener in liquid or solid foods, beverages as a substitute for conventional sugars. Sweetening agent of choice for diabetic patients.

2. LIQUORICE:

Synonyms: Yashtimadhu, Mulethi, Liquorice root.

Biological Source: These are dried peeled, unpeeled roots and stolons of plant *Glycyrrhiza glabra* of family Leguminosae.

Geographical Source: The plant is native of Mediterranean region and China. It is in cultivated France, Italy, Spain, USA, England, Asia and also in India.

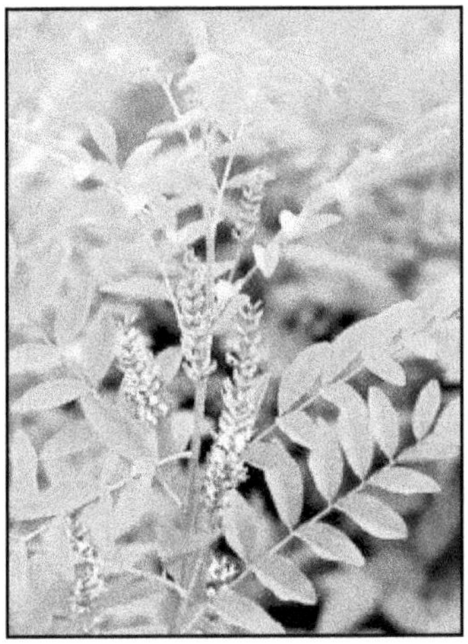

Fig. 7.6: *Glycyrrhiza glabra* plant

Constituents: Glycyrrhizin is a pentacyclic triterpenoid saponins glycoside found in the form of potassium and calcium salt of glycyrrhizic acid. Because of its sweet taste it is used as natural sweetener and flavouring agent in pharmaceutical industry. It is 100 times sweeter than sucrose. Plant consists of constituents such as Glucose (up to 4%), Sucrose (2.5 to 6.5%), Glycyramarin resins-(Bitter principle), Aspargin (2 to 4%), Fat and Flavonoids like Liquiritin and Isoliquiritin.

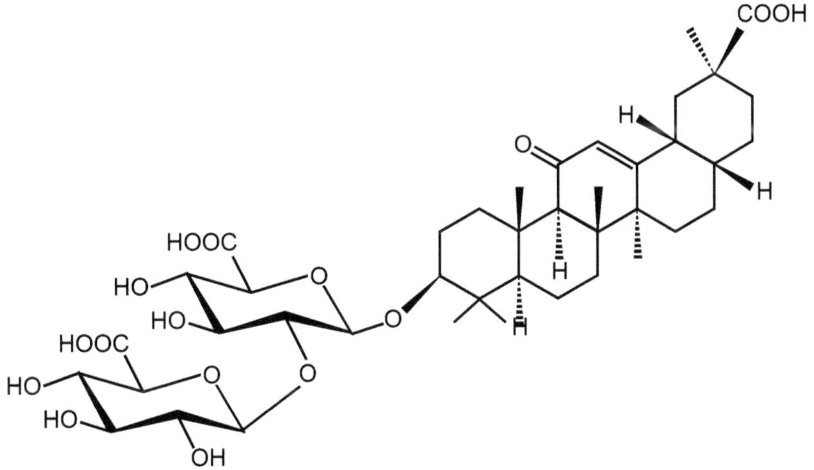

Glycyrrhizin

Description: Glycyrrhizin is freely soluble in hot water, alcohol and practically insoluble in ether.

Chemical test: With 80 % of sulphuric acid, it shows deep yellow colour.

Applications: It is used as sweetener, flavouring agent and foam stabilizer in various pharmaceutical dosage forms.

3. SERENDIPITY BERRY:

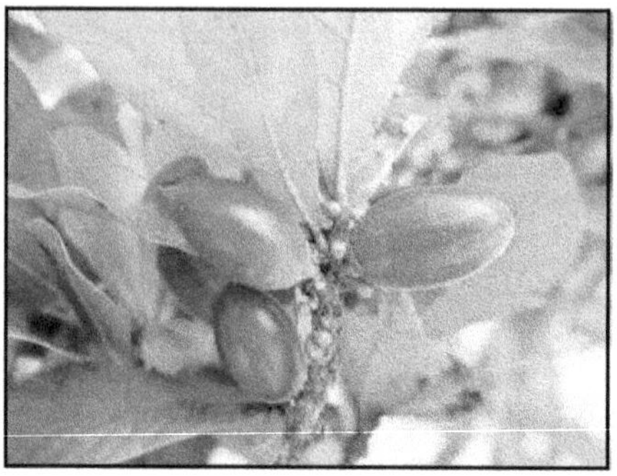

Fig. 7.7: *Dioscoreophyllum volkensii* plant

Synonym: Monellins

Biological Source: It is obtained from *Dioscoreophyllum volkensii* belonging to family Menispermaceae.

Geographical Source: Plant is native of tropical Africa.

Description: It is readily water soluble but denatures at higher temperature. Monellins is sweet taesting protein which is 1500-2000 times sweeter than 7% sucrose solution. One drawback of Monellin is it has a slow onset of sweetness and lingering aftertaste. Its sweetness is also pH dependant. It is tasteless below pH 2 and above pH 9. It is unstable at high temperature, making it unsuitable for processed food. It is readily water soluble.

Constituents: The fruit of the plant contains intensely sweet protein. Monellin is 3000 times sweeter than sucrose. It consists of two polypeptides containing 45 and 50 amino acid residues.

Uses: It is used as table top sweetener.

4. THAUMATIN:

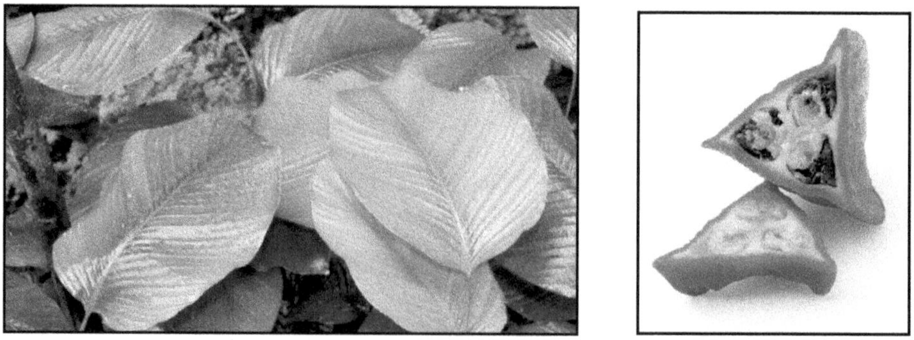

Fig. 7.8: *Thaumatococcus danielli* plant and fruit

Synonyms: Talin, Katemfe fruit.

Biological Source: It is obtained from the arils of fruits of the tropical plant *Thaumatococcus danielli* of family Marantaceae.

Geographical Source: It mainly grows in West Africa.

Constituents: Thaumatin protein occurs in two forms Thaumatin I and II which are intensely sweet. They contain 207 amino acids and two forms differ by 5 amino acids.

Description: Thaumatin is 2000 to 10000 times sweeter than sucrose. It is water and dilute alcohol soluble. Thaumatin is thermoresistent under acidic conditions. It has delayed onset of action and possesses liquorice like aftertaste.

Applications: It is acts as low calorie sweetener and flavouring agent. Thaumatin is used to mask bitter astringent taste and off flavours.

Table 7.3: List of Some Natural Sweeteners:

Sr. No.	Name of Plant	Constituents	Sweetness potency
1.	*Abrus precatoris, Leguminosae*	Abrusosides & glycyrrhizin	30-100
2.	*Cinnamomum seqlawcum, Lauraceae*	trans-Cinnamaldehyde	50
3.	*Citrus aurantium, Rutaceae*	Neo-hesperidin dihydrochalcone	1000
4.	*Cyclocarya paluirus, Juglandaceae*	Cyclocaryoside	250
5.	*Eremophila glutinosa, (Scrophulariaceae)*	Dihydroflavonols	400
6.	*Perilla frutescens, Labiatae*	Perillartine	400-2000
7.	*Periandra dulcis, Leguminosae*	Periandrin V	100-200
8.	*Symplococos paniculata, Symplocaceae*	Trilobatin	400-1000
9.	*Lippia dulcis, Verbenaceae*	Hernandulcin	1000-1500
10.	*Smilax glycyphylla, Liliaceae*	Glycyphyllin	100-200

7.3.3 Natural Binders

Binders are the excipient which binds all ingredients used in formulation to form suitable dosage form. They give plasticity and increase the interparticulate bonding strength of particles particularly in case of tablets. These are important for imparting physical strength and desired quantity to formulation. Binders are used in solid or semi-solid dosage forms. They are used in various formulations such as Tablets, Pills, Pallets, Granules, Pastes etc. Binders can be used in wet or dry form.

There are two types of binders:

(i) Solution binders: These are used in solution form after dissolving it in suitable solvent e.g. Gelatin, Cellulose.

(ii) Dry binders: Dry binders are directly added as the powder. They are used after a wet granulation step, or as part of a direct powder compression formula. E.g. Methyl cellulose, Polyethylene glycol.

Advantages of Natural Binders:

- Less toxic.
- Can be degraded naturally.
- Available easily and abundantly.
- Economic.
- Enhance stability and texture to dosage forms.

Disadvantages of Synthetic Binders:

- Synthetic binders may cause rapid overgranulation.
- Increases hardness of formulation and reduces dissolution properties.
- They need strong disintegrants to be added in formulation which increase cost of formulation.
- Sometimes synthetic polymers adversely affect formulation stability.
- Sometimes film coating appearance is observed.

1. ACACIA:

Synonyms: Indian Gum, Babul.

Biological Source: It is dried gummy exudation from the stems and branches of *Acacia arabica, Acacia senegal* belonging to family Leguminosae.

Description: It occurs as white or yellowish-white thin flakes, spherical spheres, powder, granules, or spray-dried powder. It is odourless and bland taste. Acacia is soluble in 1 in 20 of Glycerin, 1 in 20 of PEG, 1 in 2.7 of water and practically insoluble in alcohol. The bark of the Acacia gum is obtained by making incisions on tree and the exudates is allowed to dry. The dried exudates are then collected, processed and graded. The spray dried powder is also available.

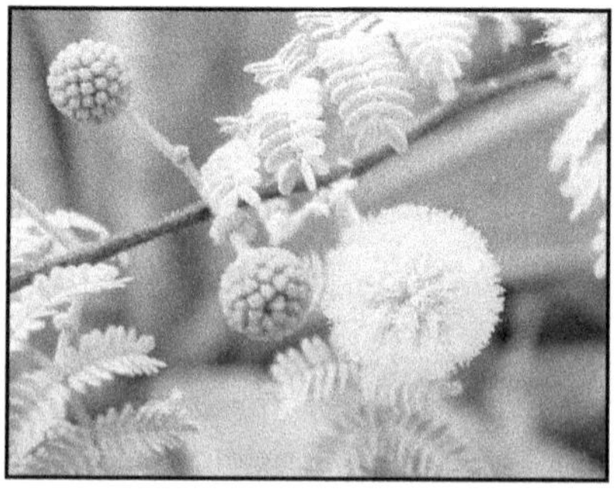

Fig. 7.9: Branch of *Acacia arabica* plant

Chemical Constituents: It mainly consists of arabinose, galactose, rhamnose and glycuronic acid.

Chemical Tests:

- When acacia powder is treated with lead sub acetate, it gelatinizes the aqueous solution.
- With ruthenium, red acacia does not yield pink colour.
- Aqueous solution of acacia powder when treated with hydrogen peroxide and benzidine in alcohol shows blue colour due to presence of oxidase enzyme.

Incompatibilities: Incompatibility is observed with ferric salts amidopyline, apomorphine, borax, basic lead acetate, aluminium chloride, cresol, ethanol, morphine, phenol, tannin, thymol, gelatine and vanillin etc.

Uses: Acacia is used as natural binder for tablets, suspending agent, emulsifying agent, thickener, as base in pastilles and lozenges. It has wide applications in cosmetics, confectionery, food industry and spray-dried flavours.

Storage: Air-tight container in a cool, dry place.

2. TRAGACANTH:

Synonyms: Gum tragacanth; Persian tragacanth.

Biological Source: It consists of dried gum obtained from plant *Astragalus gummifer* of family Fabaceae.

Geographical Source: It is found in Iraq, Iran, Syria, Turkey, Afghanistan, Pakistan, and Russia.

Description: Tragacanth has flat, lamellated, frequently curved fragments, or straight or spirally twisted linear pieces. It is white to yellowish in colour, transluscent odourless with mucilaginous taste. Tragacanth is practically insoluble in water but swells rapidly in water, also insoluble in ethanol (95%), and other organic solvents. Tragacanth gum is obtained by making incisions on stem and branches of tree. The exudates is allowed to drain and then dried. The dried exudate is then collected, processed and graded.

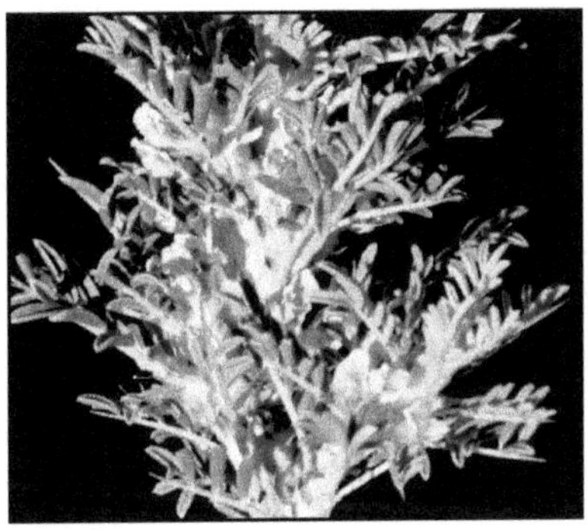

Fig. 7.10: *Astragalus gummifer* herb

Chemical Constituents: Tragacanth is made up of twoparts water-insoluble and water-soluble polysaccharides. The main water-insoluble portion is Bassorin, which constitutes 60–70% of the gum while the water-soluble material is tragacanthin. On hydrolysis, tragacanthin yields various sugars such as L-arabinose, L-fructose, D-xylose, D-galactose, and D-galacturonic acid. It also consists of cellulose, starch, protein and ash. Its approximate molecular weight is 8,40,000.

Chemical Tests:

- When strong iodine solution is added to tragacanth, it develops an olive green colour.
- When tragacanth powder is treated with 5% sodium hydroxide it develops canary yellow colour.
- After boiling tragacanth solution with 10% aqueous ferric chloride deep yellow stringy precipitate is observed.

Incompatibilities: At pH 7, it reduces the efficacy of the antimicrobial preservatives but has no effects on efficacy below pH 5. The addition of strong mineral and organic acids, alkali or sodium chloride reduces the viscosity of tragacanth dispersions.

Uses: It is used to make various pharmaceutical formulations like creams gels, and emulsions. It acts as emulsifying and suspending agent. It also acts as binder and diluents in tablet formulations. It is also used in cosmetics and food industry.

3. STARCH:

Synonyms: Amido; Amidon; Amylum

Biological Source: It is polysaccharide obtained from grains like corn (Zea mays) of family Gramineae; potato *(Solanum tuberosum)* of family Solanaceae; tapioca *(Manihot utilissima Pohl)* of family Euphorbiaceae; wheat starch *(Triticum aestivum)* and rice *(Oryza sativa)* of family Poaceae.

Description: Starch is odourless and tasteless, fine, white-coloured powder consisting of very small spherical or ovoid granules of characteristic size and shape. It is practically insoluble in cold ethanol (95%) and in cold water but it swells in water by about 5–10% at 378°C. Starch is extracted from plant by various steps such as coarse milling of plant material, repeated washing with water, wet sieving, and separation of starch by centrifugation. Then starch is dried and milled.

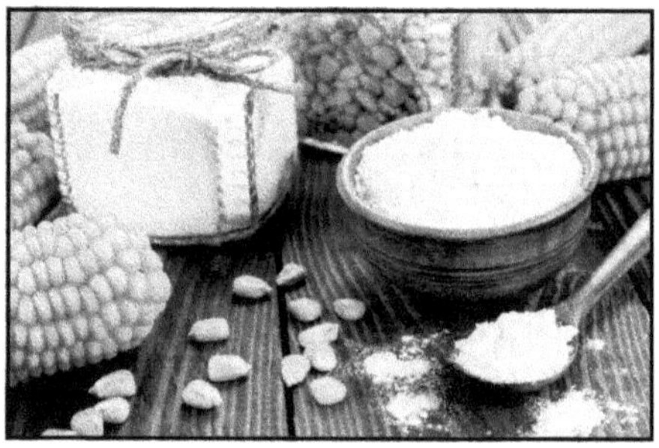

Fig. 7.11: Starch grains from various sources

Chemical Composition: Starch consists of amylose and amylopectin and α-glucose. Amylose is water soluble and amylopectin is water insoluble but swells in water.

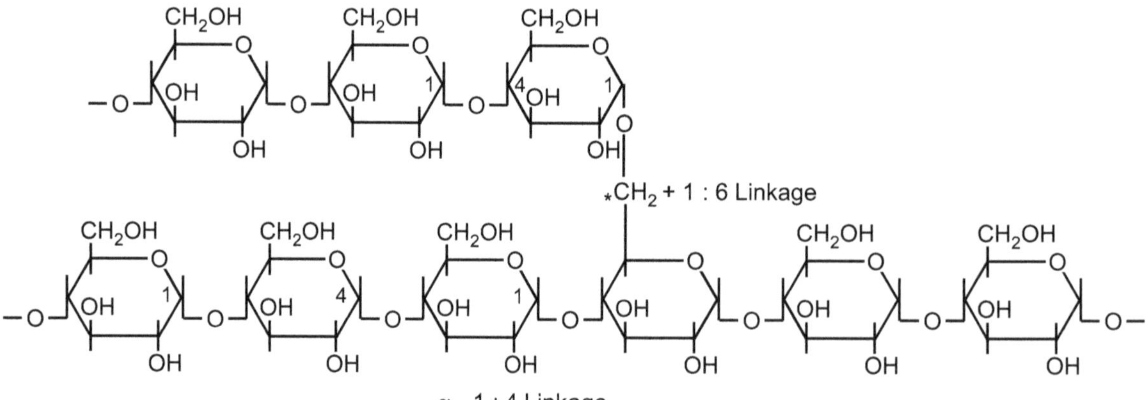

Identification Tests:

1. Starch solution is heated with hydrochloric acid and then it is neutralized by addition of sodium hydroxide. This solution is heated with Fehling's solution and brick red precipitate is produced.
2. 1 g of starch on heating with 50 ml of water, shows thin and cloudy mucilage for all types of starch except potato starch. Potato starch gives thick and more transparent mucilage.

Uses: Starch acts as diluents for preparation of standardized triturates of colorants or potent drugs. Starch is also added in dry filled capsules. Starch paste is a binder of choise in wet granulation of tablet formulation. In 3–15% w/w concentration starch acts as disintegrants. Starch has wide applications as excipient in nasal, oral, periodontal novel drug delivery systems and to get site-specific drug delivery. Starch is also used in dusting powders and ointments. It acts as the skin emollient, base of some enemas and used to treat iodine poisoning. Rice starch is used to treat dehydration caused by acute diarrhoeal diseases. It is also used as indicator in iodometric titrations.

4. GELATIN:

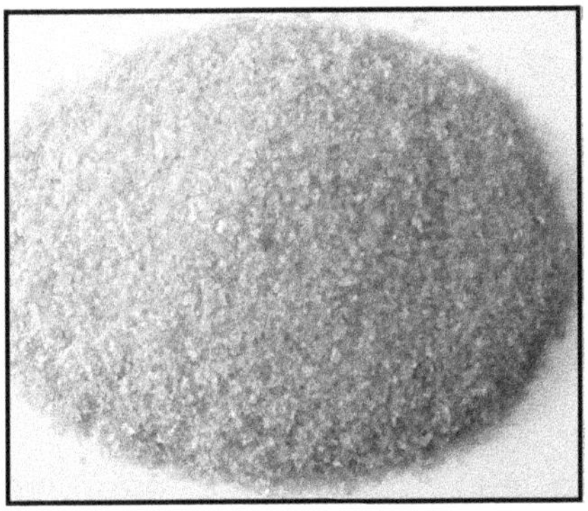

Fig. 7.12: Gelatin Powder

Synonyms: Byco; Cryogel; Gelatine; Instagel; Solugel.

Biological Source: It is protein obtained by partial acid or alkaline hydrolysis of animal collagen tissues like bone, skin, tendon and ligaments.

Description: Gelatin is faintly yellow amber coloured vitreous, brittle solid. It is practically odourless and tasteless. It occurs as flakes, sheets, shreds, powder or granules. Its gelling strength is 150-200. Gelatin is practically insoluble in water, most of organic solvents, fixed oil and volatile oils. It is Soluble in hot water, glycerol, and acetic acid. It forms gel on heating with hot water and cooling to 35-40°C.

Preparation: To prepare gelatin bones are pretreated with acid. Once the raw material is prepared, collagen hydrolysis is performed by different methods such as acid, alkali, and enzymatic hydrolysis. Acid treatment is especially carried out for pig skin collagen requires 10 to 48 hours. Alkali treatment is applied for bovine hides and requires several weeks. The gelatin prepared by acid treatment is called as type-A gelatin while gelatin obtained from alkali-treatment is known as type-B gelatin.

Chemical Constituents: Gelatin contains Glycine (25-27%), alanine, glutamic acid, proline, arginine, aspartic acid and hydroxy proline, isoleucine, leucine, phenyl alanine and tryptophan.

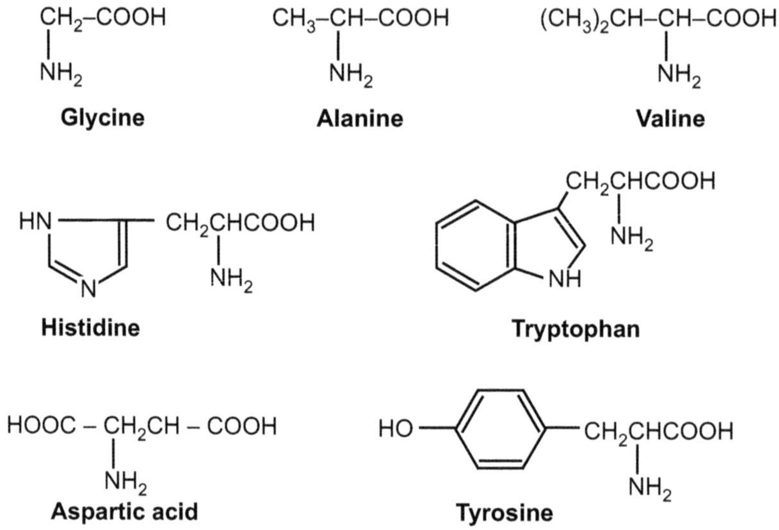

Constituents of gelatin

Chemical Tests:

- Gelatin powder, when heated with soda lime, it evolves ammonia gas.
- With picric and tannic acid it forms precipitate.
- With Million's reagent, gelatin forms white precipitate which on heating turns red-brick red.

Incompatibilities: It reacts with acids and bases. It can also react with aldehydes, aldehydic sugars, anionic and cationic polymers, electrolytes, metal ions, plasticizers, preservatives and surfactants. With alcohols, chloroform, ether, mercury salts, and tannic acid, it gets precipitated.

Uses: It is used in implantable delivery system, mainly to prepare hard and soft gelatin capsules. It is used in formulations like suppositories, pastilles, pessaries, pastes. Gelatin is tablet binder, thickener, stabilizer, coating agent and viscosity-building agent. Absorbable gelatin sponge acts as Haemostatic agent. Absorbable gelatin occurs as sterile film, ophthalmic film, sterile sponge, sterile compressed sponge, and sterile powder from sponge etc. It is good emulsifying agent and is vehicle for injection. Gelatin is also used in food industry and in photographic emulsions.

Table 7.4: List of Various Natural Binders, Disintegrating Agents and Viscosity Builders

Sr. No.	Name of Binder	Role
1.	Accroides, *Xanthorrhoea semiplana ssp.*	Binder in fireworks and flares.
2.	Candelilla, *Euphorbia antisyphilitica*, Euphorbiaceae	Binder in chewing gum.

Contd...

3.	Karaya gum, *Sterculia urens, Malvaceae*	Binder in baking and paper manufacturing.
4.	Bel (Bael) *Aegle marmelos, Rutaceae*	Binder, thickener
5.	Khaya gum, *Khaya grandifoliola,* Meliaceae	Controlled release tablets
6.	Ayoyo gum, *Cochorus olitorius, Tiliaceae*	Emulsifying agent Thickener, Binder
7.	*Prunus gum,* *Prunus domestica, Rosaceae*	Binder and tonic
8.	*Brachystegia mucilage* *Brachystegia eurycoma,* *Leguminosae-*	Emulsifer, Stabilizer Thickener
9.	Tamarind gum, from tamarind seeds *Tamarindus indica, Fabaceae*	Gelling agent, Stabilizer, Binder
10.	Almond gum, *Prunus communis, Rosaceae*	Suspending agent Thickening agent Stabilizer
11.	Shellac, *Kerria lacca* (order Hemiptera, Kerriidae,	Binder in mascara, eyeliners, fireworks and pyrotechnics.
12.	Xanthan, *Xanthomonas campestris,* *Xanthomonadaceae*	Binder in baking, laxatives and toothpaste.
13.	Gum kondagogu *Cochlospermum gossypium,* *Bixaceae*	Emulsifer, thickener
14.	Cassia gum *Cassia fistula, Caesalpiniaceae*	Binder
15.	Albizia gum, *Albizia zygia,* Leguminoseae	Tablet binder, coating materials
16.	Okra gum *Abelmoschus esculentus, Malvaceae*	Suspending agent Disintegrating agent

Contd...

17.	Moringa gum *Moringa olifera, Moringaceae*	Disintegrating agent
18.	Cassia tora mucilage *Cassia tora, Caesalpiniaceae*	Binder and disintegrating agent
19.	Hibiscus mucilage, *Hibiscus rosa-sinensis*, Malvaceae	Disintegrating agent
20.	Isapgol mucilage, *Plantago ovata*, Plantaginaceae	Disintegrating agent

7.3.4 Natural Diluents

Active Pharmaceutical Ingredients (API) having the therapeutic effect cannot be administered directly. It should be combined with suitable excipients to get a desired dosage form for patient's compliance. Natural fillers and diluents are the substances which enhance the bulk solid dosage form or may dilute liquid formulation. They provide proper structural form and assure proper weight for easy administration. They are used in solid, semisolid and liquid dosage forms such as tablets, pills, pallets, paste, solutions and suspensions etc.

In tablet formulations, diluents are added for following reasons:

- To get improved cohesion of particles.
- Helps in direct compression of drugs.
- Enhance flow properties of granules.
- To get desired tablet weight.

Advantages of Natural Diluents:

They are biodegradable, do not have side effect, and have no toxicity, easily availability, economic, no environmental damaging effects.

Disadvantages of Synthetic Diluents:

They are costly, may affect environment, may have toxic effects and may be incompatible with few ingredients.

1. CELLULOSE:

Synonyms: Arbocel; E460; Elcema; Sanacel.

Biological Source: It is polysaccharide and is structural compound found in the cells of plants, algae and few bacteria.

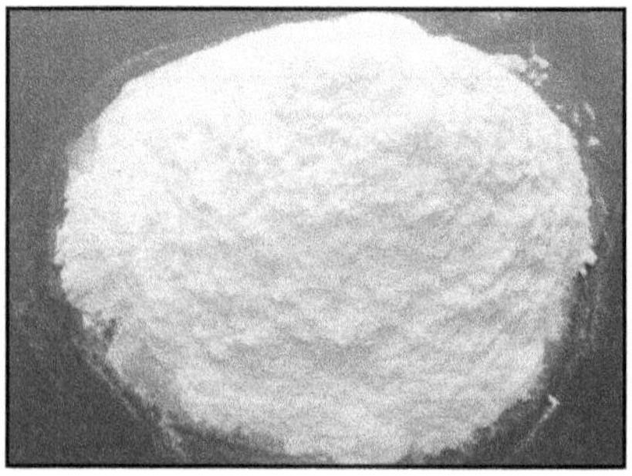

Fig. 7.13: Cellulose Powder

Description: It is white, odourless and tasteless powder varying particle sizes. It may be fine free-flowing powder or granular dense powder or coarse, fluffy and non-flouwing material. Cellulose is practically water insoluble, insoluble in dilute acids, and most of the organic solvents. It is slightly soluble in 5% w/v sodium hydroxide solution. Plant-derived cellulose consists of mixture of hemicelluloses, lignin and pectin.

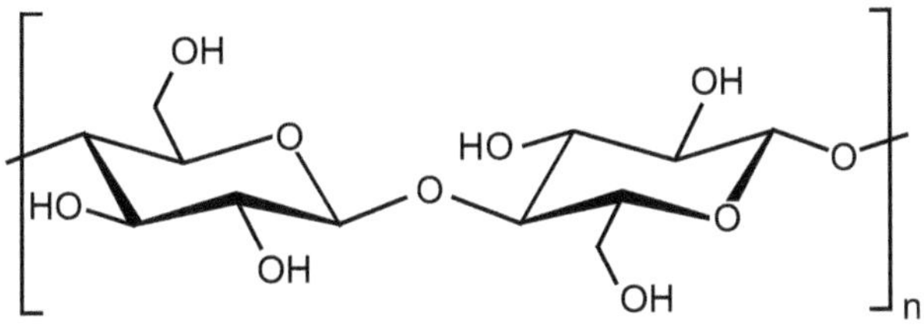

Cellulose

Chemical Test: With Schulze reagent cellulose shows purple colour.

Incompatibilities: incompatibility is observed with strong oxidizing agents.

Applications: Cellulose acts as diluents for tablets and filler for hard gelatin capsules. It helps in direct compression of granules. It is suspending agent and also used in manufacturing of suppositories. It is used in manufacturing of pellets and in cosmetics and food industry. Cellulose derivatives, like microcrystalline cellulose (MCC), acts as a stabilizer and thickening agent. CMC (carboxy methyl cellulose) is very important pharmaceutical excipient.

2. LACTOSE:

Synonyms: Milk sugar, Lactin, Lactosum.

Biological Source: It is a natural disaccharide of animal origin consisting of galactose and glucose and obtained from milk of most of mammals.

Description: It is white crystalline powder, odourless and faintly sweet taste. It is available in several forms like anhydrous α, α monohydrate and anhydrous β lactose.

Anhydrous lactose is made up of 70–80% anhydrous β-lactose and 20–30% anhydrous α-lactose. Lactose is water soluble; sparingly soluble in ethanol (95%). It is hygroscopic at high relative humidity.

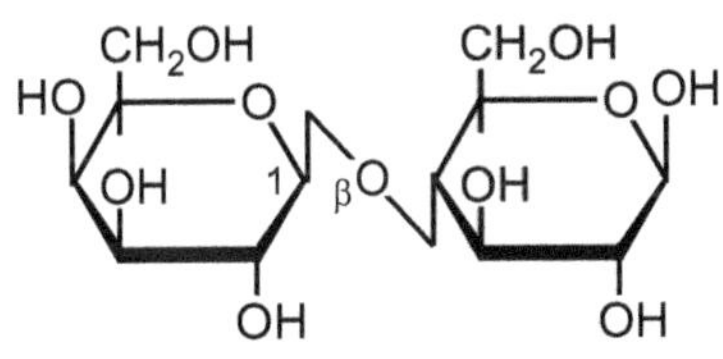

Structure of Lactose

Constituents: Lactose mainly contain O-beta-D-galactopransosyl-(1-4)-alpha-D-glucopyranose.

Chemical Tests:

- When lactose is mixed with water and heated on water bath with 10M ammonia, it shows red colour.
- When hot saturated solution of lactose is mixed with sodium hydroxide it shows yellow colour on warming and on treating with few drops of cupric sulphate, turns brownish red forming red precipitate of copper hydroxide.

Incompatibilities: Incompatible with strong oxidizers.

Uses: It acts as diluent in tablets, capsules, dry powder inhalations. It is used as coating solution with sucrose. Lactose helps in direct compression of granules. It is also used to prepare lyophilized products.

3. MANNITOL:

Synonyms: Cordycepic acid; manna sugar; D-mannite; mannite; Mannogem.

Biological Source: It is exudation from the stem of Fraxinus ornus Linn belonging to family Oleaceae.

Description: It is white, crystalline, powder or free flowing granule. It is odourless, non- hygroscopic, and sweet powder. Its sweetness potency is similar to glucose and half as sucrose. It develops cooling sensation in the mouth. In microscopy it shows orthorhombic prisms. It also shows polymorphism. It is soluble in Alkalis. Soluble in Ethanol (95%) 1 in 83, Glycerin 1 in 18 and Water 1 in 5.5. In ether, it is practically insoluble.

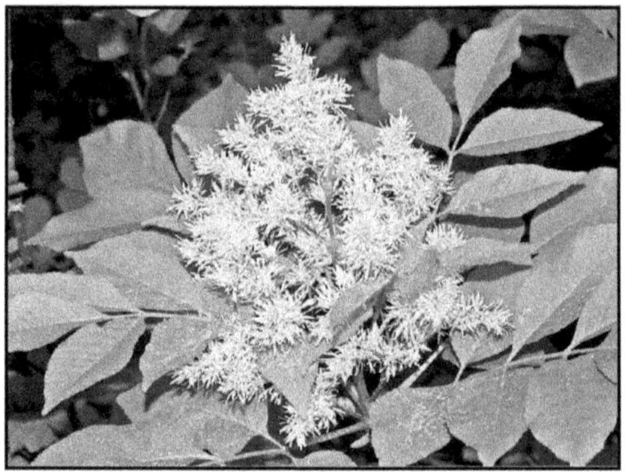

Fig. 7.14: Plant of *Fraxinus ornus*

Preparation: Mannitol is obtained from dried sap of manna and other natural sources by extracting with hot alcohol or other selective solvents. Commercially, it is prepared by the catalytic or electrolytic reduction of monosaccharides such as mannose and glucose.

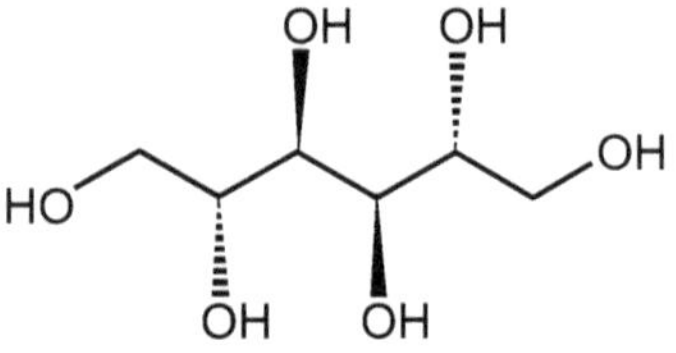

Mannitol

Constituents: Plant mainly consists of mannitol, mannotriose, mannatetrose, dextrose, mucilage and small amount of fluorescent substance Fraxin.

Incompatibilities: Mannitol is precipitated by potassium chloride or sodium chloride. It is incompatible with xylitol infusion, aluminum, copper and iron.

Uses: It acts as diluents for tablet formulation also suitable for moisture sensitive drugs. Mannitol helps in direct compression or in wet granulation. It acts as sweetening agent. As granules with mannitol dry quickly so it is suitable for formulations such as antacid preparations, glyceryl trinitrate tablets, and vitamin preparations. Mannitol is also used to manufacture chewable tablets and lyophilized formulations. It acts as thickening agent, plasticizer in soft-gelatin capsules, in sustained-release tablet formulations, and as a carrier in dry powder inhalers, as a diluent oral dispersible tablets. Therapeutically mannitol acts as osmotic diuretic, as a diagnostic agent for kidney function, as an adjunct in the treatment of acute renal failure, and to reduce intracranial pressure, in treatment of cerebral edema, and to reduce intraocular pressure.

Table 7.5: The Examples of Diluents

Sr. No.	Name of diluent	Role
1.	Calcium carbonate	Buffering agent; coating agent; opacifier; tablet and capsule diluent; therapeutic agent.
2.	Dextrates	Tablet binder; tablet and capsule diluent.
3.	Kaolin	Adsorbent; suspending agent; tablet and capsule diluent.
4.	Sodium Alginate	Stabilizer; suspending agent; tablet and capsule disintegrant; diluent, binder; viscosity builder.
5.	Sucrose	Coating agent; granulating agent; sugar coating agent; suspending agent; sweetening agent; tablet binder; tablet and capsule diluent; viscosity builder.
6.	Xylitol	Preservative; base; coating agent; emollient; humectant; sweetening agent; tablet and capsule diluent.
7.	Microcrystalline cellulose	Dry binder, diluent, tablet disintegrants, absorbent, lubricant, anti-adherent.
8.	Sorbitol	Humectant; plasticizer; sweetener, diluent.

7.3.5 Viscosity Builders

Viscosity builders are added aqueous solutions to increase its viscosity without altering properties like taste. The main functions of viscosity builders are to increase stability, to improve palatability or pourability of dosage forms, to decrease sedimentation rate.

Advantages of viscosity Builders:

- They inhibit the crystal growth.
- Improves physical stability.
- They prevent formation of stable crystal from metastable crystal.

Disadvantages of viscosity Builders:

- High viscosity may interfere with re-dispersibility of the sediments. It may slow down drug absorption. Handling and manufacturing of highly viscous formulation is difficult.

Viscosity builders or thickening agents are of following types:

- Natural gums such as acacia, tragacanth, xanthan gun, alginate.
- Cellulose derivatives such as methyl cellulose, ethyl cellulose, carboxy methyl cellulose.
- Chitosan.
- Synthetic polymers like carbomer, polyvinyl alcohol.
- Clays like magnesium aluminium silicates, bentonite etc.

1. **Xanthan gum:**

Synonyms: Corn sugar gum; Keltrol; Rhodigel.

Biological Source: It is a polysaccharide produced by fermentation using the bacterium like *Xanthomonas compestris.*

Description: Xantham gum is cream or white-coloured, odorless, free-flowing, fine powder. It is practically insoluble in ethanol and ether; soluble in cold or warm water. Temperature change does not affect viscosity of xanthan gum. In market, it occurs as potassium and sodium salts.

Preparation: After aerobic fermentation of a carbohydrate with *Xanthomonas campestris,* polysaccharide is recovered using propan-2-ol. It is dried and milled.

Chemical Nature: Chemically it is made up of D-glucose, D-mannose and D-glucuronic acid with short side chains. It is prepared as sodium or potassium salts.

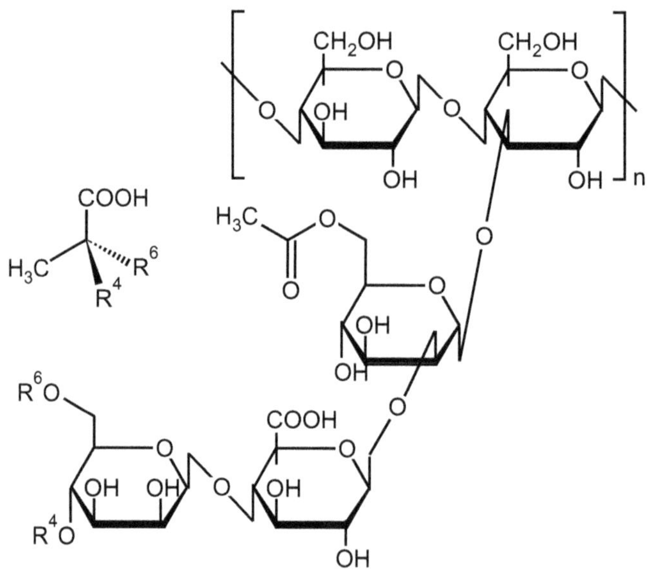

Structure of Xanthan gum

Chemical Tests:

- Xanthan gum is suspended in 0.1 N hydrochloric acid in flask. The flask is then closed with formation bulb containing barium hydroxide. It is then heated. Barium hydroxide solution shows white turbidity.
- Mixture of xanthan gum and locust bean gum is heated at 60°C with vigorous stirring for 30 min. then it is cooled to 40°C. The rubbery and firm gel is observed which is not observed in case of Xanthan gum alone.

Incompatibilities: Xanthan gum is incompatible with oxidizing agents, coatings agents, carboxymethyl cellulose sodium, dried aluminum hydroxide gel, amitriptyline, tamoxifen, and verapamil, cationic surfactants, polymers and preservatives etc.

Uses: It acts as good emulsifying agent, stabilizer and thickener, viscosity enhancer for oral and topical pharmaceutical formulations, cosmetics and foods. It can be added in sustained-release matrix and ophthalmic liquid dosage forms. It can be incorporated in spray-drying and freeze-drying processes. Xanthan gum can be also used in formulations of vaginal and colon specific drug delivery systems.

2. CARRAGEENAN:

Synonyms: Chondrus extract; Irish moss extract.

Biological Source: It is sulphated polysaccharide obtained from the red-algae *Chondrus crispus* belonging to family, Rhodophyllaceae.

Geographical Source: It is produced at North Atlantic coast of Europe, North America, France, Spain, Denmark and USA.

Description: Carrageenan is yellow-brown to white coloured, coarse to fine powder, without any taste. It is water soluble and stable at pH 9.0. There are two forms of carrageenan, one form which is extracted with cold water gives viscous solution in water. Another form is extracted with hot water forms gel on cooling.

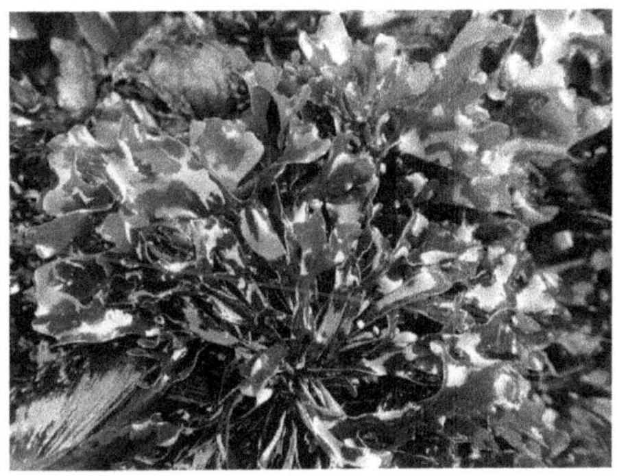

Fig. 7.15: *Chondrus crispus* algae

Chemical Constituents: It mainly consists of potassium, sodium, calcium, magnesium, and ammonium sulfate esters of galactose and 3,6-anhydrogalactose copolymers which are alternately linked at the α-1,3 and β-,4 sites in the polymer. Depending upon the position of sulphate and presence or absence of anhydrogalactose there are mainly three families.

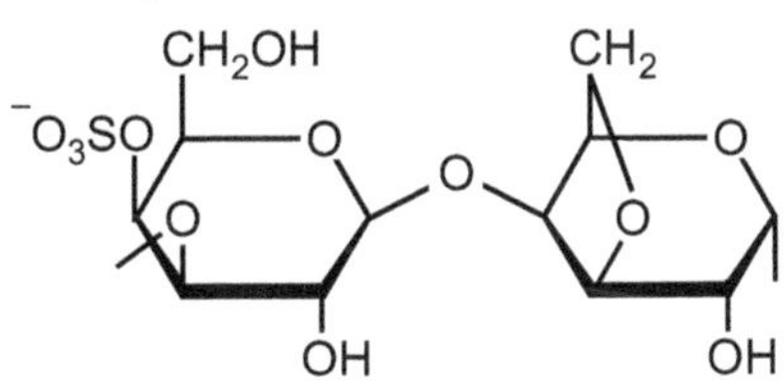

Kappa Carrageenan (KC)

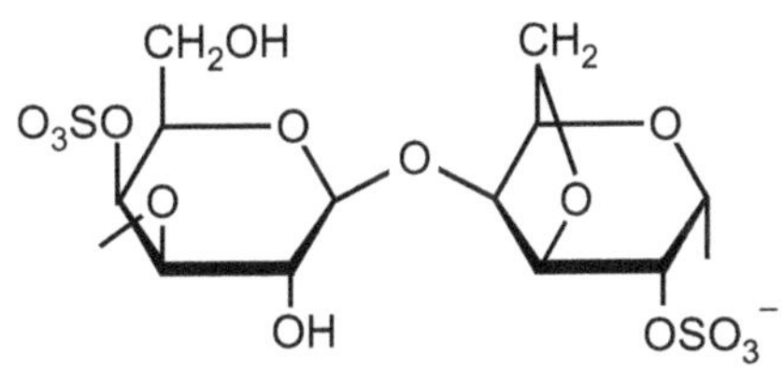

Iota Carrageenan (IC)

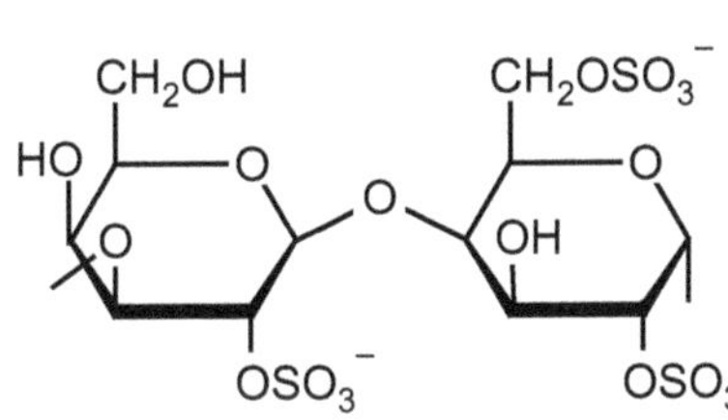

Lambda Carrageenan (LC)

Structure of Carrageenan

- Lambda-carrageenan: It is a nongelling polymer consisting of 35% ester sulfate by weight and no 3,6- anhydrogalactose.

- i-Carrageenan (iota-carrageenan) is a gelling polymer approximately consisting of 32% ester sulfate by weight and 30% 3,6-anhydrogalactose.
- k-Carrageenan (kappa-carrageenan) has helical tertiary structure and is a strongly gelling agent. It mainly consists of 25% ester sulfate and 34% 3,6-anhydrogalactose.

Preparation: The seaweed is washed several times to remove impurities and extracted with hot alkali. The extract is clarified and concentrated. From extract, carrageenan is isolated by three methods.

- **Freeze-thaw technique:** In this method, extract is converted to gel by using various salts and then it is freezed. Further, thawing is carried out to separate water and mass of carrageenan.
- **Alcohol precipitation:** Concentrated extract of carrageenan is treated with alcohol to precipitate carrageenan. The precipitate is dried and ground to the desired particle size.
- **KCl precipitation:** Hot extract is concentrated and passed through spinnerets into a cold 1.0–1.5% solution of potassium chloride. Thus, gel threads are formed which are washed with potassium chloride solution and are dried converted to carrageenan powder.

Chemical Tests:

- Carrageenan becomes translucent and gelatinous when soaked in cold water.
- Its 3 % solution in boiling water forms a thick jelly on cooling.

Incompatibility: It can react with cationic materials.

Uses: It is used to prepare various pharmaceutical such as suspensions, emulsions, gels, creams, lotions, eye drops, suppositories, tablets, capsules etc. It acts as emulsifying, stabilizing, gelling agent and viscosity builder. It is excipient of choice in oral and buccal drug delivery. It is used to make hard and soft capsule shells, toothpastes and cosmetic preparations. Carrageenan is used for microencapsulation of proteins and probiotic bacteria. According to various studies, it can cure infections due to herpes simplex virus, human cytomegalovirus, human papilloma virus; sindbis virus; vesicular stomatitis virus; and HIV. It is applied in the form of wound dressings.

3. Guar Gum:

Synonyms: Guaran, Guar flour; Jaguar gum.

Biological Source: It is galactomannan polysaccharide obtained from the endosperm of the seed of the guar plant, *Cyamopsis tetragonoloba* (L) Taub. *(Cyamopsis psoralioides)* belonging to family Fabaceae.

Geographical Source: It is mainly cultivated at India, Pakistan, U.S., Australia and Africa.

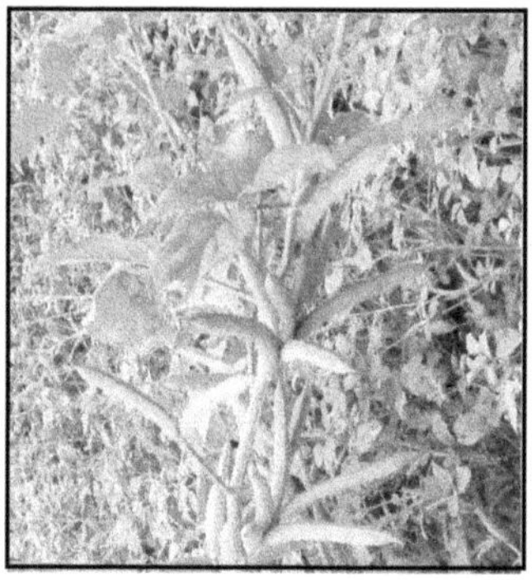

Fig. 7.16: Plant of *Cyamopsis tetragonolobus*

Composition: Guar gum is an exo-polysaccharide consisting of galactose and mannose sugars. Its backbone is made up of linear chain of β 1, 4-linked mannose, residues and galactose residues are attached by 1,6-linkage at every second mannose residues. Its molecular weight is approximately 50,000 – 8,000,000.

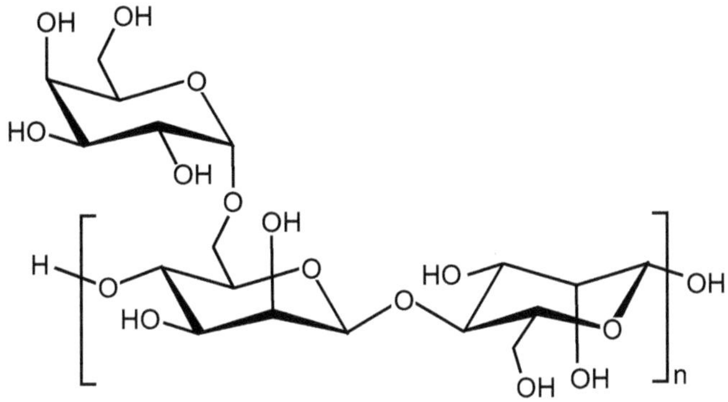

Structure of guar gum

Description: Guar gum is white to yellowish-white powder which is odourless or nearly odourless, with a bland taste. Guar gum is practically insoluble in organic solvents. In cold or hot water it swells immediately to form a highly viscous solution. It can withstand temperatures of 80 °C (176 °F) for five minutes. Its solution remain stable over pH range 5-7.

Preparation: To remove seed hull, seeds are subjected to grinding, soaking in sulfuric acid or water, or by heating. The embryo is separated by differential grinding. It is then ground to get powder of different particle sizes.

Chemical Tests:

- It does not form olive green colour with dilute iodine solution.
- Guar Gum does not form pink colour with ruthenium red.
- With 2 % lead acetate guar gum gives precipitate.

Uses: Guar gum is used as a binder, disintegrant, suspending, thickening, and stabilizing agent; and in controlled-release carrier dosage forms. It is used as a part of the diet for diabetic patients. It is commonly used in food and cosmetic industry.

Incompatibilities: It is incompatible with acetone, ethanol (95%), tannins, strong acids, and alkalis.

7.3.6 Disintegrating Agents

Disintegrating agents helps in dispersion or disintegration of tablets and release contents of capsules into smaller fragments. When added to the drug formulations disintegrating agents causes quick dissolution. They act by various mechanisms like:

- **Swelling:** Disintegrants swell and break tablet into pieces.
- **Porosity:** Water starts penetrating inside tablet by capillary action and break interparticulate bonds.

- **Deformation:** During compression, disintegrating agents deformed. When they come in contact with water, they get back to their normal structure. It felicitates break up of tablet.
- **Repelling:** Particle repel each other causing tablet to disintegrate.

Advantages of Synthetic Disintegrants:

- They are effective in lower concentrations.
- They do not affect compressibility and flowability.
- They are more effective at intragranular region.

Disadvantages of Synthetic Disintegrants:

- High cost.
- Can cause toxicity, or side effects.
- May cause environmental pollution problems during synthesis.
- Obtained from non-renewable sources.
- Less patient compliance.

1. CHITOSAN:

Synonym: Deacetylated chitin.

Source: It is a natural polysaccharide obtained from crab and shrimp shells. Chitosan is produced commercially by deacetylation of chitin present in these organisms.

Description: Chitosan is odourless, white or creamy-white powder or flakes. During precipitation chitosan may form cotton like fibre. Chitosan is sparingly soluble in water; practically insoluble in ethanol (95%), other organic solvents. Chitosan is soluble in dilute and concentrated organic acids and to some extent in mineral inorganic acids except phosphoric and sulfuric acids.

Composition: Chitosan is made up of two units mainly β-(1→ 4)-linked D-glucosamine (deacetylated unit) and N-acetyl-D-glucosamine (acetylated unit).

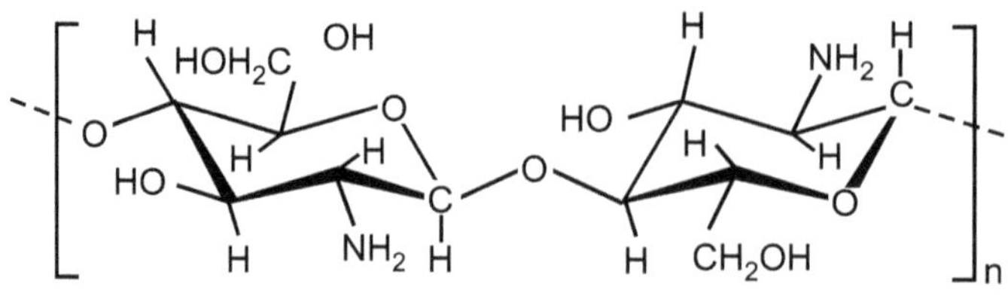

Chitosan

Preparation: The shells of crabs and shrimps are powdered. Then proteins are removed by treating with 3–5% aqueous sodium hydroxide solution. The product is neutralized and treated with aqueous hydrochloric acid 3–5% solution at room temperature to remove calcium and to precipitate chitin. The chitin is dried and N-deacetylation of chitin is carried out with an aqueous sodium hydroxide (40–45% solution) at high temperature. The precipitate thus obtained is washed with water. The crude sample is mixed with 2% acetic acid and the insoluble material is removed. To obtain purified white precipitate of chitosan the clear supernatant solution is collected and neutralized with aqueous sodium hydroxide solution. The purified product is processed to get fine uniform powder or granules.

Chemical Tests:

- With iodine and 10 % sulphuric acid solution, chitosan forms deep violet colour.
- With 50 % nitric acid, chitosans forms spherical crystals of chitosans nitrate.

Uses: Chitosan is used in various pharmaceutical dosage forms such as controlled drug delivery, mucoadhesive dosage forms, rapid release, improved peptide delivery, colonic drug delivery systems, and for gene delivery. Chitosan can be used in gels, films, beads, microspheres, tablets, and coatings for liposomes. It acts as coating agent; disintegrant; film-forming agent; mucoadhesive; tablet binder; viscosity-increasing agent.

Incompatibilities: Incompatiblilies are reported with strong oxidizing agents.

2. PREGELATINIZED STARCH:

Synonyms: Compressible starch; Instastarch; Pharma-Gel; Prejel.

Source: Pregelatinized starch is obtained from modification of potato starch.

Description: Pregelatinized starch occurs as a moderately coarse to fine, white to off-white colored powder which is odourless and has characteristic taste. It is practically insoluble in organic solvents, slightly soluble to soluble in cold water.

Composition: It mainly consists of 5% free amylose, 15% of free amylopectin, and 80% unmodified starch.

Chemical Tests:

When solution of pregelatinised starch is treated with iodine solution, it forms reddish violet to blue colour.

Applications: It is mainly used as disintegrants, binder and diluents in tablets and capsules. It is suitable binder for tablets made by dry-compression or direct compression method. It acts as disintegrating agent between 5 to 10 % concentration.

Incompatibilities: Nil.

3. MICROCRYSTALLINE CELLULOSE:

Synonyms: Avicel; Celex; Cellulose gel.

Source: It is obtained from partial depolymerisation of cellulose.

Description: It is a white, odourless, tasteless, crystalline powder having porous particles. It is commercially available in different particle sizes and moisture grades. It is slightly soluble in 5% w/v sodium hydroxide solution and practically insoluble in water, dilute acids, and most organic solvents.

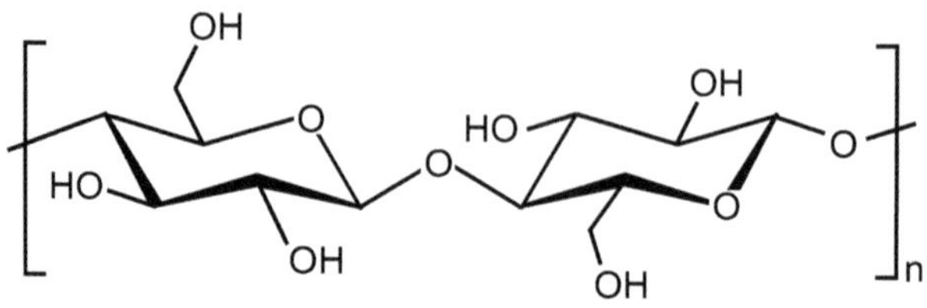

Microcrystalline cellulose

Preparation: α-cellulose, obtained as a pulp from fibrous plant materials is subjected to controlled hydrolysis with dilute mineral acid. Then solution is filtered and spray-dried to get powder of microcrystalline cellulose.

Composition: It is linear chain of β 1, 4- linked glucose residue.

Chemical Tests:

- Microcrystalline cellulose is heated with phosphoric acid and solution of catechol in phosphoric acid is added. On heating for 30 min. it produces red colour.
- With phloroglucinol and hydrochloric acid, microcrystalline cellulose does not produce red colour.

Uses: It is used as lubricant and disintegranting agents. It is applied as binder or diluent in oral tablet and capsule formulations and is suitable for both wet-granulation and direct-compression method.

Incompatibilities: Incompatiblilities are reported with strong oxidizing agents.

7.3.7 Natural Perfumes and Flavouring Agents

Natural Perfume is a mixture of essential oils or aromatic compounds, fixatives and solvents applied to the human body, animal, food objects, pharmaceutical products and living spaces. Fixatives are added to reduce the rate of evaporation of a perfume while an extender is added to increase the volume of the perfume without diluting the aroma. Perfumes are obtained from steam distillation, hydrodistillation, solvent extraction and supercritical fluid extraction.

Flavours are taste masking agents used to mask the unpleasant taste or order of dosage form and enhance the flavour of medicine and patient compliance.

Advantages of Natural Flavoring Agents or Perfumes:

- Natural flavouring agents or perfumes give the realistic flavour.
- Do not affect environment and are non-toxic.
- They are cheaper and stable.
- Readily available.

Disadvantages of Synthetic Flavours and Perfumes:

- They are toxic in nature.
- Can affect environment as they are not easily biodegradable.
- Costly.
- Highly concentrated and should be used in minimum concentration.

1. SANDAL WOOD OIL:

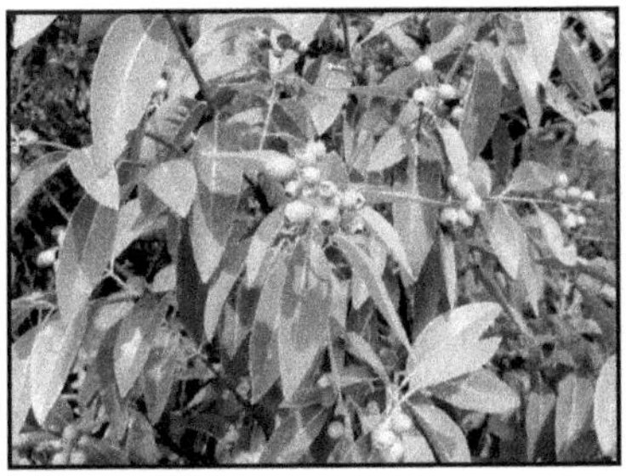

Fig. 7.17: Branch of *Santalum album* tree

Synonym: Chandan.

Biological Soruce: It is volatile oil obtained by steam distillation of heartwood of *Santalum album* and *Santalum spicatum* belonging to family *Santalaceae.*

Description: Sandal wood oil is colourless to golden yellow in colour with pleasant sweet woody persistent odour. It is oily, viscous liquid, generally affected by light. It is soluble in 5 volumes of 70% alcohol.

Chemical Constituents: Its main constituents are sesquiterpene alcohol, α and β santalol, α and β santalene, α and β santalic acid, santalone, santanone and santene.

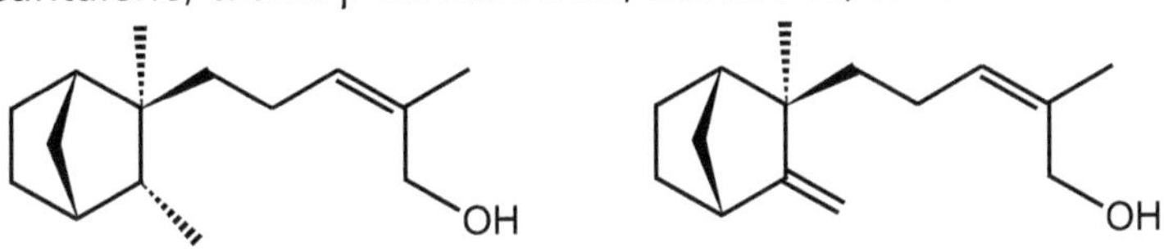

α-santalol **β-santalol**

Santalols

Uses: It is used in aromatherapy in soaps and cosmetics as perfume. Traditionally it is used to treat common colds, bronchitis, fever, urinary tract infections, and inflammation.

2. ROSE OIL:

Synonym: Otto of rose, Attar of rose, Rose essence.

Biological Source: It is volatile oil obtained by distillation of fresh flowers of Rosa damascena, Rosa centifolia, and other Rosa species, of family Rosaceae.

Description: Rose oil is colourless or yellow liquid with characteristic odour of rose. On cooling, it forms translucent, crystalline mass which may be easily liquefied by warming. Rose oil is miscible in 1 ml chloroform.

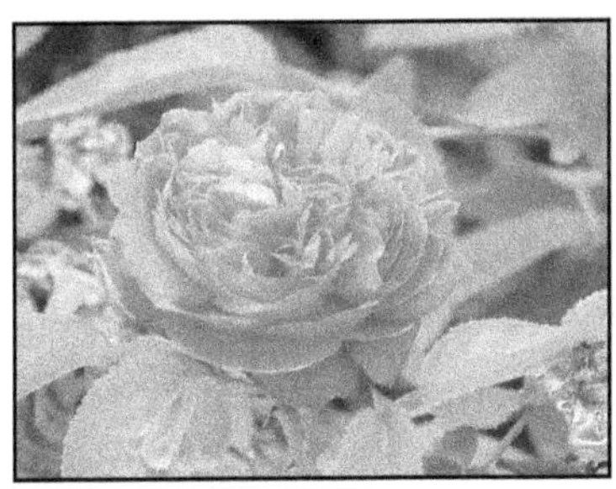

Fig. 7.18: Plant of *Rosa damascena*

Constituents: Particular perfume of rose oil is due to constituents like β-damascenone, β-damascone, β-ionone, and rose oxide. Other constituents are citronellol, geraniol, nerol, linalool, phenyl ethyl alcohol, farnesol, stearoptene, α-pinene, β-pinene, α-terpinene, limonene, p-cymene, camphene, β-caryophyllene, neral, citronellyl acetate, geranyl acetate, neryl acetate, eugenol and methyl eugenol etc.

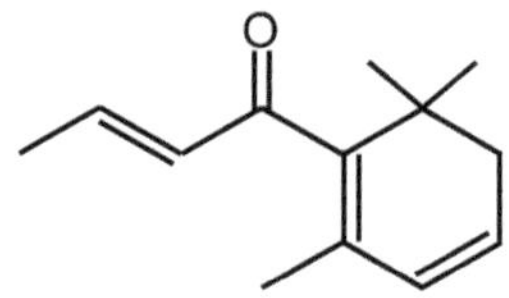

β-Damascenone

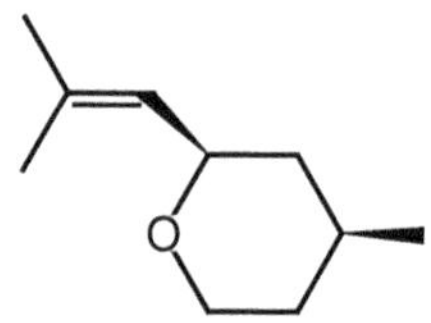

Rose Oxide

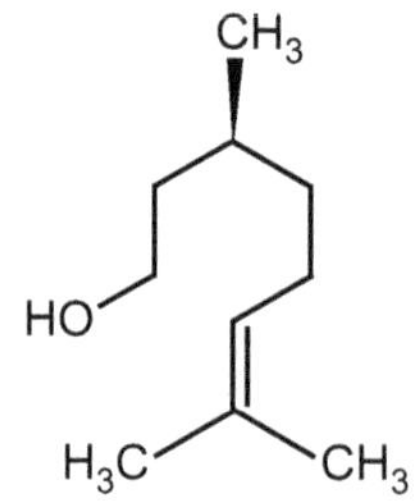

Citronellol

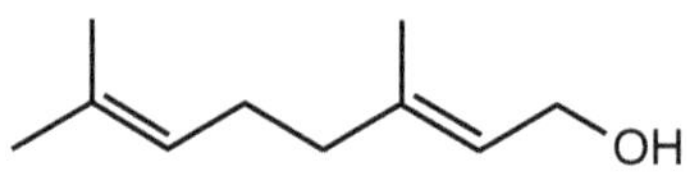

Geraniol

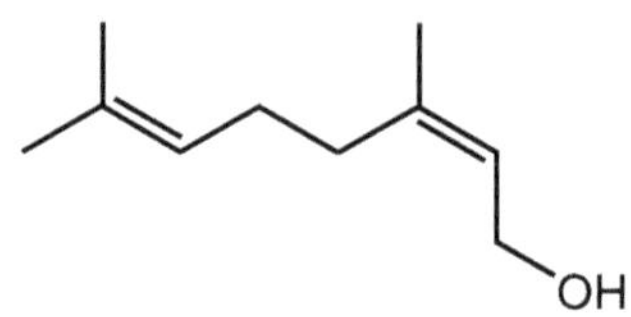

Nerol (*trans*-Geraniol)

Chemical Tests: Rose oil is mixed with equal quantity of chloroform and 90% alcohol is added. The resulting liquid is neutral or acidic. At 20^0 C it deposits crystals within 5 minutes.

Uses: It is used as flavouring agent and perfume. Also it is applied on skin to hydrate dry skin, to treat acne, reduce signs of aging, scars and help to treat eczema. Its therapeutic applications include treatment of anxiety, depression, headaches, menopausal symptoms, menstrual cramps and migraines.

3. PEPPERMINT OIL:

Synonyms: Oleum, Peppermint.

Biological Source: The volatile oil obtained by steam distillation of fresh flowering tops of plant *Mentha piperita* belongs to family Labiatae.

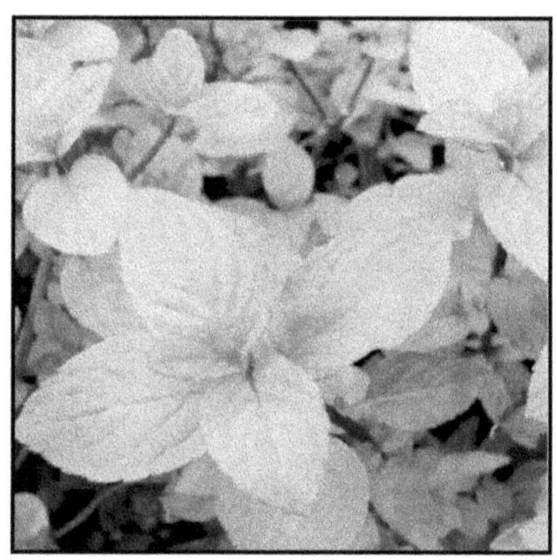

Fig. 7.19: Plant of *Mentha piperita*

Description: Mentha oil is colourless or yellowish in colour, pleasant odour, and pungent taste followed by cooling sensation. It is clear and translucent liquid. It is soluble in 70 % alcohol, ether and chloroform but insoluble in water.

Chemical Constituents: It consists of 0.3 – 0.4% of volatile oil which contains phytoconstituents such as menthol, menthone, isomenthone, menthyl acetate, menthofuran, 1,8-cineol, camphene, limonene, zasmine and menthofurone etc.

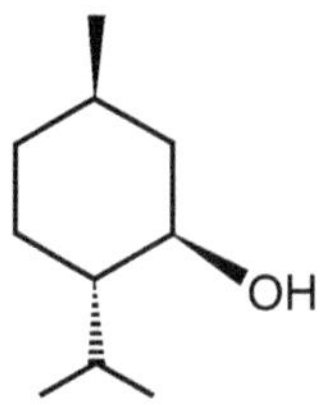

(–)-Menthol

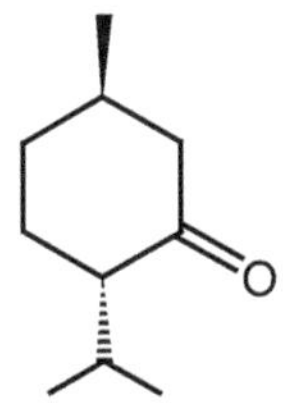

(–)-Menthone

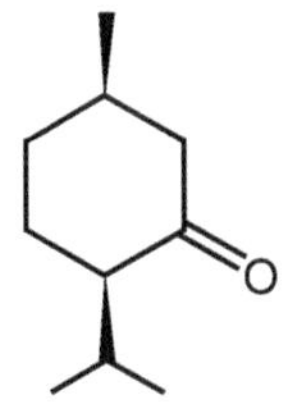

(–)-Isomethone

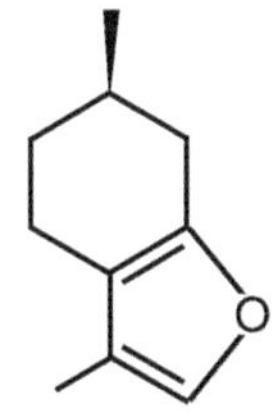

(–)-Menthofuran

Chemical Test: Peppermint oil is mixed with nitric acid solution and heated. Within 5 min. it forms blue colour, which darkens, and copper coloured fluorescence is observed. Finally golden yellow colour is observed.

Uses: It is carminative, Aromatic, Stimulant, Flavouring agent, Antiseptic and Counter irritant. Peppermint oil is used to treat various disorders such as irritable bowel syndrome (IBS), nausea, digestive issues, common cold, headaches, itching, muscle pain, and headache, as flavouring agent in foods and mouthwashes, as perfume in soaps and cosmetic products. Peppermint oil acts as flavor products such as ice cream, candy, fruit preserves, alcoholic beverages and chewing gum, toothpaste and skin care products.

4. LEMON OIL:

Synonyms: Limbu, Oleum limonis.

Biological Source: It is volatile oil obtained from fresh peel of the ripe fruits of Citrus lemon belonging to family Rutaceae.

Description: Lemon oil is pale greenish-yellow in colour with sharp, fresh smell, bitter taste and has watery viscosity. At low temperature, it turns cloudy. It dissolves in 3 volumes of alcohol and miscible with carbon disulphide and glacial acetic acid.

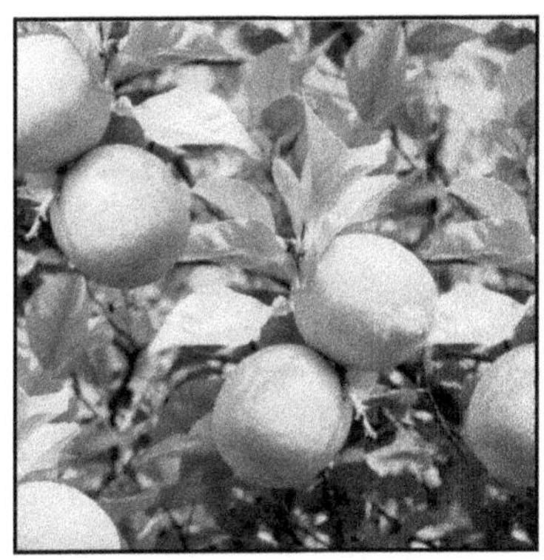

Fig. 7.20: Plant of *Citrus lemon*

Constituents: The main constituent of lemon oil includes α pinene, camphene, β pinene, sabinene, myrcene, α-terpinene, linalool, α-bisabolene, limonene, trans- α-bergamotene, nerol and neral.

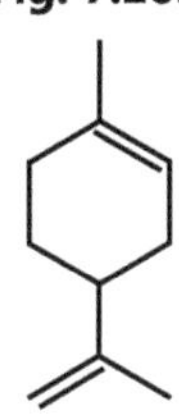

Limonene

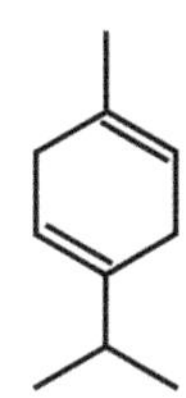

γ-terpinene

Chemical Test: Solution of lemon oil with 3 volumes of alcohol is neutral to slightly acidic in nature.

Applications: It is flavouring agent and perfume. It is used to treat fever, throat infections, bronchitis, asthma, constipation, dyspepsia and flu. It is also used in treatment of painful cold sores, mouth ulcers, herpes, insect bites and in skin and hair care cosmetics.

Table 7.6: List of Natural Flavours and Perfumes

Sr. No.	Name of flavour/ perfume	Constituents	Use
1.	Ajowan, *Trachyspermum ammi*, Apiaceae	Thymol, γ-terpinene, p-cymene	Perfume
2.	Anise oil, *Pimpinella anisum*, Apiaceae	Anethole	Flavour
3.	Balsam of Peru, *Myroxylon balsamum*, Fabaceae	Cinnamein, cinnamic acid, cinnamyl cinnamate	Flavor in foods and drinks, fragrance in cosmetics
4.	Bay oil, *Cinnamomum tamala, Lauraceae*	Eucalyptol	Flavour, perfumery and aromatherapy
5.	Cardamom oil, *Elettaria cardamomum*, Zingiberaceae	α-terpineol, myrcene	Flavour, fragrance in soaps, perfumes, aromatherapy
6.	Citronella grass *Cymbopogon nardus*, Poaceae	Citronella, geraniol and citronellol	Perfume in soaps, insect and in aromatherapy
7.	Clove oil, *Syzygium aromaticum*, Myrtaceae	Eugenol, acetyl eugenol, caryophyllene	Flavour, aromatherapy, dental analgesic
8.	Davana oil, Artemisia *pallens*, Asteraceae	Davanone, davan ether, davana furan, linalool	Perfumes of sweet and fruity fragrances
9.	Nutmeg oil, *Myristica fragrans*, Myristicaceae	d-pinene, limonene, d-borneol, l-terpineol, geraniol	Flavour and perfume
10.	Lavender oil, *Lavandula latifolia* Lamiaceae	Linalool, linalyl acetate	Perfume, for aromatherapy, and for skin applications

Table 7.7: Different Types of Excipients used in Modern Pharmaceutical Dosage forms

Sr. No.	Name of excipient	Role
1.	Okra gum *Abelmoschus esculentus,* Malvaceae	Suspending agent, disintegrant (4%) , poor sustained release tablet and colon targeted tablet formulation
2.	Locust bean gum *Ceratonia siliqua,* Leguminosae	Controlled release agent
3.	Tamarind gum, *Tamarindus indica* Fabaceae	In microspheres
4.	Hibiscus gum, *Hibiscus Rosasinensis,* Malvaceae	Sustained release agent
5.	Bavchi gum, Ocimum canum, Gigarginaceae	Suspending agent, emulsifying agent
6.	Aloe mucilage, Aloe species (Liliaceae)	Sustained release agent, gelling agent
7.	*Cordia gum,* *Cordia oblique,* Boraginaceae	Enteric-resistant and sustained release material
8.	*Behara gum,* *Terminalia bellerica roxb* Combretaceae	For microencapsulation
9.	Alginates brown sea weed, Phaeophyceae	In novel drug delivery systems such as matrix type alginate gel beads, in liposomes, gastrointestinal transit time modulation, for local applications and tissue engineering applications
10.	Khaya gum, *Khaya grandifoliola,* Meliaceae	Controlled release tablets
11.	Pectins	Microencapsulation, controlled drug delivery
12.	Saffron, *Crocus Sativus Linn,* Iridaceae	Colouring and flavouring agent

13.	Spermaceti, *Physeter macrocephalus*, Physeteridae	Emollient in cosmetics
14.	Soyabean oil, *Glycine soja*, Leguminosae	Emollient in cosmetics, in liposomes, microspheres and dry emulsions.
15.	Honey, *Apies mellifera*, Apidae	Demulcent, sweetener, antiseptic, used in creams, lotions, pills, soft drinks

QUESTIONS

1. Write an elaborative note on natural excipients.
2. Define excipients. Give advantages and disadvantages of herbal excipients.
3. Classify natural excipients. Give their functions.
4. What are ideal properties of excipients?
5. What is the role of excipients in pharmaceutical dosage forms?
6. Write a short note on natural colourants.
7. Define natural sweeteners. Write about its advantages and disadvantages. Write in brief about Stevia.
8. Discuss in detail about natural sweeteners.
9. Discuss in brief about acacia and tragacanth as natural binders.
10. What is the significance of natural diluents. Write elaborative note on natural diluents.
11. Write in detail about substances of natural origin used as viscosity modifying agents.
12. Describe in detail about natural disintegrating agents.
13. Write an elaborative note on natural products used as flavouring agents and perfumes.

❖❖❖

Chapter...8

HERBAL FORMULATIONS

Objectives

- To understand the concept of conventional and novel dosage forms.
- To learn about different conventional solid, liquid and semisolid dosage forms.
- To learn about advantages, preparation and applications of different types of novel dosage forms.

8.1 INTRODUCTION

In past three decades, there is exceptional rise in herbal drug demand in global market. According to World Health Organization about 80% of world's population uses herbal medicines as their healthcare needs. Herbal products are the products derived from whole plant, parts of plants or extracts which are used to treat various diseases. The herbal materials like unprocessed seeds and plant exudates can be used as starting materials and herbal preparations like powders or dried extracts act as intermediates in the preparation of finished herbal products or herbal dosage forms. Various commonly available herbal dosage forms are decoctions, herbal teas, tinctures, glycerites, herbal soaps, herbal tablets, herbal syrups, herbal capsules, herbal creams and ointments. Growing interest in herbal dosage forms demand for their large scale production.

Dosage forms are the means by which drug molecules are introduced in the body. As per WHO Finished herbal products consist of one or more herbal preparations made from one or more herbs. These may contain excipients in addition to the active ingredients.

Definition: According to WHO, Herbal dosage forms are physical form like liquid, solid, semi-solid products produced from herbs, with or without excipients, in a particular formulation (such as decoctions, tablets and ointments). The herbal materials such as dried roots or fresh juices or herbal preparations such as extracts are used to produce herbal dosage forms.

Challenges in Herbal Formulation:

- The toxicological, epidemiological, and other data available regarding herbal formulation is confusing.
- Authentification of herbal materials is difficult.
- Pharmacological, toxicological, and clinical documentation is tedious task.
- It is difficult to follow Pharmacovigilance guidelines in case of herbal formulations.
- There is need to study herb-drug interactions.

- Standardization, safety and efficacy measurement of herbal formulations are a big challenge.
- There are various hurdles in conduction of Clinical trial of herbal formulations.

Steps in Herbal Drug Formulation:

1. **Selection, drying and grinding of herbal drugs:** Based on medicinal properties, the specific part of the plant is selected. The plant material is then dried using sun drying, shade drying or oven drying techniques. The plant material is subjected to pulverizing and sieving.
2. **Extraction of plant material:** The powdered plant material is extracted by using different techniques like cold maceration, hot maceration or soxhlet extraction depending on chemical nature of phytoconstituents.
3. **Filtration and concentration of extract:** Extract is further concentrated using vacuum evapouration to get solid mass free of solvent. This extract can be directly used to make formulation or purified further.
4. **Powdered extract:** The extract is converted into dry powder by spray drying techniques. This powdered extract is used to make various dosage forms.
5. **Preparation of dosage forms:** Various dosage forms like tablets, capsules, ointments, creams, syrups etc. are made using dried extract or powdered extracts.

8.2 TYPES OF CONVENTIONAL HERBAL DOSAGE FORMS

The different types of conventional herbal dosage forms are disussed as follows:

8.2.1 Liquid Herbal Dosage Forms

Liquid herbal dosage forms are usually solutions, syrups, emulsions or suspensions containing one or more active substances in a suitable vehicle. As per British pharmacopoeia liquid dosage forms include oral solutions, emulsions, suspensions, powders and granules for oral solutions and suspensions, oral drops, powders for oral drops, syrups, powders and granules for syrups etc.

Different types of herbal liquid dosage forms are as follows:

(a) Decoctions: These are herbal formulations prepared by boiling the crude drug with specific volume of water for specific period of time. The extract is then cooled and filtered. Decoctions are normally intended for immediate use, or use within a 24-hour to 72 hrs. It is suitable for hard plant materials.

Dosage: 3 to 4 times a day upto 500 ml per day.

Examples: E.g. Sijunzi decoction, Chinese herbal remedy is mixture of *Panax ginseng, Poriacocos, Atractylodes macrocephala* and *Glycyrrhiz auralensis*.

(b) Infusions: Infusions are made by using cold or hot water for herbal extraction and are dilute solutions. For heat sensitive drugs, cold infusions are prepared by soaking drug in cold water for several hours. Hot infusions can be prepared by pouring boiling water on plant material. Infusion should be stored in cold and dry place. The shelf life of infusion is upto 24 hours.

Dosage: 3 to 4 times a day upto 500 ml per day.

Examples: Tea, coffee, lemon infusions.

(c) Tincture: It is an alcoholic or hydroalcoholic extract of herbal material, by using 1 part of herbal material and 5–10 parts of solvent like ethanol. Tinctures can be stored in cool, dry and dark place for 2 years.

Dosage: 5 ml diluted to 25 ml, can be taken 2 to 3 times a day.

Examples: Tincture of iodine, Benzoin tincture, Cannabis tincture.

(d) Syrups: According to WHO, syrups are viscous liquids containing high amount of sugars or other sweetening agents. They are prepared by various methods such as dissolving, mixing, suspending or emulsifying herbal extracts or decoctions in a solution of honey, sucrose or other sweetening agents. Syrups can also be prepared by using infusions. Syrups may or may not contain medicine or flavouring agent. The syrup which does not contain medication but contains only flavouring agent is called as flavoured or non-medicated syrup. Medicated syrup consists of medication and flavour to mask its unpleasant taste. Due to high sugar content syrups are susceptible to microbial contamination so they contain preservatives.

Advantages of Syrup:

- Unpleasant taste of medications can be masked.
- It is easy to swallow medication in Syrup form as they are thick. Hence only small portion of medicament comes in contact with the taste buds and remaining is swallowed as it is.
- It is easy to administer drug in pediatric patient as they are sweet in taste.
- Syrups also have a soothing effect on irritated tissues.

Preparation of Herbal Syrups:

Different steps of Herbal Syrups preparation are as follows:

- **Preparation of decoction of plant material:** Accurately weighed quantity of plant material is extracted with sufficient quantity of boiling water. The boiling is continued till the volume of solution reduces to one fourth of its original volume. Then the liquid is cooled and filtered.
- **To prepare simple syrup:** 40 gm of sucrose is dissolved in sufficient water to get 100 ml of concentrated simple syrup. Then the solution is filtered.
- To prepare final syrup, plant decoction is mixed with simple syrup in 1 : 4 ratio respectively to get 100 ml of herbal syrup.
- Preservatives, colourants and flavouring agents may be added.

Evaluation of Herbal Syrup:

The syrups are evaluated for organoleptic characters, pH, specific gravity, total solid content, thermal stability, degradation product and microbial tests.

- pH can be determined by using pH meter.
- **Determination of total solid content:** To determine total solid content accurately weighed, quantity of syrup sample is placed in the empty pre-weighed petridish. Sample is evaporated using water bath and further dried at low temperature. The final weight of petri dish is again taken. The total solid content is determined by using following formula.

$$\text{Total solid conents} = \frac{\text{Weight of petri dish after drying} - \text{Weight of empty petri dish}}{\text{Sample weight}} \times 100$$

- Ostwald viscometer is used to determine viscosity of syrup.
- Specific gravity is measured using Pcynometer 25°C.
- **Stability testing:** Stability testing of herbal syrups is carried out by storing the syrups at room temperature and accelerated temperature conditions. Then at the interval of 24 hr, 48 hr and 72 hr syrups are evaluated for physicochemical parameters, turbidity, thermal stability, degradation and homogeneity etc.

Dosage: 1 to 2 teaspoonful thrice a day.

Examples: Hempushpa syrup, Brahmi syrup, Cough syrup, Heart tonic syrup.

(e) Oral emulsions: These are liquid dosage forms consisting of two immiscible phases which are stabilized by addition of emulsifying agent. One liquid can be uniformly dispersed in another immiscible liquid in the form of small droplets using emulsification equipment such as agitators, homogenizers, colloid mills and ultrasonic devices etc.

Examples: Intralipid® emulsion, Smoflipid®, Perikabiven® etc.

(f) Aromatic waters: These are water based formulations saturated with essential oil. Aromatic water is prepared by mixing distilled water with one part of essential oil and ten parts of talcum powder. It is shaken well and then kept aside for 12 hours, and then filtered and volume is adjusted. It should be made in small quantities to protect it from decomposition.

Examples: Cardamom water, Peppermint water, Camphor water.

(g) Herbal glycerites: These are tincture like dosage forms which are prepared by extracting herbal drug with 50-60 % of glycerine as extraction medium. The shelf life of glycerites is about six months to two years. This form is suitable for preparation of pediatric medicines. Glycerin cannot be used for herbs containing gums or resins.

Examples: Goldenseal extract, Echinacea herbal extract, Rhodiola extract.

(h) Oxymels: These are sweet and sour formulations containing honey and small amount of vinegar as carrier.

Examples: Oxymels are used for intense herbs like Garlic, Cayenne, and Lobelia.

8.2.2 Solid Herbal Dosage Forms

(a) Herbal tea bags: These bags contain mixture of single or more herbs sufficient for single dose for making infusion. Herbal materials such as dried roots or leaves or flowers are packed into paper or cloth bags. These bags should be free of bleach, gluten and dioxin. The boiling water should be poured on tea bags for making infusion.

(b) Dried powder: Herbs are dried and pulverized to make coarse or fine powder. Traditionally it can be administered directly by mixing it with warm water. It can be available in capsule or sachet form.

(c) Dry extract powders: Dry Plant extract is prepared by evaporation of the solvent used for extraction. Powdered extract can be prepared by spray-drying or freeze-drying of a fluid extract with or without using an adsorbent, or made by drying and milling to produce a powder. It may contain excipients, stabilizers and preservatives. Dry extracts can be incorporated into capsules, tablets or granules.

(d) Herbal mixtures: Herbal mixtures are combination of two or more plants. The plants are dried and pulvarised. Then plant powders are mixed in specific proportions to get herbal mixtures. These are also prepared by mixing dried powdered extracts in specific proportions. Herbal mixtures are generally used to treat various ailments or as health supplements. Examples: herbal mixture for pain, herbal mixture for fever.

(e) Granules: Granules are agglomerations of small spherical particles made from dried fluid extracts. They can be administered after reconstitution with water as solution or suspensions.They can be used for making tablet compression or capsule filling. To prepare granules dried liquid extract is mixed with diluents, binders or other suitable excipients, and then solvent is added to promote agglomeration. Then the wet mass is dried and sized to yield the desired product. Examples: Vasawlehachurna granules, chyavanprash granules, Gastrobeet oral dispersible granules.

(f) Pills: Pills are spherical dosage forms larger than granules made from dried herbal extracts or herbal materials. Pills are made by triturating dried powdered herbs or dry extract with excipients to form mass. Examples: Madhunashinivati, Chandraprabhavati, Khadiradivati etc.

(g) Capsules: These are solid dosage forms containing drug and appropriate filler enclosed in a gelatin container. The dry powdered herbal ingredients or granules are enclosed in hard gelatin capsules while herbal oils and oil soluble herbal ingredients are available in soft gelatin capsules.

Advantages of capsules are:

- They mask unpleasant taste of medicines.
- Provide uniformity of dosage.
- Stability of herbal capsule is relatively better than aqueous herbal preparations.
- Capsules release the content rapidly than tablets.

Examples: Fenugreek capsules, Chlorella capsules, Pudinhara, Moringa capsules etc.

(h) Tablets: Tablets are solid dosage forms made up of the herbal extract powder, plant powder or granule is blended with excipients such as binders, glidants, disintegrating agents, diluents etc. and compressed to form a defined shape and size. Tablets are coated or uncoated. Tablets are coated to mask unpleasant taste of drug and to protect the contents from acidic environment of stomach.

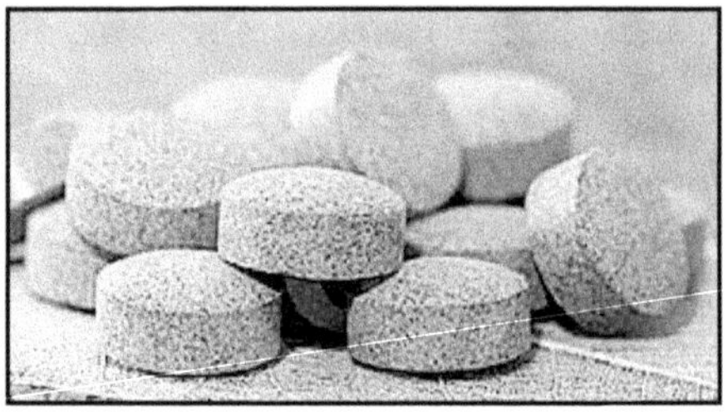

Fig. 8.1: Herbal tablets

Tablets can be prepared by following methods:

(i) Direct compression method: In this method, herbal ingredients are accurately weighed and mixed with appropriate excipients. Then by using tablet compression machine all the ingredients are directly compressed to form tablets.

(ii) Wet granulation method: In this method, accurately weighed herbal extracts are triturated with excipients and binder solution of desired concentration. The wet mass thus obtained is then passed through sieve to obtain granules. Then granules are dried, sieved and mixed with lubricants. These granules are punched by tablet compression machine into desired size and shape.

(iii) Granulation by preliminary compression: This method is used for moisture sensitive drugs. First dry extract powder is compressed to form large slugs or tablets. Then these slugs are break into small pieces and sieved through specific sieve to obtain granules. These granules are mixed with lubricating and disintegrating agents and compressed to form tablets.

Coating of tablets:

Coating is done to mask undesirable colour, odour and taste, to protect from moisture or to make sustained release product. It is carried out using pan coating or press coating method.

Evaluation:

According to various pharmacopoeias tablets are evaluated for pre-compression parameters such as bulk density, tapped density, Hausner's ratio, Carr's index and angle of repose. Post compression evaluation parameters such as hardness, thickness, friability, weight variation and content uniformity should be checked.

Hardness of tablets can be measured by using Monsanto hardness tester or Pfizer hardness tester.

Friability is checked by using friabilator apparatus. It is necessary to evaluate tablets ability to withstand wear and tear.

All tablets in a batch should have uniform weight. So uniformity of weight is determined by weighing 20 tablets randomly and calculating average weight. The individual tablet weight is compared with average weight which should be within prescribed limits given in Pharmacopoeias.

Content of drug in tablet should be uniform and within prescribed limits mentioned in pharmacopoeias.

Disintegration time determines rate of absorption of tablet. It can be determined using disintegration test apparatus.

The dissolution test is carried using dissolution test apparatus. It is important to know rate at which drug will be available for absorption in body.

Examples: Spirulina tablets, Rheumatil tablets, Orthocare tablets, Vitamin C tablets.

(i) Lozenges:

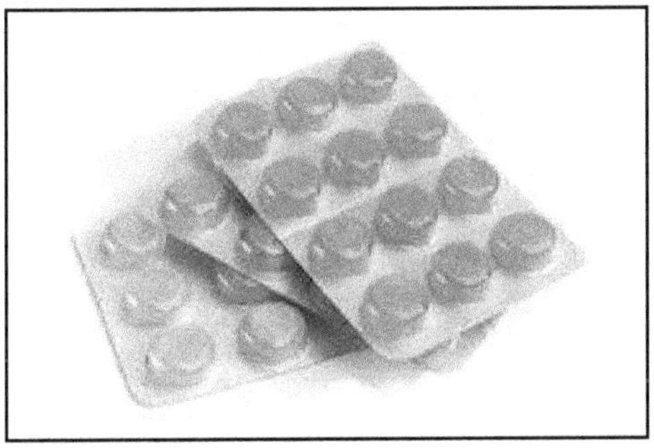

Fig. 8.2: Lozenges in strip pack

These are solid dosage forms which slowly and pleasantly release medication in mouth. It can give local or systemic action. Lozenges contain excipients like flavouring agents and sweetened bases. To make lozenges herbal extract is boiled with sucrose and water. Then colouring and flavouring agents are added during cooling. The molten mass is added into moulds to get lozenges of desired shape.Lozenges are generally used to treat throat infections.

Examples: Zecuf, Koflet lozenges, Herbal cough lozenges etc.

8.2.3 Other Herbal Dosage Forms

(a) Ointments:

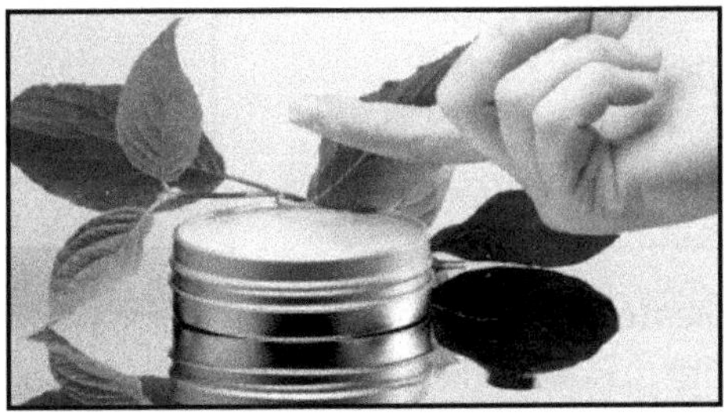

Fig. 8.3: Ointments

These are semi-solid, greasy preparations containing anhydrous immiscible base generally used for skin, rectum or nasal mucosa. Herbal ointments are prepared by mixing finely powdered herbs or extracts with oily base and emulsifying agents. The process of making ointment involves heating of oil phase and aqueous phase separately and then mixing of both the phases while constant stirring until the mixture get congealed.

The ointment bases are as follows:

(a) Hydrocarbon bases like hard or soft paraffin.

(b) Absorption bases like wool fat, bees wax.

(c) Neutral oil bases like olive oil, almond oil.

Examples: Calendula ointment, Herboheal ointment, Pilex, Pain care ointment etc.

(b) Herbal balms: These dosage forms are like ointments used to relieve pain. These are made by mixing herbs having analgesic and anti-inflammatory effect with ointment base.

Examples: Tiger balm, Herbal pain balms, Lip balms.

(c) Herbal creams: Creams are semi-solid dosage forms containing herb in hydrophilic base. Herbal creams are prepared by mixing finely powdered herbal drug or an extract in cream base. It has relatively shorter shelf life as compared to ointments.

Examples: Herbal fairness cream, Baby creams, Acne control creams.

(d) Inhalations: Inhalations are preparations intended to be used in bronchial tubes or lungs in the form of aerosols. These are of two types dry powder inhalers or inhalation liquid preparations. Traditionally steam inhalation method is used to administer volatile substances from herbal drugs.To prepare dry powder inhalers dry extracts are pulverized into fine particles. Then it is mixed with excipients to make homogeneous mixture. For liquid Inhalation preparations dry herbal extracts are mixed with a vehicle to form solution or suspension and pH is adjusted.

Examples: Astha aid drops, Karvol plus inhalation capsules.

(e) Plasters and patches: These are made by spreading soft or dry herbal extract on support made up of fabric or synthetic resin. Plasters and patches are intended to use topically on the skin and deliver the active ingredients through the skin, usually to get relief of pain, backache or sore muscles. Example: Herbal pain relieve patch, Capsicum patch, Herbal medicated plasters etc.

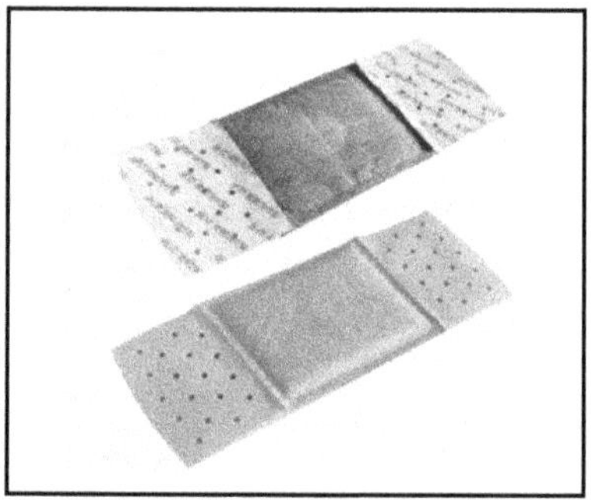

Fig. 8.4: Plaster and Patches

(f) Medicated oils: Medicated oils are prepared by mixing, macerating or boiling herbal drug, extract of fresh juice with suitable fixed oil. The drug is boiled with oil to remove water completely, then filtered and cooled. Medicated oils are mostly used topically or sometimes orally.

Examples: Indulekha oil, Tea tree oil, Sesa oil, Peppermint oil etc.

(g) Herbal soaps: These are prepared by incorporating herbal drugs having antifungal or antimicrobial properties with detergent base.

Examples: Neem and turmeric soap, Herbal care soap, Papaya skin whitening soap.

(h) Herbal pastes: These are similar to ointment which contains 50% of drug powder incorporated in fatty base. For topical use herbal ingredients are dispersed in fatty base while for oral use they are dispersed in aqueous base. Herbal pastes are less greasy than ointments.

Examples: Dantkanti toothpaste, Miswak, Aloevera toothpaste, complete care toothpaste.

(i) Herbal suppositories and Herbal pessaries: Herbal suppositories are made by mixing finely powdered herbs or extracts with cocoa butter base. Herbal suppositories are used to treat inflammation of the nasal mucosa, and membranes and used as laxative. Herbal pessaries meant for vaginal use are made by incorporating herb powder or extract in glycerated-gelatin base. Examples: Tea tree pessaries, neem oil suppository, Herbal vaginal pessaries.

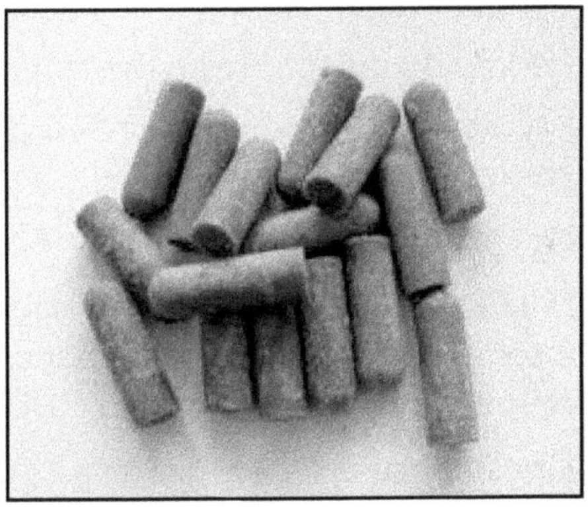

Fig. 8.5: Suppositories

(j) Herbal liniments: Herbal liniments are used in treatment of soreness in muscles and ligaments and pain. They should not be applied on cut or broken skin. Liniments are prepared by using oil or alcoholic extracts of heat producing herbs like cayenne.

Examples: Liniment plus, penil, pain fighter liniment.

8.3 NOVEL DOSAGE FORMS

Various conventional dosage forms release the drug immediately causing blood level fluctuations. Hence maintain drug levels in therapeutically effective range novel dosage forms are developed. Novel Drug delivery System (NDDS) means the approaches, formulations, technologies, and systems to transport a pharmaceutical compound in the body so that it can safely achieve its desired therapeutic effects. NDDS is nothing but the combination of advanced techniques and new dosage forms in which drug is delived by the system other than conventional drug delivery system. It has various advantages over conventional dosage forms.

Advantages of Novel Dosage Forms:

- Solubility and bioavailability of phytoconstituents is enhanced.
- Distribution and pharmacological activity is enhanced.
- Drugs can be released at predetermined rate and deliver the drug at the site of action.
- Produce less toxicity as novel dosage forms avoid accumulation of drug to non-target areas.
- Stability of phytoconstituents can be improved.
- Easily administered to pediatric and geriatric patients.

- Phytoconstituents are susceptible to acidic environment and undergo liver metabolism. Novel dosage forms avoid degradation or presystemic metabolism of drug.
- Sustained drug delivery can be achieved.

Disadvantages Dosage Forms:

- Conventional dosage forms cannot exert effect for longer period of time.
- Phytoconstituents cannot be released at desired site of action.
- Desired therapeutic response cannot be achieved.
- Phytoconstituents have limited solubility and bioavailability when administered as conventional dosage forms.

8.3.1 Types of Novel Dosage Forms

Different types of novel dosage forms are mouth-dissolving tablets, liposomes, phytosomes, pharmacosomes, nanoparticles, microspheres, transfersomes, ethosomes, transdermal drug delivery system (TDDS), and proniosomes etc.

1. Liposomes:

Liposomes are microparticulate or colloidal carriers, having 0.05–5.0 μm diameter. Liposomes consist of polar liquid and have hydrophilic and lipophilic groups. Liposomes are artificial microscopic vesicles containing one or more phospholipid layers enclosing an aqueous core. In liposomes, hydrophilic heads are orient towards the water compartment while the lipophilic tails orient towards the center of the vesicle, thus they form a bilayer. They are used to convey vaccines, drugs, enzymes or other substances to target cells or organs.

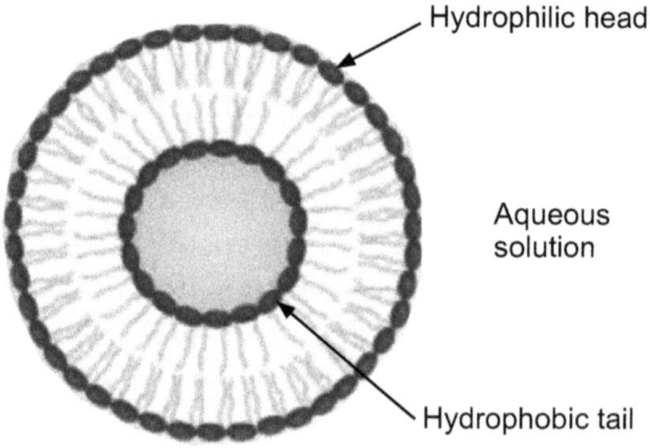

Fig. 8.6: Liposome drug delivery system

Preparation: It is prepared by basic steps like:

- Lipids are isolated using organic solvent.
- Lipids are dispersing in the aqueous media. Drug loading is carried out by active and passive loading techniques.
- Purification and evaluation of liposome.

Advantages:

- They are highly biocompatible.
- They are biodegradable, biologically inactive, non-immunogenic in nature.
- Easy to prepare.
- Acts as carrier for hydrophilic, amphiphilic, and lipophilic compounds
- Their pharmacokinetic properties can be easily modulated.
- It can be used to produce controlled release or sustained release formulations.

Examples:

- Therapeutic efficacy of anticancer drug ampelopsin is improved.
- Paclitaxel, anticancer drug liposome, shows pH sensitivity and improved entrapment efficiency.
- Antioxidant and chemopreventive Catechins shows increased permeation through skin.
- Quercetin and rutin liposomes shows enhanced haemoglobin binding property.
- Capsaicin liposomes shows prolong action and enhanced permeation.
- Usnic acid liposomes shows enhanced solubility and prolong action.

2. Phytosomes:

The term phyto means plant and some means cell like. Phytosomes are novel dosage forms of standardized plant extract or water soluble phytoconstituents which are entrapped into phospholipids to produce lipid compatible molecular complexes. It shows enhanced absorption and bioavailability.

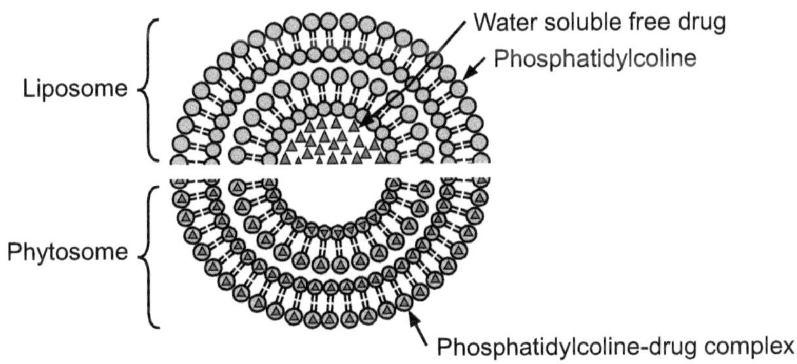

Fig. 8.7: Comparison of Phytosomes and Liposomes

Preparation: To prepare phytosomes, phospholipids are dissolved in organic solvent. Then extract of phytoconstituents like flavonoids or terpenoids are mixed in above solution in 1:1 ratio. The isolation of phytosomal complex can be carried out by precipitation with solvents containing aliphatic hydrocarbons or by lyophilization or by spray drying. Phospholipid like phosphatidylcholine isolated from soybean is commonly used in preparation of phytosomes. Phytoconstituents attach phospholipid by forming a chemical bond.

Advantages of Phytosomes:

- Phytosomes can give protection against destruction of herb by digestive secretions and gut bacteria.
- Proper drug delivery at site of action.
- The nutrient safety of herbal drugs is retained.
- Reduction in dose, enhanced absorption and bioavailability of active principle.
- Entrapment efficiency is high and predetermined.
- Better stability due to the formation of chemical bonds.
- Phosphatidylcholine used in process acts as a carrier, hepatoprotective and nourishes the skin.
- Superior toliposomes in skin care products.
- Have greater clinical benefit.

Difference between Liposomes And Phytosomes:

To prepare Liposomes water soluble phytoconstituents are mixed with phosphatidylcholine in a definite ratio under suitable conditions like phytosomes. The number of phosphatidylcholine molecules surrounds the drug molecule and there is no chemical bond formation. But in case of phytosomes phytoconstituents get attached to phospholipid by forming a chemical bond. Due to lesser phospholipid content, absorption and bioavailability of phytosomes is more than liposomes.

Evaluation of Phytosomes:

Efficiency of phytosomes depends on physical size, membrane permeability, percentage of entrapped solutes, and chemical composition of materials. The phytosomes are evaluated for vesicle size and zeta potential, entrapment efficiency, transition temperature and surface tension. The spectroscopic evaluation is also carried out to study bond formation.

Applications of Phytosomes:

- Silymarin phytosome showed increase bioavailability due to enhanced lipophilicity and therapeutic effects than silybin. Silymarin phytosome also exhibited better hepatoprotective activity than silymarin. As per one study, absorption of silybin from silybin phytosome was found to be seven times greater as compared to the absorption of silybin from regular milk thistle.
- Green tea contains therapeutically significant polyphenols which have problem of poor bioavailability. Phytosomes of green tea polyphenols showed improved bioavailability and better antioxidant effects.
- Quercetin phytosomes exhibited improved hepatoprotective effect.
- Grape seed phytosomes showed improved antioxidant and cardio protective effects.
- Antioxidant activity of cucumin phytosomes was enhanced.
- Naringin phytosomes exhibit better antioxidant activity, prolonged duration of action, due to decrease in the rapid elimination than pure drug alone.
- Ginkgo phytosomes show improved effects against asthma.

3. Nanoparticles:

Nanoparticles are the nano-sized particles, ranging from 10–1000 nm, containing synthetic or semisynhthetic or herbal drugs. These are used as carrier for hydrophilic and hydrophobic drugs. In nano-spheres, active ingredient is dispersed in a matrix type structure whereas the nanocapsules contain drug enclosed in a polymeric membrane. Nanoparticles are prepared with the objective to control particle size, surface properties of drug and to achieve the site-specific action of the drug.

Preparation: Nanoparticles are prepared from dispersion of polymers by different techniques like nanoprecipitation, emulsification /solvent diffusion, salting out, dialysis and supercritical fluid technology etc.

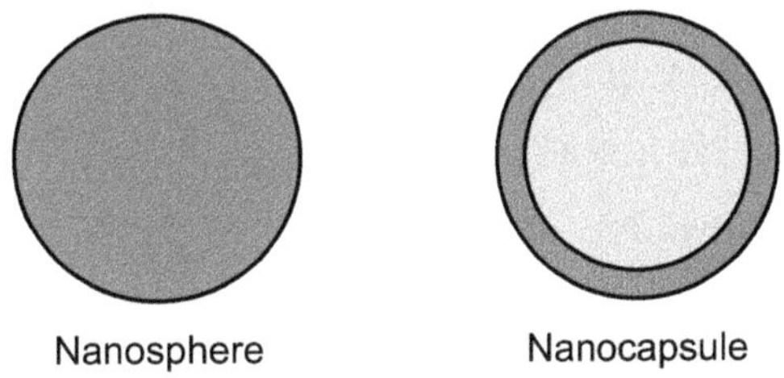

Fig. 8.8: Nanoparticle drug delivery system

Advantages:

Nanoparticles can enhance compound solubility, reduce doses, can deliver drug to site of action and improve absorbance.

Examples:

- Artemisinin nano capsules showed sustained drug release anticancer activity.
- Curcuminoids solid lipid nanoparticles are anticancer and antioxidant agent and showed prolonged release of the curcuminoids.
- Improved bioavailability was observed in Glycyrrhizic acid and naringenin nanoparticle.
- Prolonged blood circulation and high accumulation in tumors was observed in Camptothecin encapsulated nanoparticle.
- Enhanced bioavailability and sustained drug release was observed in case of anticancer Taxel nanoparticle.

(4) Microsphere:

Microsheres are spherical micro particles having diameter of 1-1000 mm. They are made up of biodegradable polymers like polylactic acid, copolymer of lactic acid, glycolic acid, albumin dextran sulfate and fibrinogen.

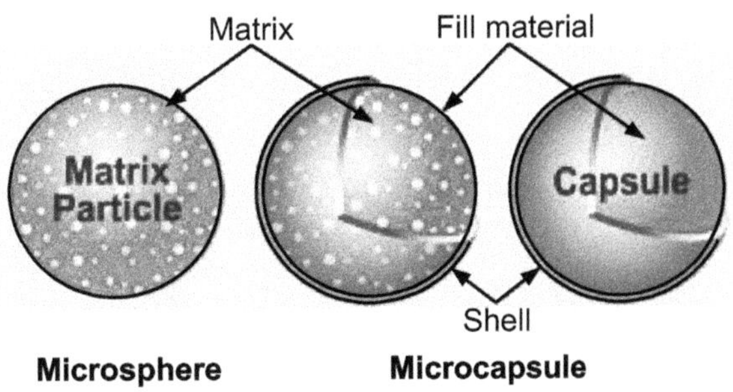

Fig. 8.9: Microsphere drug delivery system

Preparation: Microspheres are prepared by different techniques such as Spray drying, Solvent evaporation, Single and double emulsion technique, Phase separation coacervation technique, Solvent extraction and quassi emulsion solvent diffusion.

Advantages of Microsphere:

- Microspheres can be ingested or injected. So the administration of medication via micro-particulate system is more advantageous.
- It is easy to get desired release profiles and site-specific delivery of drugs.
- Easy drug release from the formulation.
- Do not affect drug activity.

Examples:

- Rutin-alginate-chitosan microcapsules able to target cardiovascular and cerebrovascular regions.
- Quercetin microspheres showed significant decrease in dose.
- Zedoary oil microsphere showed higher bioavailability and sustained release action.
- Camptothesin loaded microspheres showed prolong drug action.

(5) Ethosomes:

Ethosomes are nano-vesicles made up of phospholipids and have high content of ethanol i.e. 20%-45%. These are for transdermal delivery of drugs. Due to high ethanol content ethosomes can disrupt the membrane barrier of skin, penetrate deeper skin layers and thus enhances the solubility and permeability of drug.

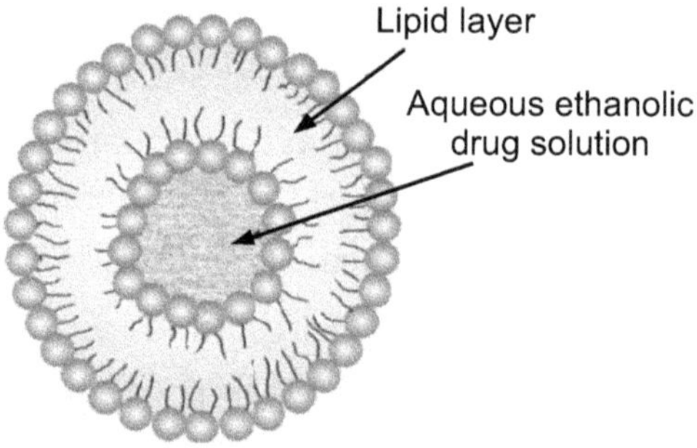

Fig. 8.10: Ethosomal drug delivery system

Preparation: Ethosomes are prepared by Cold method, Hot method and Classic mechanical dispersion method.

Advantages of Ethosomes:

- They helps to improve transdermal permeation of drug through skin.
- Ethosomes can be used for drug delivery of wide variety of drugs.
- As it is in semisolid form, provides improved patient compliance.

Examples:

- Liquorice ethosomes showed improved anti-inflammatory activity and sustained release action.
- Cannabis ethosomes showed improved patient compliance and increased skin permeation.
- Improved bioavailability was observed in case of curcumin ethosomes.
- Improved permeability is observed in case of *Sophora alopecuerides* ethosomes.

(6) Transferosomes:

These are also vesicular system consisting of phospholipids, 10-25% surfactant and 3-10% ethanol. Tranferosomes can deliver the drug in upper layers of skin. It exhibit its action by using the hydration and osmotic properties of skin. It has advantages similar to ethosomes.

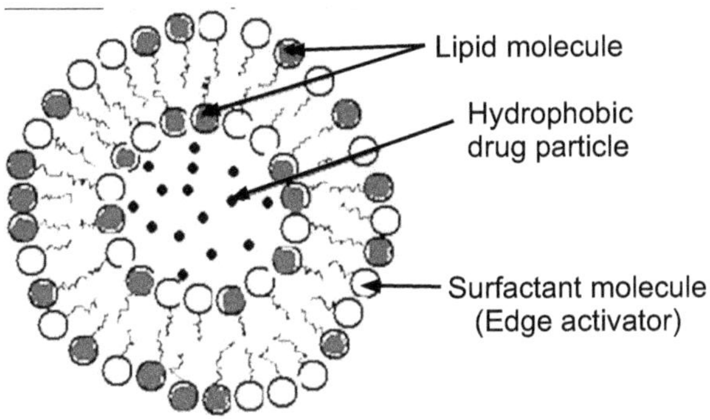

Fig. 8.11: Transfersomes drug delivery system

Preparation: Transfersomes are prepared by thin film hydration method and modified hand shaking, lipid film hydration technique.

Examples:

- Capsicum transfersomes showed enhanced skin penetration.
- Increase in permeability observed in case of vinca and turmeric transfersomes.
- Colchicum transfersomes exhibited reduced GIT effects.

(7) Niosomes:

Niosomes are also multilamellar vesicles similar to liposomes and made up of non-ionic surfactants like alkyl or dialkylpolyglycerol ether group and cholesterol. Liposomes have certain disadvantages like they are expensive, their ingredients are chemically unstable, their handling requires special training and difficult to purify. Niosomes do not exhibit such problems.

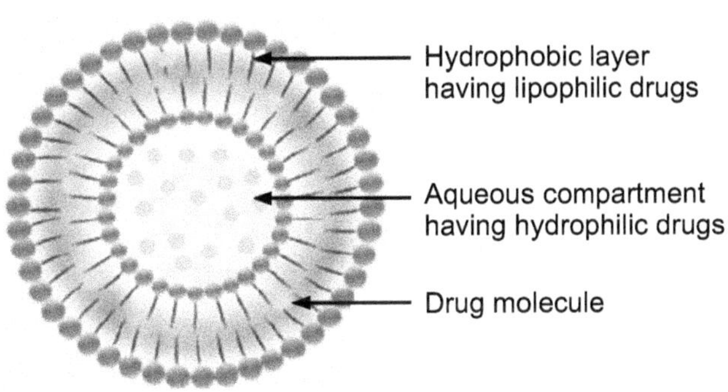

Fig. 8.12: Niosomes drug delivery system

(8) Proniosomes:

Proniosomes are water soluble carrier particles coated with surfactant. Before use, these are hydrated to form niosomes by agitation. These are gel formulation.

Examples: Levonorgestrel proniosomes gel or patch, Indomethacin oral proniosomes.

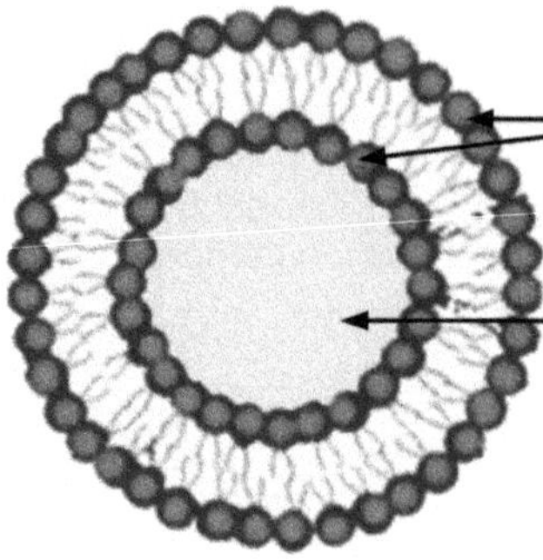

Fig. 8.13: Proniosomes drug delivery system

(9) Emulsion:

Emulsion is a biphasic system containing oily phase and aqueous phase. One phase is dispersed in the other phase in the form of minute droplets having diameter from 0.1 μm to 100 μm. Emulsion may be ordinary emulsion [0.1 – 100 μm], micro-emulsion [10 – 100 nm] and sub-micro-emulsion [100 – 600 nm]. Lipophilic drugs form o/w or o/w/o emulsion while water soluble drug form w/o or w/o/w emulsion.

Preparation: Emulsions are prepared by various techniques such as Phase inversion method, Sonication, High pressure homogenizer, Micro fluidization and using high amplitude ultrasound.

Advantages of Emulsion:

Emulsions are made with the objectives to get sustained release action, improve stability, improve penetration, to reduce drug's stimulus to tissues and to get easy intramuscular or subcutaneous drug delivery.

Examples:

- *Silibummarianum* exhibited increase in therapeutic action and better drug solubility.
- Residence time and absorption of berberis was improved in emulsion formulation.
- Emulsion containing colchicum showed better oral bioavailability.
- Curcuma *zedooria* emulsion showed improved aqueous dispersibility, stability and oral bioavailability.
- *Genistatinctoria* exhibited improved skin permeation.

(10) Transdermal Drug Delivery Systems (TDDS):

It is novel drug delivery system in which drug is delivered in the form of patches through the skin. By TDDS drug can be administered into systemic circulation at a predetermined rate over a prolonged period of time.

Preparation: The basic components of TDDS are polymer matrix or drug reservoir, drug, permeation enhancers, pressure sensitive adhesive, backing laminates, release liner and excipients like plasticizers and solvents etc. It can be prepared by following methods:

- **Polymer membrane permeation-controlled TDDS:** In this system, the drug reservoir is enclosed between an impermeable backing layer and a rate controlling membrane. The drug is released only through the rate controlling membrane.
- **Matrix diffusion controlled TDDS** is prepared by dispersing the drug homogeneously in a hydrophilic or lipophilic polymer matrix.
- **Micro reservoir controlled TDDS** is a combination of reservoir and matrix-dispersion systems.

Advantages of TDDS:

- It eliminates first pass metabolism.
- Improved therapeutic efficiency.
- Frequency of drug administration can be reduced.
- Less side effects and improved patient compliance.
- Load on digestive tract and liver is reduced.
- Convenient to administer.

8.4 DIFFERENCE BETWEEN CONVENTIONAL HERBAL DOSAGE FORMS AND NOVEL DOSAGE FORMS

Sr. No.	Conventional Herbal Dosage Forms	Novel Dosage Forms
1.	Drug is rapidly and completely released immediately after administration.	Drug release can be modified for extended period.
2.	Absorption is rate limiting step.	Rate limiting step is drug release.
3.	Blood level of drug fluctuates.	Constant blood level can be achieved.
4.	There is risk of overmedication or under medication.	Risk of overmedication or under medication is reduced.
5.	Less patient compliance.	More patient compliance.
6.	Dosage adjustment is difficult.	Dosage adjustment is easy.
7.	More total dose is required during the course of therapy.	Less total dose is required.
8.	More GIT side effects.	Less GIT side effects.

Contd...

9.	Not suitable for drugs having short half life.	No problems for drugs with short half life.
10.	Not suitable for chronic diseases due to risk of symptom breakthrough.	Can be used to treat chronic diseases.

QUESTIONS

1. What are herbal dosage forms? Discuss about different types of herbal solid dosage forms.
2. Explain in detail about herbal formulation: Syrup.
3. Describe in detail about various liquid herbal dosage forms.
4. Discuss in detail about formulation and evaluation of herbal tablets.
5. Write an elaborative note on herbal semisolid dosage forms.
6. What are novel herbal dosage forms? Give their advantages.
7. Discuss in detail about Liposomes.
8. Write in detail about advantages, preparation and applications of phytosomes.
9. Explain in detail about different types of Novel dosage form.
10. How liposomes differ from phytosomes?
11. Differentiate between Conventional and Novel herbal dosage forms.

❖❖❖

UNIT-IV

Chapter...9

EVALUATION OF DRUGS

Objectives

- To learn about concept of WHO and ICH guidelines for the acessment of herbal drugs.
- To understand concept of stability tesing of herbal drugs.

9.1 WHO & ICH GUIDELINES FOR THE ASSESSMENT OF HERBAL DRUGS

Introduction

Quality is conformance to requirement. When product matches with stated or implied labelled claim, then product is said to be of good quality. In case of herbal drug, quality refers to identity, purity, safety and finally efficacy. **Evaluation is checking of quality, purity and efficacy of drug.** It also involves determination of adulteration. So evaluation of herbal drugs involves checking of various parameters which gives idea regarding quality of drug.

Table 9.1: Basic Evaluation of Crude Drug

Sr.	Type of Evaluation	Criteria Involved	Examples
1.	Morphological / organoleptic evaluation	Sensory characters like colour, size, shape, taste, odour or other morphological features.	Characteristic smell of umbelliferous fruit, colour of barks like Cinchona, Cinnamon.
2.	Microscopic evaluation	Microscopic characters like type and number of stomata, stomatal index, vein islet number, vein termination number, trichomes.	Unicellular lignified trichome present in *Nux vomica*, paracytic stomata in Senna.
3.	Chemical evaluation	Chemical nature or contents are checked with various tests.	Presence of alkaloid can be checked with Dragendorff's reagent, presence of protein can be checked with Millen's, biuret, Ninhydrin test.

Contd...

4.	Physical evaluation	Physical properties like ash value, moisture content, melting point, solubility, can be checked with different instruments.	Viscosity, melting point, solubility, moisture content, volatile matter, specific gravity, density, optical rotation, refractive index, bitterness value, hemolytic activity, swelling index, foaming index, ash value and extractable by hot extraction or cold maceration.
5.	Biological evaluation	This includes the estimation of crude drugs or preparations on living organisms or animals.	Checking of hepatoprotective, hypoglycemic, anti-inflammatory activity on different animals.
6.	Chromatographic evaluation	Use of chromatographic techniques for separation and purification.	TLC, HPTLC, HPLC, GC, GLC Techniques.
7.	Spectro-photometric evaluation	Used for determination of structure of compound.	UV, IR, NMR, MASS, X ray diffraction methods.

Role of ICH in Assessment of Herbal Drugs:

ICH is the 'International Council for Harmonisation of Technical Requirements for Pharmaceuticals for Human Use'. ICH is non-profit association started in 1990 to co-ordinate regulatory bodies and pharmaceutical industry. ICH brings together experts from all fields to discuss scientific and technical aspects of drug registration. The mission behind ICH is to achieve greater harmonisation worldwide for safe, effective, and high quality medicines. ICH brings uniformity through the development of guidelines via a process of scientific consensus with different experts from regulatory field and industry. These guidelines bring uniformity throughout world and avoid confusion. ICH does not give separate guidelines only for herbal drugs as such. But all herbal drug industries follow these guidelines in all aspects whichever applicable to them. So now-a-days, drug development, formulation, analytical method development, stability testing, clinical trials and other activity related to herbal drugs are done according to ICH guidelines. This has resulted in good quality of herbal drugs.

ICH guidelines are divided into four types: QSEM (Quality guidelines, Safety guidelines, Efficacy guidelines and Multidisciplinary guidelines).

- Quality guidelines include stability, analytical validation and quality of biotechnological product, GMP, pharmaceutical development, development and manufacture of drug substance.

- Safety guidelines of ICH include guidelines to uncover potential risks like carcinogenicity, genotoxicity and reproductive toxicity. It also includes pharmacology studies, immunotoxicity studies, photo safety evaluation and non-clinical paediatric safety.
- Efficacy guidelines mainly covers the design, conduct, safety and reporting of clinical trials. It also covers Good Clinical Practices, novel types of medicines derived from biotechnological processes and the use of pharmacogenetics/ pharmacogenomics techniques.
- Multidisciplinary guidelines are important for areas other than quality, safety and efficacy. These guidelines cover the ICH medical terminology (MedDRA), the Common Technical Document (CTD). The development of Electronic Standards for the Transfer of Regulatory Information (ESTRI), gene therapy, mutagenic impurities, bioanalytical method validation is also addressed by these guidelines.

Role of WHO in Assessment of Herbal Drugs:

As ICH is mainly related with pharmaceutical industry, World Health Organization (WHO) as name indicates is more related with health and disease. The World Health Organization is specialized agency of the United Nations. It was established in 1948 for international health matters and public health. World health Organization has wide area and several functions including provision of reliable information and advice in the field of human health. WHO deals with diseases as well as give guidelines for traditional and herbal medicine. According to WHO survey, more than 60% of world population use one or either form of traditional medicines.

Herbal medicine is the oldest form of healthcare used from many centuries. Herbs had been used worldwide by all cultures throughout history. The plants have provided us food, clothing, shelter and most importantly medicine. Much of the medicinal use of plants may be developed through observations of wild animals or by trial and error. Conventionally use of herbal drugs was limited. Many of the plant species are used in only particular area of the world, but because of the globalization, now used all over the world. Herbs and plants can be processed and used in different ways and forms. One can use the entire herb, extracts, teas, syrups, essential oils, ointments, liniments, capsules, and tablets. The growing demand for herbal drugs has forced large scale manufacturing as a routine thing. Large scale production comes with different issues related to quality of herbal drugs because of longer storage times and possible product deterioration. Therefore, the need for the quality assurance and stability of the product become important. Herbal drugs are also required to maintain their identity, strength, quality, and purity throughout the shelf life. Commonly-available herbal dosage forms mainly include herbal tablets, herbal capsules, herbal creams, ointments, decoctions, herbal teas, tinctures, herbal soaps and other forms. Herbal drugs vary in chemical constituents so the herb extracts. Apart from this, processing conditions also affect the finished product. Different extraction conditions like solvent, temperature, extraction time, and type of extracts also make difference. Herbal products may be defined as plants, parts of plants or extracts from plants that are used in healthcare or in combating the disease. To avoid confusion with culinary herbs, herbs and plant extracts that have some association with medical uses are referred to as 'herbal medicinal products'.

Concept of traditional medicine according WHO includes different health practices, approaches, knowledge and beliefs. It also covers plant, animal and/or mineral drugs, spiritual therapies, manual techniques and exercises to maintain well-being, as well as to treat, diagnose or prevent illness. Natural products obviously include drugs from plants, animals as well as minerals. Among these plants serve as most valuable source for curing many ailments.

WHO Guidelines:

In order to provide affordable and accessible medicines to world, WHO is promoting natural products. In order to ensure good quality medicine WHO has also provided different guidelines. These guidelines are the most widely used and accepted by the industries, academics, research institutes etc. Along with Good Manufacturing Practices, Good Laboratory Practices, the latest of WHO guidelines are Good Agricultural and Collection Practices (GACP). In general, it provides the basic criteria for evaluation of safety and quality of herbal medicines. According to these guidelines, the safety and quality of drugs derived from medicinal plants depend on many factors. There are several factors like methods of cultivation, harvesting, processing, transport and storage can have an impact on the quality of herbal products.

The guidelines are divided into five sections.

Section 1: Gives a general introduction.

Section 2: Discuss good agricultural practices for medicinal plants.

Section 3: Disucss good collection practices for medicinal plants.

Section 4: Describes common technical aspects of good agricultural practices for medicinal plants and good collection practices for medicinal plants.

Section 5: Considers other relevant issues.

Guidelines to carry out the standardization of crude as well as finished herbal products are also provided by WHO. These guidelines include various parameters like foreign matter, organoleptic evaluation, ash values and extractive values, volatile matter, moisture content determination, toxic contaminants, microbial contamination, pesticide residues, radioactive contamination and heavy metals.

The salient features of WHO guidelines are: (i) Quality assessment (ii) Stability (iii) Safety assessment (iv) Assessment of efficacy. Thus, these guidelines are helpful in quality control of herbal medicines right from collection of raw drug material up to the processing and obtaining the finished product. These guidelines for the assessment of herbal medicines help government regulatory authorities, scientific bodies and industry.

Herbal or natural does not mean it is always safe. Adverse effects or toxicities of herbal medicines can arise because of the wrong identification of medicinal plants, incorrect dosing and errors while using by consumers, interactions with other medicines, and use of adultrated products contaminated with hazardous substances.

Therefore WHO has developed guidelines for safety monitoring of herbal medicines which includes:

- Expanding the source of case reports.
- Establishing a system for the exchange of regulatory and quality information on herbal medicines among national pharmacovigilance centres and national drug regulatory authorities.
- Strengthening capacity to carry out monitoring of herbal medicines at national pharmacovigilance centres.
- Developing a standard classification and/or coding system for herbal medicines, with standardized terms and definitions.
- Strengthening communication and awareness at all levels (global, regional, national, local and community) and among key players (international bodies, regulatory authorities, national pharmacovigilance centres, health-care providers and consumers).

It is not a mandatory guideline for any country, but it is a model or a sort of checklist which any country can use to make their own national regulations. On this background, it is beyond doubt that WHO addressed **most valuable and important issue of natural products**.

WHO Guidelines describes different quality assessment parameters for herbal drugs:

- Control of quality of herbal drugs.
- Assessment of safety based on experience or toxicological studies.
- Assessment of efficacy through biological activity evaluations.
- Stability assessment and shelf life.

Three major steps to assure quality in herbal drugs as per WHO/ ICH guidelines are:

1. Identification/ ensuring genuinity.
2. Purity/ ensuring safety.
3. Ensuring efficacy.

Herbal drugs are primarily evaluated based on their efficacy and safety to ensure quality. Being complex in nature with different groups of primary and secondary metabolites, assessment of quality is equally important. In addition to this intrinsic complexity, other contaminants are critical to their efficacy and safety of herbal drugs. Raw material sourced from right geography, collected in the suitable season, properly authenticated, documented appropriately and processed with stringent systems of manufacturing can **ensure good quality of medicine**.

Assessment of Quality:

Quality of herbs used in the formulation start with identification and procurement. Sourcing should comply with Good Agricultural and Collection Practices (GACP) as per WHO guidelines. Main objectives of GACP are to assure the quality of plant material used as the source for herbs. This also helps to encourage and support the sustainable cultivation and collection of plants of good quality. This also helps in the conservation of plants and also the environment. Good Agricultural and Collection Practices (GACP) also provides assurance about quality. Creation of Standard Operating Procedures (SOPs) is first step for Good agricultural and collection practices. It starts with SOPs for collection, post-harvest treatments and maintaining traceability. An expert taxonomist can be used for this certification. Plant authentication can be also carried out by macroscopic, microscopic character sets and their phytochemical (secondary metabolites) profiles. Monographs are most useful for identification of herbs based on morphological and anatomical characters. In phytochemical profiling, the chromatographic finger print of the sample developed using a validated analytical method is compared with a botanical reference material of the same species. Apart from chemical fingerprints in addition to above conventional methods, modern methods based on genomic profiling and DNA barcoding can be used as complementary techniques for correct botanical identity.

Pharmaceutical Assessment:

- Pharmaceutical assessment includes all important aspects of the quality assessment of herbal medicines. It should be sufficient to make reference to a pharmacopoeia monograph if one exists.
- Availability of monograph is very important and official pharmacopoeia should contain such monograph for checking of quality.
- All procedures should be in according to the code of good manufacturing practices.

Crude Plant Material:

- Correct identification of a plant should be done with botanical identification including definition, including genus, species and authority.
- Description of drug should contain the part of the plant (root, stem, leaves, bark) from which the medicine is prepared. It should contain information regarding condition of material like fresh, dried or traditionally processed.
- The active and characteristic constituents or marker should be specified with content limits.
- Possible impurities, foreign matter, and microbial content or load should be defined or limited for reference.
- Voucher specimen number or herbarium number, from each lot of plant material need to be authenticated by a qualified botanist. This record should be stored for at least a 10-year period for future reference.

Plant Preparations:

- Plant preparations are powdered plant materials, extracts, tinctures, fatty or essential oils, expressed juices and preparations whose production involves different processes like fractionation, purification or concentration.
- Detail method of preparation should be described. All other substances added should be mentioned in the manufacturing procedures.
- Identification method should be available for plant preparation like assay of the plant preparation. If assay is not available, or assay of an active principle is not possible, 'chromatographic fingerprint' should be used to assess quality of the preparation.

Finished Product:

- Detail manufacturing procedure and formula; amount of excipients used should be described. A finished product specification should be mentioned in detail.
- When single active constituent identification or quantification is not possible, 'Chromatographic fingerprint' should be used to check quality of the preparation. The finished product should meet specified requirements for particular dosage forms.
- For imported finished products, confirmation of the regulatory status in the country of origin should be followed. In this case, WHO Certification Scheme on the Quality of Pharmaceutical Products Moving in International Commerce should be used.

Stability:

- WHO has given guidelines for checking physical and chemical stability of the product in the container in which it is to be marketed. Stability should be tested under defined storage conditions and the shelf life should be established.

Assessment of Safety:

- Safety assessment of herbal drugs should cover all relevant aspects. With the growing market demand on herbal products, there are still concerns associated with their safety. Surprisingly, not more than 10% of herbal drugs in the global market are actually standardized to known active marker. At the same time, toxicity data is not available. Checking purity also attribute to impurities in herbal drugs. Impurities include heavy metal, pesticide residues, and aflatoxins/mycotoxins. Herbal drugs may contain heavy metal because of several reasons including contamination from soils. Heavy metals like Pb, Hg, As and Cd are tested in herbal products with help of Atomic Absorption Spectroscopy (AAS), inductively coupled plasma Mass Spectrometry (ICP-MS). The allowable limits for these metals are prescribed by WHO and individual herbal monographs of British and US pharmacopoeias. Pesticide residues from fungicides, insecticides, and weedicides like organochlorines, organophosphorus, carbamates, benzimidazoles, dithiocarbamates, and amino acid herbicides are used in plant cultivation. There is limit prescribed by guidelines. Toxins from different fungi like aflatoxins, ochratoxin A, fumonisins, zearalenone, and deoxynivalenol are also have neurotoxic, carcinogenic, immunotoxic, and teratogenic effects. This is serious concern about safety. Toxicity testing using harmonized guidelines from WHO, ICH, OECD, schedule Y in a Good Laboratory Practice (GLP) can minimise risks which are associated with use of herbal drugs.

- In case of traditional medicine, as drugs have been in use without harm, no specific restrictive regulatory action should be undertaken unless new evidence demands a specific risk.
- A review of the relevant literature about safety should be provided with original articles or references to the original articles. If official monograph/review results exist, reference can be made to them.
- Health hazards associated with long term ise of some herbal medicines are very crucial. In recent years, there is much concern about the long-term hazards of some herbal medicines.
- Pharmacovigilance of herbal medicines also properly documented.

Toxicological Studies:

- Assessment of herbal drug should contain toxicological studies also with required literature.

Documentation of Safety Based on Experience:

- For assessment of safety, documentation of a long period of use should be important. When there are no detailed toxicological studies, documented experiences of long-term use without evidence of safety problems should form the basis of the risk assessment.
- Even if herbal drugs are used for over a long period, chronic toxicological risks may be possible. In such case, period of use, the health disorders treated, the number of users and the countries with experience should be specified. In case of known toxicological risk, necessary toxicity data must be submitted.
- Dose dependant or independent risk should be documented. In case of dose dependant risk, the dosage specification must be an important part of the risk assessment. Nature of risk should be explained.
- Documentation should be carried out with respect to potential for misuse, abuse and drug dependence. If documentation of long-term traditional use is not possible, doubts on safety, toxicity data should be submitted.

Assessment of Efficacy:

- Assessment of efficacy should cover all important aspects related to activity, clinical use and traditional use. A review of the relevant literature including research studies should be taken into account. Bioactivity-based detection of marker(s) can provide valuable information about phytochemicals responsible for biological effects. The connection of biological effects with the identification and quantification of phytochemicals is critical for addressing quality. Also, synergy or additive activity can be checked through biological activity. Efficacy studies can be carried out to check levels of efficacy. Identification of the bioactive molecule and its qualitative and quantitative analysis is required for good quality herbal drugs.

Activity:

- The pharmacological/therapeutic and clinical effects of the active ingredients and constituents with therapeutic activity should be specified or described.
- Evidence required supporting indications.
- The indication or use of the medicine should be specified. In the case of traditional medicines, the requirements for proof of efficacy should depend on the kind of indication.
- For minor diseases and also for prophylactic use some relaxation can be given after considering traditional use. Individual experiences recorded in reports related to efficacy from physicians, traditional health practitioners or treated patients should be taken into account.
- Where traditional use has not been established, appropriate clinical evidence should be required.

Combination Products:

- Generally, herbal remedies are sold as a combination of several active ingredients along with traditional remedies. In this case, assessment should differentiate between old and new combination products. This clearly means, there should be proper assessment of old and new combinations separately.
- In case of herbal drugs from traditional medicine, classical texts of Ayurveda, traditional Chinese medicine, Unani, Siddha and experience can be used as evidence of efficacy.
- Whenever new combinations are used, explanation should be given about effective dose ranges and compatibility. In such case, additional documents should be provided in addition to the documentation of traditional knowledge of each single ingredient.
- Herbal drugs containing new ingredients should require clinical studies to show efficacy.

Quality Assessment Parameters:

Parameters of quality control and assessment of herbal drugs:

1. **Definition:** The name of the herbal drugs and content of active substances.
2. **Characters:** Appearance, taste, odour, solubility.
3. **Identification:** Macroscopic and microscopic examination, TLC.
4. **Tests:** Water, loss on drying, total ash, foreign matter, insoluble matter, extractable matter, swelling index, microbial contamination, bitterness value, broken drug.
5. **Assay:** Essential oils, tannins, declared active substances (GC, LC, UV/VIS).

Table 9.2: Parameters of Quality Control and Assessment of Herbal Preparations

Parameter	Dry extracts (extractum siccum)	Liquid extracts (extractum fluidum)	Tincture (tinctura)	Essential oil (aetheroleum)
Definition	Standardized dry extract, content of active substances	Liquid extract produced from plant parts	Tincture produced from plant by using alcohol as solvent	Essential oil obtained by distillation
Production	Methods of extraction and solvents	Method of extraction and solvents	Method of extraction and solvents	Method of extraction and solvents
Characters	Appearance.	Appearance, taste, odour	Appearance, taste, odour	Appearance, odour, solubility.
Identification	TLC	TLC	TLC	TLC, chromatographic profile (GC and GC-MS).
Tests	Loss on drying, total ash, microbial contamination	Ethanol, methanol and 2-propanol, loss on drying, microbial contamination	Ethanol, methanol and 2-propanol, dry residue, microbial contamination	Relative density, refractive index, optical rotation, chromatographic profile
Assay	Declared active substances (LC)	Declared active substances (LC, UV/VIS)	Declared active substances (LC, UV/VIS)	Active substance by GC

Parameters of quality control and assessment of phytopreparations:

A) Mono-component tea and tea mixture:

1. Identification
2. Appearance
3. Verification of components, declared mass ratio of components
4. Verification of package weight
5. Microbial contamination

B) Liquid herbal preparations (liquid extracts, tinctures, and mixtures of extracts or tinctures), herbal drops, solutions, syrups:

1. Identification.
2. Appearance.
3. Loss on drying.
4. Content of ethanol.
5. Relative density.
6. Refractive index.
7. Verification of package weight.
8. Qualitative and quantitative analysis.
9. Microbiological contamination and/or complete health safety control.

C) Semi-solid forms (herbal gels, cream, and unguent):

1. Identification.
2. Appearance.
3. Verification of package weight.
4. pH value.
5. Microbiological contamination and/or complete health safety control.

D) Solid-dosage forms (capsules, tablets etc.):

1. Identification.
2. Appearance.
3. Declared mass of single-dose preparations.
4. Disintegration.
5. Qualitative and quantitative analysis of the declared active components.
6. Microbiological contamination and/or complete health safety control.

9.2 STABILITY TESTING OF HERBAL DRUGS

World Health Organization/ ICH guidelines for herbal drug stability:

Concept of Stability:

According to modern medicine system, stability is the capacity of a specific formulation in a particular container/closure system to remain within its prescribed limits like physical, chemical, microbiological, toxicological, therapeutic specifications.

Stability is defined as, *"the capacity of a drug to remain within established specifications limits to maintain its identity, strength, quality, and purity throughout the retest or expiration dating periods"*.

The shelf life of a product can be defined as, "the time duration up to which it is expected to retain 90% of its active ingredients (label claim) when stored in recommended condition". Stability testing provides us the evidence of how the quality of a pharmaceutical product changes within particular time. There is impact of a variety of environmental factors, like temperature, humidity and light. Apart from outside factors there are product-related factors like container closure system, storage conditions and packaging materials.

Stability Testing Advantages:

- Help in determination of shelf life and storage conditions.
- Help in selection of suitable formulations, excipients and container closure systems for a product.
- Wellbeing of the patient and manufacturer by ensuring the good product quality and enhance patient confidence in herbal drugs and improve compliance.

As per USP, different types of stability study are performed and represented in the below table.

Table 9.3: Types of Stability Study as per USP

Sr. No.	Type of stability	Conditions to be maintained throughout the shelf life of drug product
1.	Physical	The original physical properties, namely, appearance, uniformity, palatability, dissolution, and suspendability are maintained.
2.	Chemical	Each and every active ingredient retains its chemical integrity as well as potency specified on label, within the specified limits.
3.	Microbiological	Sterility or resistance to microbial growth is maintained as per the specified requirements.
4.	Therapeutic	The therapeutic effect remains unaltered.
5.	Toxicological	No valid increase in toxicity occurs.

Stability of Herbal Drugs:

The concept of stability is of the critical importance when it comes to herbal drugs. For stability studies of herbal drugs as till date, no specific comprehensive guidelines are available. Stability of herbal drugs is very challenging as plant extract contain many different compounds in different quantities. International Conference on Harmonization (ICH) and the World Health Organization provides details regarding parameters for stability study of pharmaceutical products but ICH guidelines from Q1 to Q11 are generally followed throughout world. For modern medicine, a proper stability protocol with selection of batches and samples, test attributes, analytical procedures, acceptance criteria, storage conditions and period, testing frequency, sampling plan, container closure and various types of stability study and stability testing methods are available and followed. Currently, pharmaceutical product is generally assayed using a validated stability indicating analytical method. Protocol to calculate an expiry date is based on the predicated period from date of manufacture to more than 10% deterioration in the active molecule is available. The general concept of stability for herbal drugs or modern medicine remains same but the parameters used to assess the stability may vary from product to product.

Use of standardized extract in herbal drugs is becoming popular, now-a-days. However, during manufacturing and the extraction process for herbal drugs, the drug molecules or components are exposed to temperature, oxidation, hydrolysis, microbial attack and other environmental degradation which can cause a problem of stability. So checking concentration of the bioactive constituents is extremely vital as it also affects the quality, efficacy and shelf-life of the herbal drugs. Herbal drugs have gained wide acceptance in both developing and advanced countries and are being produced in commercial quantities.

EMA guidelines for stability of herbal drugs:

- The herbal substance or herbal preparation in its entirety is regarded as the active substance. Because of this stability of whole preparation, along with other ingredients is necessary. Determination of the stability of the constituents with known therapeutic activity is not sufficient.
- The stability of other substances present in the herbal substance or in the herbal preparation, apart from active ingredient also needs to be demonstrated.
- Chromatographic fingerprint can be used for this purpose.
- Most of the time, the herbal medicinal product contains many phytochemicals and combinations of several herbals preparations. In this case, it is not possible to determine the stability of each active ingredient. Chromatographic fingerprint should be used to determin stability of such herbal medicinal products.
- Other methods of assay and physical and sensory tests or other appropriate tests can be used in addition to chromatographic fingerprint.
- When herbal medicinal product contain a constituent which is known for therapeutic activity the variation in content during the proposed shelf-life should not exceed ± 5% of the declared assay value.
- In the case of constituents with known therapeutic activity are unknown, a variation in marker content during the proposed shelf-life of ± 10% of the initial assay value can be allowed.
- When traditional herbal medicines are used as vitamins and/or minerals, the stability of the vitamins and/or minerals should be demonstrated.

Specifications Criteria:

A specification is defined as. "a criteria or list of tests, references to analytical or biological procedures, and appropriate acceptance criteria, which are numerical limits, ranges, or other criteria for the tests described". It establishes the set of criteria or limits to which herbal drug should conform to be considered acceptable for its intended use. 'Conformance to specifications' includes the herbal drug when tested according to the listed analytical procedures, will meet the listed acceptance criteria or limits. Specifications are legally binding for compulsory quality standard requirements. The setting of specifications for a herbal drug is part of an overall control strategy which includes control of raw materials and excipients, in-process testing, process evaluation/validation, stability testing and testing for consistency of batches.

The following points can be taken into consideration when establishing specifications criteria for herbal drugs:

- Botanical characteristics of the plant (genus, species, variety, chemotype; usage of genetically modified organisms), parts of the plants.
- Macroscopy and microscopy of plant, phytochemistry, marker compounds, toxic constituents (identity, assay, limit tests).
- Biological/geographical and other types of variation.
- Cultivation/harvesting/drying or processing conditions (microbial levels, aflatoxins, heavy metals etc).
- Pre-/post-harvest chemical treatments (pesticides, fumigants).
- Profile and stability of the constituents.

Different Stability Testing Methods:

- **Real time (long-term) testing:** This type of testing is normally performed for longer duration to allow significant degradation of the product under specified storage conditions.
- **Accelerated testing:** In this testing, the product is subjected to a several conditions including high temperatures, humidity, light intensity. This accelerates degradation and the amount of heat required to degrade the product is determined so as to predict the shelf life. This is one sort of forced study to predict future stability of drug. This study is based upon Arrhenius equation which describes the relationship between storage temperatures and deterioration rate.
- **Intermediate testing:** It is designed to moderately increase the rate of degradation for a drug intended to be stored long-term at 25°C. These are mainly conducted when the accelerated studies for general case failed to meet the acceptance criteria.
- **Stress testing:** It is carried out to check the effect of temperature, humidity (e.g., ≥75% RH), oxidation, photolysis and hydrolysis on drug and its stability.
- **Forced degradation testing:** This study is carried out to check stability assessment of the drug, to elucidate the possible degradation pathways by identifying the likely degradation products.

Protocol for Stability Testing:

The protocol is a document describing the basic components of a stability study. Protocol of testing is selected depending upon nature of drug, country and its climatic zone where drug is going to launch.

Typical Stability Protocol:

- **Selection of batches and samples:** Generally, random sampling can be done from one or 2-3 batches.
- **Test selection:** The tests that monitor the quality, potency, purity, and identity that are selected for stability checking.
- **Analytical procedures:** If available, procedures given in the official compendia are followed. The method used need to be duly validated.
- **Acceptance criteria:** This can be determined in the form of statistical limits for the results manifested in computable terms and pass or fail for qualitative tests.
- **Storage conditions:** These are selected depending upon marketing climatic zone of the drug as depicted in following table 9. 3.
- **Testing frequency:** It can be selected depending upon the stability profile of the drug. Test schedules for different types of stability testing are shown in Table 9.5.
- **Storage period:** Storage period generally extend from minimum of 3 or 6 months. Stress testing is carried out up to 12, 18, or 60 months in on-going or follow-up stability testing.
- **Sampling plan:** This involves devising for the number of samples to be placed in the stability chambers. Sample from this is taken for study.
- **Container closure system:** In this study effect of actual containers and closures used is checked for entire duration of storage.
- **Evaluation:** The data is analysed to determine the time duration and acceptance limit.
- **Statements, labelling:** A storage statement summary, retest period, and re-test date based on the stability evaluation of the drug substance should be established at the end.

Climatic Zones for Stability Testing:

World has been divided into four zones for checking stability as per different environment conditions shown in the table given below:

Table 9.4: Climatic Zones and Long-term Stability Conditions according to ICH and WHO

Climatic Zone	Climate	Countries	MAT/MAPWP*	Long-term Testing Conditions
I	Temperate	UK, Northern Europe, US	<15°C /<11hPa	21°C/45%RH
II	Subtropical and Mediterranean	Japan, Southern Europe	>15-22°C/>11-18hPa	25°C/60%RH

Contd...

III	Hot and dry	Iraq, India	>22°C/<15hPa	30°C/35%RH
IVa	Hot and humid	Iran, Egypt	>22°C/>15-27hPa	30°C/65%RH
IVd	Hot and very humid	Brazil, Singapore	>22°C/>27hPa	30°C/75%RH

MAT: Mean annual temperature measured in open air, **MAPWP:** Mean annual partial water vapour pressure, **ICH:** International Conference on Harmonization.

Table 9.5: Stability Testing Storage Conditions for Drugs as per ICH and WHO

Intended Storage Condition	Stability Test Method	Test Temperature and Humidity (Period in months) as per ICH	Test temperature and Humidity (Period in months) as per the WHO
Room temperature	Long term	25 ± 2°C/60 ± 5% RH	25 ± 2°C/60 ± 5% RH 30 ± 2°C/65 ± 5% RH 30 ± 2°C/75 ± 5% RH
	Intermediate	30 ± 2°C/65 ± 5% RH	30 ± 2°C/65 ± 5% RH
	Accelerated	40 ± 2°C/75 ± 5% RH	40 ± 2°C/75 ± 5% RH
Refrigerated	Long term	5°C/ambient	5 ± 3°C
	Accelerated	25 ± 2°C/60 ± 5% RH	25 ± 2°C/60 ± 5% RH 30 ± 2°C/65 ± 5% RH
Freezer	Long term	−20°C/ambient	−20°C ± 5°C

ICH: International Conference on Harmonization, **WHO:** World Health Organization.

Table 9.6: Test Schedule for Stability Testing of New Products according to ICH guideline

Sr. No.	Method and Climatic Zone	Environment	Time Points for Sampling
1.	Long term for climatic Zones I and IV	25°C/60% RH	3, 6, 9, 12, 18, 24, 36 months
2.	Long term for climatic Zones III	30°C/35% RH	3, 6, 9, 12, 18, 24, 36 months
3.	Long term for climatic Zone IVa/intermediate for Zones I and II	30°C/65% RH	3, 6, 9, 12, 18, 24, 36 months
4.	Long term for climatic Zone IVb/intermediate for Zones I and II	30°C/75% RH	3, 6, 9, 12, 18, 24, 36 months
5.	Accelerated condition for all zones	40°C/75% RH	3, 6 months

Table 9.7: Shelf Life of Ayurvedic Medicine as per D and C Amendment Rules, 1945

Sr. No.	Name of the Group of Ayurvedic Medicine	Shelf Life
1.	Arka, eye drops.	1 Year
2.	Churna, Kwath Churna, DantManjan powder, Dant Manjan paste, Varti, Shweta Parpati, Ear/Nasal drops, Dhoopans (inhalers), Ghrita.	2 Years
3.	Gutika tablet containing Kasthaushadhi, Avleha, Taila, LepaChurna, LepaGuti, LepaMalahar, Ghana Vati, Soft gelatin capsules containing Kashta- Aushadhi, Syrup, Granule/Khand, PravahiKwath.	3 Years
4.	Rasa Gutika, Guggulu, Dravaka, Lavana, Ksara, Naga Bhasma, Vanga Bhasma, Tamra Bhasma, Hard gelatin capsules.	5 Years
5.	Mandura- Lauha.	10 Years
6.	Rasaushadhies, Asava Arista, Kupipakva, Parpati, Pisti and Bhasma, Swarna, Rajata, Lauha, Mandura, Abhraka, Godanti, Shankha Bhasma.	10 Years

Evaluation of Stability Data:

- Stability data can be evaluated from the physical, chemical, biological, and microbiological tests, including particular attributes of the dosage form. Solid oral dosage forms can be evaluated for dissolution rate.
- The stability study is used for determination of shelf file. For this reason minimum two or three batches need to be evaluated. The degree of variability of individual batches should be within specification throughout its shelf life.
- For more safety, the overall shelf life should be based on the minimum time a batch can be expected to remain within acceptance criteria.
- The evaluation should involve not only the assay but also the degradation products and other appropriate attributes.
- Selected markers and possible degradation products should also be checked with time in order to help determine the shelf-life of the products.
- Chromatographic techniques like TLC, HPLC, HPTLC, UV-Visible spectrophotometry can be used to quantification of markers as well as determine the levels of degradation products.
- All listed tests are not necessary for each formulation, but depending upon type of formulation, tests can be selected. Table 9.7 presents some recommended stability tests for various herbal dosage forms.

Table 9.8: Recommended Stability Tests for Different Herbal Dosage Forms according to WHO

Sr. No.	Type of Dosage Form	Recommended Stability Tests
1.	Decoctions (oral), Glycerites, Aceterites, oxymels	Change in colour, odour, taste, formation of a precipitate, clarity, specific gravity, total solid residue, pH, viscosity, extractable, phytochemical constituents, microbial contamination, preservative efficacy/challenge tests, and toxicity/safety.
2.	Tablets	Change in colour, pH, total water or solvent extractive, phytochemical constituent, dissolution (or disintegration, if justified), water content, hardness, friability, swelling, crakes and clumping (coated tablets), microbial contamination, preservative efficacy/challenge tests, toxicity/safety.
3.	Capsules	Change in colour, pH, total extractive, phytochemical constituent, brittleness, hardening or softening of shell, dissolution (or disintegration, if justified), water content, microbial contamination, preservative efficacy/challenge tests, toxicity.
4.	Alcoholic beverages, Tinctures Extracts	Clarity, pH, specific gravity, alcohol content, extractable, change in colour, odour, taste, the formation of a precipitate, total solid residue, extractable, phytochemical constituents, microbial contamination, toxicity.
5.	Teas and powders	Change in odour, moisture content, pH, total water extractive, formation of hard mass, caking, Phytochemical constituents, microbial contamination and toxicity.
6.	Ointment, balms	Change in colour, odour, homogeneity, pH, consistency, grittiness, excessive bleeding, phytochemical constituents, microbial contamination and toxicity.
7.	Oils	Rancidity, change in colour, odour, pH, phytochemical constituents, microbial contamination, toxicity.
8.	Pastes and creams	Change in colour, odour, homogeneity, pH, consistency, grittiness, cracking, shrinking due to evaporation of water, phytochemical constituents, microbial contamination, preservative challenge tests (where preservatives are used), toxicity.
9.	Soaps	Change in colour, odour, homogeneity, pH, phytochemical constituents, microbial contamination, preservative challenge tests (where preservatives are used), toxicity/skin sensitivity tests.
10.	Suppositories and Pessaries	Softening, hardening or drying, dissolution.

Microbial Tests:

Microbial contamination of finished product is one of the most important factor for determination of stability and shelf life. Several factors affect the efficacy of the antimicrobial activity of biocid. Preservatives added are the active ingredient, excipients, storage conditions, the container and its closure. While preparing formulation, not only current microbial load but possible proliferation of microorganisms need to be considered. Analyses of such parameters with time allow the tracing of stability of the product and subsequent prediction or estimation of shelf-life. These tests need to carry out according to Pharmacopoeia methods (British Pharmacopoeia, United States Pharmacopoeia, European Pharmacopeia.), WHO methods, or any other internationally recognized methods.

The important microbial tests need to conduct are: Total viable aerobic plate count; contaminating fungus (yeast and mould); Salmonella spp.; *Escherichia coli* and *Staphylococcus aureus*. Table 9.8 shows the Pharmacopoeia acceptance criteria for microbiological testing of herbal products.

Table 9.9: Acceptance Criteria for Microbiological Tests as per USP

Sr. No.	Microbiological Quality	Criteria A	Criteria B	Criteria C
1.	Total aerobic microbial count	Not more than 5×10^7 CFU per g or per ml	Not more than 5×10^4 CFU per g or per ml	Not more than 5×10^5 CFU per g or per ml
2.	Total yeast and mould count	Not more than 5×10^5 CFU per g or per ml	Not more than 5×10^2 CFU per g or per ml	Not more than 5×10^4 CFU per g or per ml
3.	Bile-tolerant gram negative bacteria	Not more than 10^2 CFU per g or per ml	Not more than 10^2 CFU per g or per ml	Not more than 5×10^4 CFU per g or per ml
4.	*Salmonella spp.*	Absent in 10 g or 10 ml	Absent in 25 g or 25 ml	Absent in 25 g or 25 ml
5.	*Escherichia coli*	Absent in 1 g or 1 ml	Absent in 1 g or 1 ml	Absent in 1 g or 1 ml

Criteria 'A' is herbal medicinal product containing herbal drugs, with or without excipients, intended for the preparation of infusions and decoctions using boiling water (for example herbal teas, with or without added flavourings).

Criteria 'B' is for herbal medicinal products containing, extracts and/or herbal drugs, with or without excipients, where the method of processing (for example, extraction) or, where appropriate, in the case of herbal drugs, of pre-treatment, reduces the levels of organisms below to those stated for this category).

Criteria 'C' is for herbal medicinal products containing, extracts and/or herbal drugs, with or without excipients, where it can be demonstrated that the method of processing (for example, extraction with low strength ethanol or water that is not boiling or low-temperature concentration) or, in the case of herbal drugs, of pre-treatment, would not reduce the level of organisms sufficiently to reach the criteria required under B.

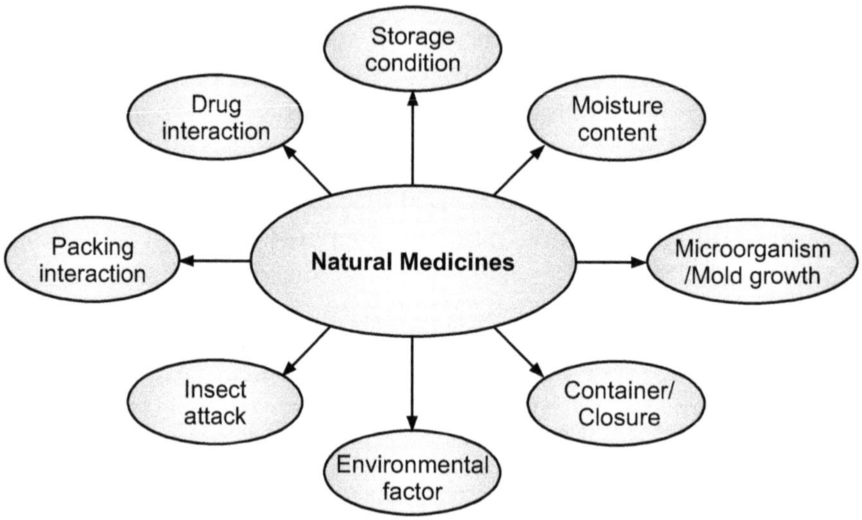

Fig. 9.1: Factors affecting stability of natural medicines

Issues Related to Stability of Herbal Drugs:

Herbal drugs may have many active constituents as alkaloids, glycosides, tannins, flavonoids or other chemicals. Each component is having different stability conditions and nature. Hence, actual stability condition for the herbal formulation is different than its individual component. Stability of herbal drug should be taken as overall stability of all components of formulation not as single component. Determination of storage condition is difficult for herbal drugs. Stability of finished herbal drug is dependant on stability of all constituents.

Physical Instability:

- Herbal drugs have problem of physical instability due to the presence of moisture, impurities. This can result in interaction with the container, growth of the microorganisms, affect the secondary metabolites and chemical composition. There can be volatile active components, or other chemicals which decrease activity after storage.

Processing Environment:

- Processing environmental conditions, storage conditions, different harvesting procedures, time and method of collection, manufacturing processes such as selecting, drying, purifying, extracting, and genetic variability can create substantial variability in the product.

Chemical Instability:

- Herbal drugs can degrade during storage. Chemical instability may be because of oxidation, hydrolysis, crystallization, emulsion breakdown, enzymatic deterioration and chemical reactions between different componemts like the additives and excipients. Temperature and moisture are the two major reasons behind chemical instability of the herbal product. At the same time, moisture can result in early degradation in case of susceptible drug. .

Complexity:

- Herbal drugs are too complex mixtures of different chemical components. One plant may contain up to hundred different chemicals. Each component has different chemical nature, shelf-life, activity, concentration and consistency.

Drug Interactions:

Moisture content, mould growth, interaction with packaging material, interactions of active component with the other ingredients of formulations used such as additives can affect stability of product.

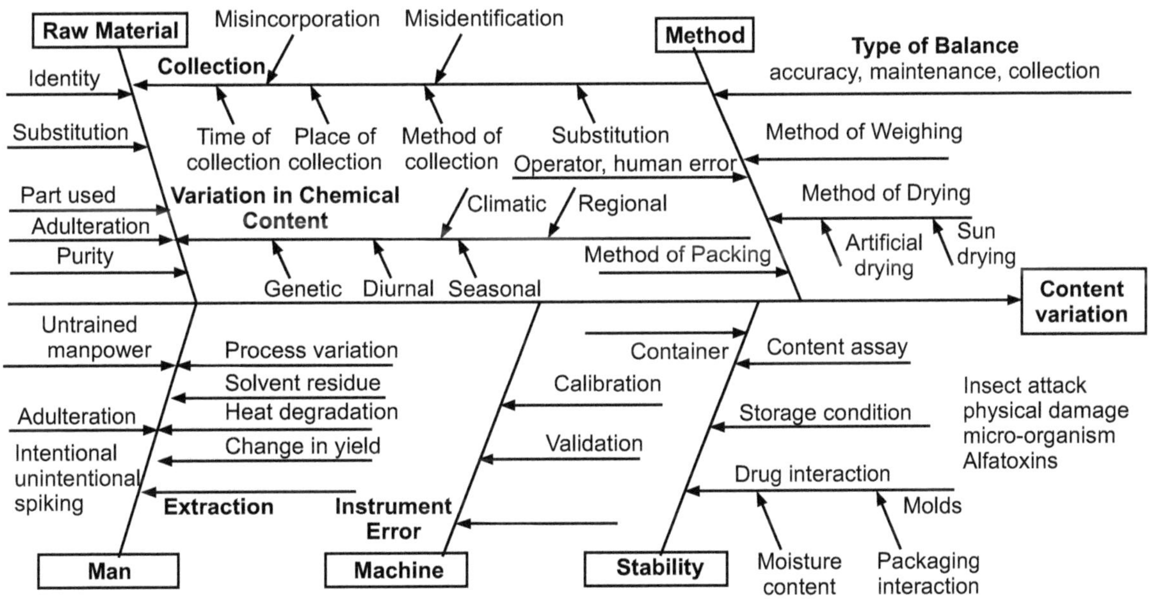

Fig. 9.2: Ishikawa Cause and Effect Diagram for Content Variation in Herbal Drugs

QUESTIONS

1. Explain WHO guidelines for accessment of herbal drugs.
2. Which are different parameters for quality control of herbal preparations?
3. What is stability? Explain stability testing of herbal drugs.

4. Explain different shelf life of Ayurvedic medicine as per Drug and Cosmetic Amendment rules, 1945.
5. Which are different issues related to stability of herbal drugs?
6. Which are different recommended stability tests for herbal dosage froms as per WHO?
7. Which are different climatic zones as per ICH for stability study of drugs?
8. Which are different methods for stablity testing?
9. Explain role of WHO and ICH in accessment of herbal drugs.
10. What is evaluation of crude drugs?

❖❖❖

Chapter...10

PATENTING AND REGULATORY REQUIREMENTS OF NATURAL PRODUCTS

Objectives

- To learn about concept of intellectual property right and patent.
- To understand farmers right, breeders right related to natural products .
- To understand bioprospecting and biopiracy.
- To understand different patenting aspects of traditional knowledge and natural products.
- To understand case study of Curcuma and Neem.

10.1 INTELLECTUAL PROPERTY RIGHTS

Intellectual property (IP) is the property possessed by virtue of one's intellectual creativity. **Intellectual property rights (IPR) are exclusive rights to make, use, and sell a new product or technology for a limited period.** Scope and area of IPR is becoming very important day by day. Intellectual property right protects inventor and indirectly benefit country or society. IPRs are meant to reward innovators, inventors and researchers for fast growth of industry.

There are different types of intellectual properties which can be protected by law:

Table 10.1: Types of IPR

Sr. No.	Type of IPR	Law	Protection given	Application/ Example	Duration in years
1.	Patents	Indian Patent Act, 1970	Discoveries and inventions	Drugs, medicine, scientific discovery	20 years after filing, can't be renewed
2.	Trademarks	Trademarks Act, 1999	Phrases, symbols, and designs	Business, branding	10 years duration can be renewed for again 10 years

Contd...

3.	Copyright	Copyright Act, 1957	Musical, literary, and artistic works	Books, drama, literature	Lifetime of author or artist and 60 years after death
4.	Industrial design	Design Act, 2000	Design of machined, equipment etc.	Manufacture of equipment, industries	Initial 10 years can be extended 5 more years
5.	Plants	The Plant Variety Protection Act of 1970	Plant variety, farmers right, trees	Farmer	15 years from date of registration
6.	Geographical goods	The Geographical Indications of Goods (Registration and Protection) Act, 1999	Certain goods	Basmati rice, Banarasi silk, Madhubani Painting	Initial 10 years can be extended for another 10 years

Intellectual property is intangible property, once upon a time was considered as safe. Now-a-days, ideas or inventions can be stolen for monetary benefit. Therefore, intellectual property needs to be protected from piracy. From all above type of intellectual properties, patents and trademarks are more important for pharmaceutical industries. **A patent is a set of exclusive rights granted by a state (national government) to an inventor or their assignee for a limited period of time.** Patent is purely territorial right and there is no world patent. Patent is valid in country or particular region only.

In pharmaceutical industry, whenever there is discovery of new chemical, first thing done is filing of patent. This patent will prevent other companies to work on particular molecule. Generally, patent protection is for twenty years. That drug may require ten more years after filing to come in the market. After the expiry of patent, molecule becomes open to all other companies and low price generic version comes to market. Thus, company practically has only ten years to recover the huge amount that has been invested on research and development and to gain profit. Obviously, there is cutthroat competition for filing of patent and protecting own rights. The procedure for granting patents, the requirements and the exclusive rights also vary widely according to national laws of each country and international agreements.

Drugs obtained from natural resources are fundamental to new drug discovery and development. Natural products have proved their metallic presence in the process of drug discovery and development. Issues related to regulatory aspects of natural products are as complex as natural product itself. Because of tremendous competition and high money turnover, these issues are of utmost importance. Till date because of loopholes in regulatory guidelines, there was exploitation of natural products.

When it comes to natural product, protection of intellectual property becomes very difficult and challenging. Natural products are derived from plant, animal, mineral and have entirely different back ground as compared to synthetic drugs. Now-a-days, natural products are becoming more popular throughout world. So there is increased awareness about issues related to IPR and natural products. Due to globalization, trade between countries is also changing dynamically, so natural product regulations. As natural medicine expands and evolves, intellectual property (IP) protection is playing a bigger role in its existence. Because of these complexities of natural product, there is necessity of different rules and laws for better regulation.

IPR issues related to natural product are important because of following reasons:

- Natural products have inherent variation in chemical constituents and therapeutic effect.
- Laws related to patent and IPR issues are different according to country or region.
- Some natural product may come under traditional medicine making regulation more difficult.
- Natural products are related with ecological issues like over harvesting, biodiversity, bio piracy.

While filing of patent, a patent application must include one or more claims defining the invention which must be new, inventive, and useful or applicable. In simple words, it should have novelty, non-obviousness and industrial applicability. There were certain incidents which involve, collecting information from tribal healers on variety of plants and using it for commercial benefits. Many pharmaceutical corporations are misusing traditional knowledge and making huge profits in form of what is known as biopiracy. Most people might assume there is no IP protection for herbal medicines. In countries like India, to manage cost of IP protection, many small scale herbal industries prefer trade secret. It does not require registration with government and is not bound by time. Most famous example of trade secret is formula of Coca Cola. Company is successful to keep their formula as trade secret for many years. But this concept is not suitable and applicable in medicine.

WTO (World Trade Organization) was formed on 1st January 1995 to regulate trade among all over world. Most of the countries including India become member of this international organization. WTO has four different organization structures:

1. Council for trade in goods,
2. Council for Trade-Related Aspects of Intellectual Property Rights (TRIPS),
3. Council for Trade in Services works with GATS (General Agreement on Trade related Service)
4. Trade Negotiations Committee (TNC).

All of above organizations and agreement including TRIPS came into force from 1st January 1995. But developing countries were given 10 years window period to amend their laws. From 1st January 2005, TRIPS become mandatory for India. Indian laws were amended accordingly to conform to TRIPS. Because of this reason, last two decades have seen lot of changes in regulatory issues.

10.2 PATENT

A patent is a set of monopoly rights given to patentee by government that excludes others from making, using, selling or importing particular invention for limited period of time.

A patent can be granted for an invention which may be related to any process or product. The word "Invention" has been defined under the Patents Act 1970 as amended from time to time. "An invention means a new product or process having industrial application and involving an inventive step". A patent may be granted only for an invention in respect of which the following conditions are satisfied:

(a) The invention is new;

(b) Involves an inventive step; and

(c) Is capable of industrial application or utility.

Important points related to patent:

- A patent is a statutory right for an invention granted for a limited period of time. Currently, patent granted is for 20 years from the date of filing of application.
- Patentee has to fully disclose his invention for grant of patent.
- Patent is territorial right means there is no world patent. One has to apply in respective country to receive patent for that country.
- Patent is sort of negative right. For a patentee, after grant of patent, use of that invention is not mandatory. It excludes others making, using, selling, and importing the patented product.
- India has four patent offices located which are located at Kolkata, New Delhi, Mumbai and Chennai.

Table 10.2: History of Indian Patent System

Year	History
1856	The act VI of 1856. The objective of this legislation was to encourage inventions of new and useful manufactures and to induce inventors to disclose secret of their inventions.
1859	The act modified as act XV.
1872	The Patents & Designs Protection Act.
1883	The Protection of Inventions Act.

Contd...

1888	Consolidated as the Inventions & Designs Act.
1911	The Indian Patents & Designs Act. This Act brought patent administration under the management of Controller of Patents for the first time and replaced all previous acts.
1972	The Patents Act (Act 39 of 1970). This act replaces patent act of 1911.
1999	First amendment of 1970 act: Patents (amendment) Act, (1999) came into force from 01-01-1995.
2002	Second amendment of 1970 act: The Patents (Amendment) Act 2002 came into force from 20th May 2003.
2005	Third amendment of 1970 act: The Patents (Amendment) Act 2005 effective from 1st January 2005.
2016	Patent (Amendment) Rules, 2016. On May 16, 2016, India brought in various changes to the Patent Rules, 2003. This includes changes like mandatory e-submission and video-conferencing for faster examination.

(Source: http://www.ipindia.nic.in/history-of-indian-patent-system.htm)

The patent system has been introduced and known in India since 19th century. The first patent act came into effect in the year 1856. It was based on British patent law of 1852. This act granted exclusive rights to inventors for period of 14 years. Later, the patent law was amended from time to time.

Patent document is divided in following section:

Writing of patent is art as well as skill. Ideal patent writer can write patent documents in such a way that even single word cannot be deleted without changing meaning of main text.

1. **Title:** The title document demonstrates and gives idea of the invention for the grant of patent.
2. **Abstract:** It gives the precise or detail description of the invention. Abstract also contain the technical information in brief covering all important points.
3. **Description:** It describes an invention with the help of words, drawings and diagrams. The aim is to provide enough detail that a person with ordinary skill in the area of the invention would understand and recreate the invention. The description part must be comprehensive and precise, leaving no ambiguity or confusion. In short, it should contain all relevant details about the invention.
4. **Claims:** This is the backbone of patent document. It describes the inventive concept(s) of an invention. They recite which concepts described in the detailed description are inventive. When a patent is granted, the claims are the only part of the patent that is enforceable. In a patent application, patent holder can only prevent others from using or practicing the concepts presented by the claims. Any part which is not recited in claim remains unprotected. It means patentee can debar you from making, selling or manufacturing the things that are described in the claims.

Advantages of Good Patent System:

1. It saves time and energy by making available current literature and technology to other inventers reducing duplication.
2. Identification of technology, transfer, licensing, alternative or substitute of existing technology and new research is possible because of good patent system.
3. Knowledge on the latest technologies in desired field of expertise is available.
4. One can plan more effective and better technology after current patent search.
5. Sharing of ideas, knowledge, and innovation is possible to benefit country and mankind.
6. Know about the commercial applicability for the invention in the field of expertise.
7. Ease of doing business is achieved because of good patent system.
8. Inventor can benefit from money while possible infringement can be avoided.
9. One can legally object grant of patent, if it conflict with particular invention/ claim.
10. Expired patents are pool of knowledge which is open to all free of cost.

Patent and Natural Products:

Patent comes under IP, patents may provide the strongest IP protection, but to get the IP protection for natural or herbal medicines is very difficult. To qualify for a patent, an invention must be novel, useful and not obvious. Most natural or herbal medicines have been used or practiced from more than hundreds of years, thus, their novelty comes into question. Also, the product being patented cannot have been publically used or known, as most herbal medicines are known from ages. So most natural products come under prior art.

Several common ways to obtain patents for herbal medicines:

- Finding new uses or therapeutically completely different action for an existing herb.
- Isolation of a new active ingredient not previously reported.
- Significant improvement in the method for extraction/separation of the active ingredient(s).
- Claiming entirely new uses for old compounds.

The following inventions are not protected under patent act:

(a) Naturally occurring micro-organisms and their components, animals, plants or extracts from animals or plants.

(b) Scientific or mathematical rules or theories.

(c) Computer programs.

(d) Methods of diagnosis, treatment or cure of human and animal diseases.

(e) Inventions which are hazardous and contrary to public order, morality, health or welfare.

Access to Affordable Medicines and Patent System:

Patent system plays dual role. It rewards inventor and also make availability of affordable medicine to common man. The issue of public health and patents is much debated. The exorbitant prices of branded or patented drugs have led to emergence of a global campaign for access to affordable medicines over the last few years. In 2019, USFDA have approved Novartis's drug named 'Zolgensma' which single dose costs about 2.1 million dollar. Prices of branded or patented drugs are often far higher than prices of similar products by alternative or generic sources. Where generic alternatives are available, the price of the patented drug drops. Patent protection helps in profit maximization through elimination of competition from generic producers and maintenance of market monopoly. A decade ago, millions of people suffering from HIV/AIDS could not afford the price of antiretroviral (ARV) drugs. The cost has come down from 4 to 5 lakh per annum to 4 to 5 thousand. Compulsory License is one important concept for affordable medicine in emergency. In case of epidemic or threat to humanity, government can give permission to any company for large scale manufacture of particular drug.

It is now recognized that, the current patent regime being 'globalised' by the World Trade Organization. By shutting out competition, TRIPS gives drug companies the ability to charge high monopoly prices for their drugs. The core of the issue is how to make medicines more affordable to more people who need them. HIV drugs can be considered as one good example. Drugs for cancer, tuberculosis, cancer, asthma, diabetes and Parkinson's disease are costly, unaffordable because of patents.

According to The Patent Second Amendment Act, 2002, process patents are allowed on microbiological, biochemical and biotechnological processes. Because of this, methods of genetic engineering, processes in the pharmaceutical industry using microorganisms and related processes are patentable.

According to Second Amendment of Patent Act, 2002 following things are not patentable:

- Plants, animals in whole or any part.
- Seed or varieties of plant.
- Biological processes for the production of plants and animals.
- Microorganisms can be claimed for a patent provided if they are not only discovery of organisms existing in nature.
- Methods for rendering plants free of diseases or to increase their economic value will be patentable.

As per the Act of 2002, it is mandatory to deposit the biological material mentioned in the specification with a depository notified in the Gazette of India. This also requires the source and geographical origin of the biological material to be disclosed in the specification.

In U.S., there are three types of patents. These consist of utility patents, design patents, and plant patents. Utility patents are the most common of the three and cover the invention of any new and useful process, composition of matter, machine, or article of manufacture.

The plant patents are those covering new plant varieties. But there are some stipulations or conditions with plant patents. Plants that have been bred are acceptable, while plants growing naturally in the wild are not patentable. Plants that are sexually reproduced are not patetable. If the plant is produced by asexual method like cutting, layering, grafting then it can be patentable.

In fact, the objective of The Patents (Amendment) Bill 2005 was to meet India's World Trade Organization (WTO) under the TRIPS. This has introduced three new definitions, viz, inventive step, new invention and pharmaceutical substance. The bill also defines the term 'new invention'.The bill defines the inventive step as "a feature of an invention that involves technical advance as compared to the existing knowledge or having economic significance or both that makes the invention not obvious to a person skilled in the art. According to the bill 'Pharmaceutical substances' are "any new entity involving one or more inventive steps". India has established patenting of GMO (Genetically Modified Organisms) including genes of animals and plants. TRIPS allows member countries to exclude certain subject matters provided under article 27.3 from patentability which includes essentially biological processes, however member countries can decide on their patentability. Plant patents in US can be granted to person who invents or discovers and asexually reproduces any distinct and new variety of plants. This can be mutants, hybrids and newly found seedlings except tuber, propagated plant or uncultivated plant.

10.3 PROTECTION OF PLANT VARIETIES AND FARMER'S RIGHTS ACT, 2001 (PPVFR ACT)

Need:

Increased bioprospecting and use of plants by human in recent years is increased enormously. This necessitate requirement of international as well as local laws for protection of plants and related IPR issues. International Union for Protection of New Plant Varieties of Plant (UPOV) is an intergovernmental organization established according to International Convention for the Protection of New Varieties of Plants. This convention was adopted in 1961 and later revised in the year 1972, 1978 and 1991. As India become signatory to WTO/TRIPS, it becomes mandatory to give protection to plants. According to article 27.3b of TRIPs introduction of some intellectual property protection for plant varieties was needed. Instead of protecting plants by giving patent, India carefully choose *Sui generis* system in favor of small farmers and tribal people. The Protection of Plant Varieties and Farmers' Rights Act, 2001 is an act brought into force for the protection of plant varieties, the rights of farmers and plant breeders and to encourage the development of new varieties of plants.

Prior to this law, India was having Indian Patent Act of 1970. This law was not sufficient to protect plants, agriculture related problems. Seed Act of 1966 was also for seeds and has many limitations. Countries like India almost 50% people rely on farming or agriculture related business. So for the protection of plant varieties through means of IPR are an important step for small farmers, breeders. Traditionally new plant variety was created by crossing or hybridization. But with arrival of genetic engineering, biotechnological tools, it becomes necessary to give protection to new plant variety.

Main Objectives:

- To protect rights of farmer by conserving plant genetic resources.
- To protect breeder right and stimulate research and development.
- To facilitate growth of seed industry.
- To comply the regulation as per article 27.3b of TRIPs.

The detail act contains 11 chapters and is divided in 97 clauses. Chapter one contain title and the definitions involved in this law. The last chapter is related to miscellaneous. The remaining nine chapters deal with PPVFR authority, registration of plant varieties, duration and effect of registration and benefit of sharing, surrender and revocation of certificate, farmer's rights. This also contain different provisions including compulsory license, plant varieties protection appellate tribunal, finance, accounts, audit, infringement, offences and penalties etc. for better protection. Indian act has provided for farmers' rights, breeders' rights, researchers' rights and equity concerns in the one legislation making this act as a unique act, when compared to other countries.

Table 10.3

No. of Chapter	Clauses	Provisions Made in Act
1.	1 and 2	Short title, extension, commencement and definitions
2.	3 to 13	Establishment of authority and registry, meeting, committee, delegation, power of authority
3.	14 to 23	Application of registration
4.	24 to 32	Duration and effect of registration and benefit sharing
5.	33 to 38	Surrender and revocation of certificate and rectification and correction of register
6.	39 to 46	Farmers right
7.	47 to 53	Compulsory license
8.	54 to 59	Plant variety protection appellate tribunal
9.	60 to 63	Finance, accounts and audit
10.	64 to 67	Infringements, offences, penalties and procedures
11.	68 to 97	Miscellaneous

Main Features of PPVFR Act 2001:

- **Important definitions according to this law:**
  'Breeder' means a person or group of persons or a farmer or group of farmers or any institution which has bred, evolved or developed any variety.

'Farmer' means any person who — (i) cultivates crops by cultivating the land himself; or (ii) cultivates crops by directly supervising the cultivation of land through any other person; or (iii) conserves and preserves, severally or jointly, with any other person any wild species or traditional varieties or adds value to such wild species or traditional varieties through selection and identification of their useful properties.

- The Central Government will establish 'Protection of Plant Varieties and Farmers' Rights Authority' for implementation of this act by notification in the Official Gazette. This authority will have chairman and fifteen members. This authority will meet periodically to function as per provisions in the act.
- Any person, who meets the criteria mentioned in the act can apply for register of any variety. Plant variety must be new or novel, distinct from other plants, uniform or homogeneous and stable means characteristics of plants must be reproducible or transferable to next generation.
- Other person within three months from the date of advertisement can file opposition to this registration. In such case, decision will be carried out as per provisions made in act.
- If there is no opposition, registrar shall register this variety and will give certificate of registration.
- Protection to all type of plants except microorganism was given. For trees and vines 18 years protection is given. For all other plants and extant varieties 15 years protection was given as per section 5 of the seed act 1966.
- This law has provisions for researchers, scientists and breeders to have free access to registered varieties only for research purpose. The registered variety can also be used for the purpose of creating new varieties. Other breeders can always use the registered variety to breed new crop varieties except when the registered variety needs to be used repeatedly as a parental line. If it needs to be used as a parental line, then in that case, authorization is required.
- Issues related to this law will be addressed by the tribunal established by a gazette notification by the Government to exercise jurisdiction, powers and authority conferred on it under this Act. The rules and working of this tribunal is also prescribed in this act.
- Central government will provide grant and fund to this as authority fund.
- Suit for infringement of this law can be filed in district court having jurisdiction. After which opinion of scientific advisor can be taken.
- Penalty for violation of this law is minimum three months to two years imprisonment or fine of minimum 50,000 to 5, 00,000 rupees or both. Penalty for selling false varieties is not less than six month imprisonment which can be extended to 2 years with above mentioned fine. Other offences also have different penalties.

Farmer's Right:

In chapter VI of this **PPVFR act**, Farmers' Rights are also given from clause number 39 to 46.

According to section 39, Farmers' rights have made following provisions to the farmers:

(i) A farmer who has bred or developed a new variety shall be entitled for registration and other protection in like manner as a breeder of a variety under this Act;

(ii) The farmers' variety shall be entitled for registration if the application contains declaration as specified in clause (h) of sub-section (1) of section 18.

(iii) A farmer who is engaged in the conservation of genetic resources of land races and wild relatives of economic plants and their improvement through selection and preservation shall be entitled in the prescribed manner for recognition and reward from the Gene Fund.

Provided that, material so selected and preserved has been used as donors of genes in varieties registrable under this act.

(iv) A farmer have right to save, use, sow, re-sow, exchange, share or sell his farm produce including seed of a variety protected under this act in the same manner as he was entitled before coming into force of this act. But the farmer can not sell branded seed of a variety protected under this act. This clearly means, branded seeds are the seeds packed in container and labelled.

- Any one person or group of persons, government or non-governmental organization (NGO) can make claim.
- There is provision for protection of innocent infringement of law in case farmer is unaware of provisions in this act.
- The Central Government shall constitute a Fund to be called the National Gene Fund for the sharing of benefit to farmers.
- After three years from registration of variety, if needed, government can issue compulsory license for production, distribution, and sale of seed or other propagating material of that variety.

10.4 THE GEOGRAPHICAL INDICATIONS OF GOODS (REGISTRATION AND PROTECTION) ACT, 1999

This act provides facility for registration and better protection of geographical indications relating to goods. This act extends to whole of India. Any agricultural, natural or manufactured goods or any goods of handicrafts or of industry include food stuff, can be considered as Good according to this act. Indication can be any name, geographical or figurative representation or any combination of them conveying or suggesting the geographical origin of goods to which it applies.

Registration of GI can be done at Registrar of Geographical indication. Any person or organization can file application. There is scrutiny of application and it is published in GI journal within three months. If there is no opposition, GI status is given. The Registrar of Geographical Indications maintains a register of Geographical Indications Agents with the entire details including name, address of the place of residence, address of the principal place of business, the nationality, qualifications and date of registration.

Main concept behind GI is some products can be produced only in a certain geographical region and they are unique to that place. They become reputed because they have certain quality or attributes or traits like in the case of Champagne or Basmati rice, Assam tea or Nagpur oranges. Champagne is sparkling alcoholic beverage produced in Champagne region of France. So any beverage produced anywhere in world cannot be named as Champagne, irrespective of similarities. In production of these products, typical geography of that region plays an important role. There is link between their quality characteristics and the geographical attributes of the region. Such products are mostly agricultural commodities like wine, cheese, rice, fruits, and coffee but may be handicraft items such as silk clothes, art, like traditional paintings, even herbal medicines or food such as Neem, Rice, and Turmeric. Unique geo-climatic characteristics or traditional skills render a unique value to the product and make replication of these goods elsewhere impossible.

Examples:

Dargeeling tea was first example of GI and today there are more than 300 GI products.

Examples of GIs registered in India during 2003-08: Kolhapur Jaggery, Paithani Saree Madhubani Painting, Basmati Rice, Hyderabadi Haleem, Nagpur Orange, Mysore Sandalwood Oil, Coorg Orange, Kangra Tea, Spices-Alleppey Green Cardamom, Coorg Green Cardamom, Monsooned Malabar Robusta Coffee. This act has made successful contribution to protect some of the specific geographical natural products.

Duration: GI protection is for ten years initially, which can be extended.

10.5 BIOPROSPECTING AND BIOPIRACY

Bioprospecting:

The process of finding new chemicals or drugs from various natural resources is called as bioprospecting. **Bioprospecting is 'the process of discovery and development of new molecules from different biological resources'.** Different fields like pharmaceuticals, agriculture, bioremediation, nanotechnology and biotechnology need new chemical compounds for different purposes. Bioprospecting is finding and using these new candidates for commercial purpose. Bioprospecting is branch of science which is required for new drug discovery and development. But along with bioprospecting, there are certain issues that need to be addressed. Use of indigenous knowledge of people is also becoming part of bioprospecting. Despite indigenous knowledge being intuitively helpful, in recent years, bioprospecting includes incorporate such knowledge in focusing screening efforts for new bioactive compounds. Many multinational companies started to tap these resources to develop new molecules. More than 200 companies and research organizations worldwide are screening plant and animal compounds for possible new drug candidates. Because of high throughput technologies, screening of new chemical has become easy and many candidates can be screened within short time. More than 20% of our pharmaceutical drugs and related compounds are coming from such biological resources. During 1980 to 2010, one third of all small molecule new chemical entities approved by the U.S. Food and Drug

Administration (FDA) were directly or indirectly derived from natural products. This part of venturing into the rainforest and screening for medicinal properties "bioprospecting" – is under criticism throughout world.

Biopiracy is one sort of theft. Biopiracy mainly focuses on the use of biological resources and/or knowledge of indigenous tribes or communities without giving those benefits. Biopiracy can be considered as economic exploitation of the resource/knowledge of people. **Biopiracy is an injustice relating to patent or intellectual property related to biological materials and traditional knowledge without sufficient authorization and/or compensation.** The terms and conditions related to bioprospecting have huge loopholes. As there is lack of an appropriate definition of biopiracy. Various international organizations like the Secretariat of the United Nations Convention on Biological Diversity (CBD), the World Intellectual Property Organization (WIPO) and the World Trade Organization (WTO) are associated with this issue. Incidents related to biopiracy are not necessarily related with money but also pride of country and people. Above organizations deal with these issues related to bioprospecting and biopiracy by avoiding conflicts with the help of international laws administered by the CBD and the WTO. The term "biopiracy" was coined in 1993 by Pat Mooney. Biopiracy means the use of intellectual property to legitimize the exclusive ownership and control of biological resources and knowledge, without giving any benefit or compensation to indigenous contributors.

India is country with rich biodiversity, traditional knowledge and enormous wild resources. There is huge pool of the genetic diversity of agriculturally important plants and animals. In India, for example, peasant producers cultivate some 50,000 varieties of rice, developed through traditional practices. In last decades, the Protection of Plant Varieties and Farmers' Rights Act of 2001 (PPVFR) and The Biological Diversity Act of 2002 (BD) are important laws related to biodiversity, introduced in India. Some loopholes in these laws are responsible for biopiracy. International efforts are made through United Nations Convention was signed by more than 150 countries except United States in 1992. This convention was regarding to "the conservation of biological diversity, the sustainable use of its components and the fair and equitable sharing of the benefits arising out of the utilization of genetic resources." The Convention legitimizes a market for owned genes and thereby diminishes biodiversity. These varieties arose from subtle differences in soil and climatic conditions due to mutation and evolution. The farmers are prohibited from harvesting and reusing the seed of any rice variety that has been patented. Lack of access to seed stocks will cause the abandonment of much of India's biologically diverse agriculture. Conservation of biological diversity regulates access to biological resources through National Biodiversity Authority and through State Biodiversity Boards. Indian citizens can freely and easily find access to biological resources for research purpose, for use in traditional systems of medicine, for example: Vaidyas & Hakims and protection of Indigenous knowledge. The property-rights theory states that "the rights of disposal of a resource should belong to those who have physical control over the resource". Conventions on biodiversity speak of the same national rights of disposal in the sense of a "national patrimony". The property rights should belong to the national governments and their local representative institutions for it are their responsibility to plan and manage areas which can be used for to preserve the biodiversity. The incentive of countries of origin to maintain biological resources rises accordingly to the amount of returns these countries get from selling their resources.

Some Important Points Related to Bioprospecting and Biopiracy:

- Bioprospecting have attracted attention of vast number of multinational companies. This has resulted in growing concerns about the collection and conservation of plants, animals, biological materials and ecosystem.
- Also at the same time, issues related to intellectual property or ownership over these biological resources needs to be addressed.
- Because of biotechnological advances or manipulation of biological resources through recombinant DNA technology, or genetic engineering issues related to ownership have become more complicated necessitating new regulations.
- Regulations related to bioprospecting and biopiracy have found difficult to control as there is absence of one single international treaty or agreement that fully captures all the issues involved. Rather most laws are country specific. Farmers, indigenous tribal peoples and local communities have different ethical, economic, cultural and political problems.
- Some cases of biopiracy involve the grant of a patent over some product or derivative from biological resources and/or traditional knowledge. At the same time, there are some cases where patent protection is not present; these atypical cases are called as 'non-patent biopiracy' incidents.
- Biopiracy can have direct as well as indirect implications, like loss of income, traditional knowledge.
- International treaties and conventions like the ITPGRFA and CBD is important while treating global cases involving intellectual property rights, genetic resources and traditional knowledge.
- Recent cases related to biopiracy have resulted in development of 'defensive' and 'positive' protection of traditional knowledge and/or biological resources by providing documentation. The IP/C/W/493 submission to the TRIPS Council by Peru on 19 September 2007 reflects the dissatisfaction of the government with recent international trends of 'biopiracy'.
- The Nagoya Protocol is an important part in these regulations. This protocol involves access to Genetic Resources with equal benefit sharing. Thos protocol can be considered as a supplementary agreement to the Convention on Biological Diversity. This protocol gives a transparent legal framework for implementation of the CBD: the fair and equitable sharing of benefits arising out of the utilization of genetic resources.
- The Nagoya Protocol was adopted on 29 October 2010 in Nagoya, Japan and came into force on 12 October 2014. The main objective behind this is sharing of benefits arising from the utilization of genetic resources, thereby contributing to the conservation and sustainable use of biodiversity.

Role of CBD in Biopiracy:

Prior to TRIPS, the Convention for Biological Diversity (CBD) was established in 1992 as an international IPR agreement to give some protection to indigenous people. According to the CBD provisions, source nations should receive some compensation or benefit for sharing knowledge and resources with corporations or multinational companies wanting to use the biodiversity. According to the CBD every country or states have sovereign rights and power to protect own resources and that those resources are no longer freely available to others. So efforts for conservation and sustainable use are of critical importance. Clearly, rich nations and multinational companies are not much interested in giving benefits to poor countries or people having resources. The CBD differs substantially from other treaties in that it takes a comprehensive approach to the conservation and sustainable use of biological resources.

The Convention on Biological Diversity (CBD) establishes important principles, rules and regulations for the protection of biodiversity while recognizing the vast commercial value of the planet's store.

Some important focus areas of CBD are:

1. Genes, species and ecosystems all these three levels are considered under the convention.
2. The Convention aims to address the causes rather than the effects of threats to biodiversity.
3. Conservation and sustainable use of bio resources are considered to be inseparable.
4. It does not set any standards for protection but outlines the goals and policies to be pursued by countries through their own legislation. But only few countries have realized the importance of natural resources and traditional knowledge and enacted the legislation.

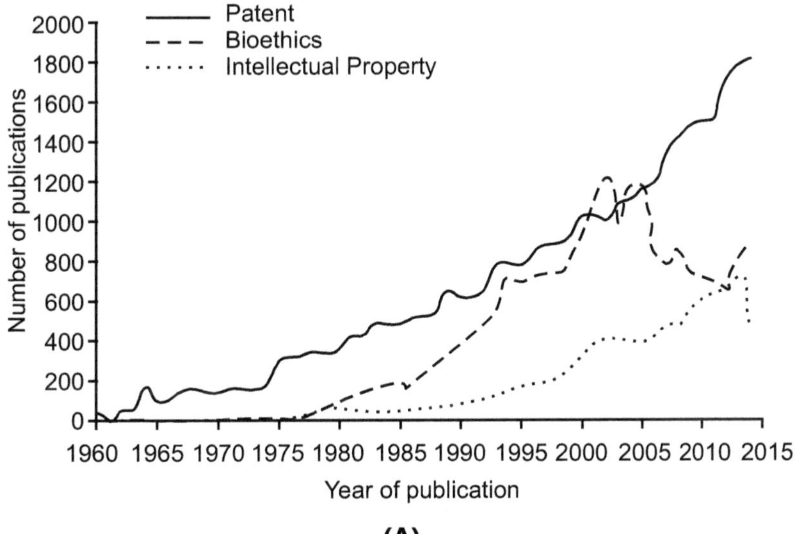

(A)

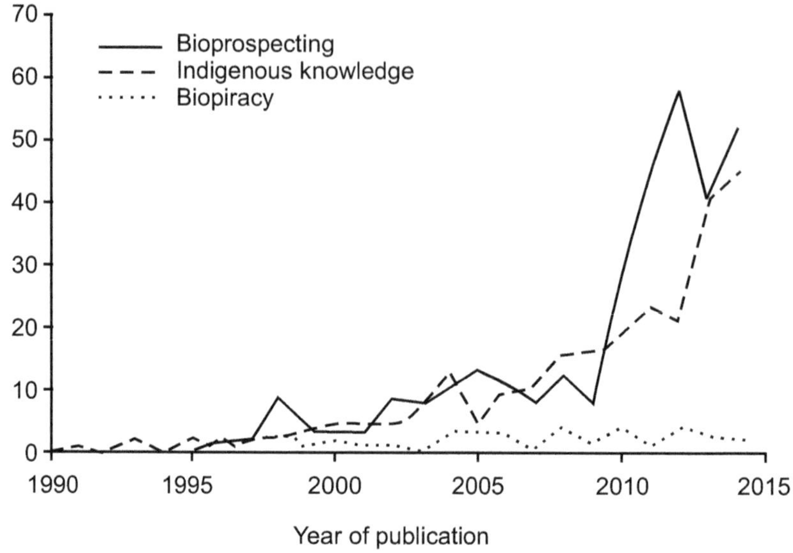

(B)

Fig. 10.1: Biopiracy of Natural Product

(**Source:** Thomas Efferth et. al. Biopiracy of natural products and good bioprospecting practice, phytomedicine)

Recent Information of Biopiracy of Natural Products:

Other case studies of biopiracy:

- **Basmati case:** This was one of the important cases from Indian perspective. The United States Patent office has granted the patent to company called 'RiceTec' on September 2, 1997. According to this patent, this company can grow aromatic rice in America and call that rice as Basmati. India objected to this patent. This patent covered 20 claims covering not only novel rice plant but also various rice lines; resulting plants and grains, seed deposit 2 claims, method for selecting a rice plant for breeding and propagation. In claim number 15-17 a rice grain having characteristics similar to those from Indian Basmati rice lines was claimed. According to Geographic indication, only rice grown in particular part of India can be called as Basmati. Basmati is grown from centuries, traditionally. This was violation of GI provisions coming under protection of intellectual property. After opposition from India these claims were withdrawn.
- French multinational company has patented the use of Kava to reduce hair loss and stimulate hair growth. Kava is one of the plants used traditionally in many countries. More than 100 varieties of Kava are grown in the Pacific region, especially in Fiji and Vanuatu, where it was first domesticated thousands of years ago.
- For generations, Shamans (traditional healers) of indigenous tribes throughout the Amazon basin are using the bark of *B. caapi* Mort. to produce a ceremonial drink known as 'Ayahuasca' which means "wine of the soul". Ayahuasca is used in traditional medicine and cultivated for that purpose for generations. The Shamans use Ayahuasca in religious

and healing ceremonies to diagnose and treat illness, meet with spirits, and divine the future. American citizen, Loren Miller obtained US Plant Patent (no. 5, 751 issued in 1986). This allowed him rights over the variety of *B. caapi* Mort. This plant was collected from a domestic garden in Amazon and called as 'Da Vine'. The plant has many potential medicinal properties. The patent claimed that Da Vine represented a new and distinct variety of *B. caapi.* Mort., mainly because of the flower colour. This patent was opposed by the Co-ordinating Body of Indigenous Organizations of the Amazon Basin (COICA), which represents more than 400 indigenous tribes in the Amazon region. Clearly this was prior art and nothing innovative or new. On reexamination, USPTO revoked this patent in November 1999. However, after successful defense from the inventor USPTO restored the rights of the innovator in April 2001.

- Quinoa is a type of staple food crop for millions in the Andes. People liken Quechua and Aymara have successfully bred a multitude of quinoa varieties. In 1997, two professors from Colorado State University, have US patent numbered 5,304,718 on *Quinoa chenopodium Quinao.* Main claim of this patent was the variety of male sterile cytoplasm is key to developing hybrid quinoa. The patent claims any Quinoa crossed with male sterile Apelawa plants. Because of this patent they have exclusive monopoly over male sterile plants of this variety. This could be used to create other hybrid varieties. The male sterility of in varieties of Quinoa is actually traditional knowledge in Chile, Peru, Bolivia and other neighbouring countries.
- For thousands of years, African tribesmen used to eat the Hoodia cactus to satisfy hunger as well as thirst on long hunting trips. The Bushmen who lived around the Kalahari desert in southern Africa used to cut-off a stem of the cactus as food. Hoodia was in news because of the bio-piracy. In 1995, South African Council of Scientific & Industrial Research (CSIR) patented Hoodia's appetite-suppressing element (P57) and hence, its potential cure for obesity. In 1997, they licensed P57 to British Biotech Company, Phytopharm. In 1998, Pfizer acquired the rights for development and marketing of P57 as a potential slimming drug and cure for obesity. This drug was having the market worth more than £ 6 billion. The San people came to know about this exploitation of their traditional knowledge, and in June 2001. After which they launched legal action against South African CSIR and the pharmaceutical industry on grounds of bio-piracy. This case was violation of traditional knowledge. Prior informed permission of tribal people and original discoverrers was not taken. This was considered as violation of the rules of the Convention on Biodiversity. Finally, the two sides entered into negotiations for a benefit-sharing agreement.
- To cite some more examples of biopiracy, the plant *Phyllanthus amarus* Schum.et Thonn. is used for Ayurvedic treatment for jaundice, a US patent has been taken for use against Hepatitis B. The plant *Piper nigrum* Linn. is used for Ayurvedic treatment for vitiligo (a skin pigmentation disorder). A patent has been taken in UK for the application of a molecule from *Piper nigrum* Linn. for use in treatment of vitiligo.

- In 2015, a French NGO accused researchers from the Institute de Recherche pour le Dévéloppement (IRD) of biopiracy. This case involves a plant named as *Quassia amara L.* (Simaroubaceae). Researchers had applied for a patent for a natural bioactive molecule against malaria and cancer, the Simalika lactone E, isolated from this plant. In this case, researchers were accused of misconduct, stealing the traditional knowledge of indigenous people. These accusations were made according to the Nagoya Protocol, French law on biodiversity, nature and landscapes.

The appropriation of elements of this collective knowledge of societies into proprietary knowledge for the commercial profit of a few is one of the concerns of the developing world. An urgent policy and action is needed to protect these knowledge systems through national as well as international policies. At the same time, focus on community knowledge, innovation, enterprise and investment is needed.

The local communities or individuals do not have the knowledge and awareness regarding protection of their property of cultural values and origin. The communities have knowledge about their flora and fauna in detail. So it is natural justice to give local people their share. This matter is regarding the use and commercialization of the biodiversity. A suitable policy which will help the progress of knowledge and gives adequate intellectual property protection as well as sustainable use is needed. This will also ensures equal benefit sharing to those who deserve it.

10.6 PATENTING ASPECTS OF TRADITIONAL KNOWLEDGE AND NATURAL PRODUCTS

Traditional Knowledge:

Traditional knowledge refers to ideas, knowledge, innovations and peculiar practices developed from experience gained over centuries and adapted to the local people, culture and environment. It is mostly information held in human memories and not written down. Traditional knowledge system acts holistic way by considering mind and body. Traditional knowledge includes experiences, philosophies, politics, and technologies practiced by the indigenous people. The traditional wisdom is mostly not written and transfer from one generation to next in the form of oral communication. This knowledge is vast and covers agricultural, medicinal, biodiversity-related, experiences, and different expressions of folklore in the different forms like music, dance, song, handicraft, designs, stories and artwork.

The traditional medical knowledge of indigenous people throughout the world is being used in the health care system from times immemorial. It has played a crucial role in identifying biological resources worthy of commercial exploitation. Ethno biological data has provided a good way in exploring new pharmaceuticals from nature's store of biological material. Pharmaceutical, biotechnology and personal care companies have focused their attention and their advertising, upon plants and animals which have been demonstrated by indigenous people to have beneficial qualities. This has saved those companies at considerable expense in obtaining that knowledge through their own research. In India, traditional medicines are governed by the Drugs and Cosmetics Act of 1940 and the Drugs and Cosmetics Rules of 1945. They regulate the import, manufacture, distribution and sale of drugs and cosmetics. In 1959, Drug and cosmetic Act was modified by the Government of India to include drugs which are derived from traditional Indian medicine. Products under traditional systems are not permitted to be manufactured without a licence. The licence for the same should be obtained from the State Drug Control Authorities. Patent and proprietary medicines derived from the traditional systems must contain ingredients which are mentioned in the recognized books of the traditional systems, as specified in the Drugs and Cosmetics Act. Special committee and an advisory board for Ayurvedic, Siddha and Unani drugs gives advise to the Government.

The Traditional Medicines Congress (TMC) was formed in the year 2004. The Traditional Medicines Congress (TMC) is proposing federal regulation that will affect everyone involved with herbs. The TMC proposal would violate the intellectual property rights of both cultures and culturally empowered individuals who hold cultural knowledge of medicinal plant use. This violates UNESCO (United Nations Educational, Scientific and Cultural Organization) and WIPO (World Intellectual Property Organization) guidelines.

There are two important international conventions that have bearing on intellectual property rights in indigenous knowledge systems. These are the World Trade Organization's Trade-Related Aspects of Intellectual Property Rights (TRIPs) and the Convention on Biological Diversity (CBD). The CBD is the only major international convention that gives ownership of biodiversity to indigenous communities and individuals. This ensures their right to protect this knowledge.

Intellectual property rights are basically a mechanism to allocate ownership of knowledge and distribute benefits from it among competing claimants.

IPR for protection of traditional knowledge and community resources is difficult of following reasons:

- Traditional knowledge is not individual or personal but collective right which belongs to a country or society.
- IPR protection is given when there is a specific act of 'invention'.
- IPR issues are related to commercial or market values, whereas traditional knowledge is for health and wellness.
- IPR issues are related to economic powers and manipulation and difficult to monitor and enforce. These issues are expensive, complicated and time-consuming also.

According to TRIPs (1994), concept called as 'Traditional Resource Rights: De Facto Self-determination for Indigenous Peoples'. This is proposed as a specific example of a *sui generis* system of legal rights. Sui generis is many 'bundles' of rights existing and being developed which can be utilised for the protection of traditional knowledge and resources.

The TRR concept can form the basis for *sui generis* systems. Apart from this, it also includes environmental protection, IPR for promotion and protection of culture, heritage and recognition of other issues.

Indian Scenario:

- India has a rich traditional knowledge and wisdom to treat different diseases afflicting people. This plethora of knowledge has generally been passed down by word of mouth from generation to generation. This knowledge is not owned by any single person and collective efforts from centuries.
- According to WHO survey more than 60% of population is directly or indirectly using drugs from natural origin including traditional system.
- India fought successfully objected Turmeric and Basmati patents granted by United States Patent and Trademark Office (USPTO) and Neem patent granted by European Patent Office (EPO). This has created lot of awareness about traditional knowledge and IPR issues.
- Indian Government has started the Department of Ayurveda, Yoga & Naturopathy, Unani, Siddha and Homoeopathy - (AYUSH) for quality research on traditional medicine. After Turmeric, Basmati and Neem cases, need for documentation of Indian Traditional knowledge became very critical. To address this issue, Traditional Knowledge Digital Library (TKDL) project was initiated in the year 2001. Department of Indian System of Medicine and Homoeopathy (ISM&H) constituted an inter-disciplinary Task Force, for creating an approach on this issue.
- As most of the traditional knowledge is in local language, not in English. Therefore documentation of this existing traditional knowledge has become mandatory. This also ensures protection from being inappropriate use in the form of patents. This was one approach to avoid biopiracy of traditional knowledge and national pride.
- TKDL provides information on traditional knowledge existing in the country can be used by different patent examiners at International Patent Offices (IPOs). This would prevent the grant of patents involving biopiracy related to traditional knowledge. TKDL thus helps the patent examiners at international level.
- TKDL is a database containing codified literature from Indian Systems of Medicine. TKDL contains more than 2.08 lakh formulations from the texts of traditional medicine systems of India which are Ayurveda, Unani and Siddha.

10.7 CASE STUDY OF CURCUMA

- Turmeric is common household remedy known as *Curcuma longa* traditionally used as a spice in Indian food. In India, rhizomes of turmeric are used as spice during cooking from many centuries. Wide ranges of biological activities including antibacterial, anti-inflammatory, anti-oxidant and anti-cancer are shown by this plant. So there is logical basis for its traditional use in foodstuff. It is commonly used as a blood purifier, in treating the common cold, and as an anti-infective for many skin infections.

- In 1995, two Indian scientists named as Dr. Suman K. Das and Dr. Harihar P. Kohli working at the University of Mississippi Medical Centre was granted a US patent (number 5, 401,504) on use of turmeric in wound healing. In this patent, they made six patent claims covering the oral and topical use of turmeric powder for healing of surgical wounds and ulcers.
- Dr. Mashelkar, from The Council of Scientific & Industrial Research (CSIR), India filed objection to this patent. They filed re-examination case with the US patent office challenging the patent on the grounds of existing of prior art and traditional knowledge.
- According to CSIR claim, turmeric has been used for thousands of years for healing wounds, rashes. This case is do not have novelty. The traditional knowledge claim was supported by documentary evidence including ancient Sanskrit text and a research paper in the Journal of the Indian Medical Association published in 1953. Despite an appeal by the patent holders, the US patent office accepted the CSIR objections and cancelled the patent.
- This was first case considered as a landmark judgment of patent based on the traditional knowledge of a developing country. The US Patent Office revoked this patent in 1997, after ascertaining that there was no novelty; the findings by innovators having been known in India for centuries. After this case, all traditional knowledge is documented in the form of TKDL (Traditional Knowledge Digital Library) to avoid such cases in future.

10.8 CASE STUDY OF NEEM

- Neem (*Azadirachta indica,* family Meliaceae) is very common tree found throughout India.
- Different parts of Neem including seeds, extracts are used in India from several centuries against hundreds of pests and fungal diseases that attack food crops. Neem parts have been widely used in traditional medicine as contraceptive and cosmetics for variety of skin problems.
- In 1994, European Patent Office (EPO) granted a patent (EPO patent No. 436257) to the US Corporation W.R. Grace Company and US Department of Agriculture. This patent claimed for a method for controlling fungi on plants by the aid of hydrophobic extract of Neem oil.
- A group of international NGOs and representatives of Indian farmers filed legal opposition against the patent next year.
- The evidence was submitted for the fungicidal effect of extracts of Neem seeds had been known and used for centuries in Indian agriculture to protect crops. So there was lack of novelty as this is in use for centuries in India, both in curing dermatological diseases in humans and in protecting agricultural plants form fungal infections.
- The main chemical involved is Azadirachtin, which is a natural compound found in the seeds of the Neem tree. Synthetic form of a naturally occurring compound may be patentable, because the synthetic form in this case is possible to prepare. Traditionally

people in India, smash Neem seed, soak overnight and scoop emulsion part for spraying on crops. So the claim made in this patent was already known publically.

- In 1999, the EPO determined this case as prior art because of all the evidence. Finally, this patent was found lack of an inventive step. The patent granted was finally revoked by the authority in May 2000.
- In March 2006, EPO even rejected the challenge made in 2001 by the USDA and the chemicals multinational, W. R. Grace to the EPO's previous decision to cancel their patent on the fungicidal properties of the seeds extracted from the Neem tree.

In future, bioprospecting and biopiracy cases can be avoided with the help of certain things like:

- Traditional knowledge, natural products need better harmonized and uniform IPR laws.
- Technologically rich countries need reform in their patent laws for better benefit sharing.
- All traditional knowledge should be public domain where transfer of knowledge and technology is better.

QUESTIONS

1. What is patent? Explain concept of IPR.
2. Which are different types of intellectual properties? Give examples.
3. Define patent. Describe different parts of patent document.
4. Which are different advantages of good patent system?
5. Explain patenting of natural products.
6. Explain main features of Farmer's Right Act.
7. What is geographical indication? Explain GI Act 1999.
8. What is biopiracy? Write different cases of biopiracy of natural products.
9. Describe patenting aspects of traditional knowledge and natural products.
10. Explain case study of Curcuma.
11. Describe case study of Neem.

❖❖❖

Chapter...11

REGULATORY ISSUES

Objectives

- To learn different regulations regarding ASU (Ayurvedic Siddha Unani) drugs in India including ASU DTAB (Drug Technical Advisory Board) and ASU DCC (Drug Consulative Committee).
- To understand regulation of manufacture of ASU drugs/ schedule Z of drugs and cosmetic act for ASU drugs.

11.1 NEED FOR REGULATION

1. Regulations provide protection to natural products users and nature also.
2. It improves use of natural products and encourages research.
3. It establishes system for control of all activities like manufacturing, sales and use of medicines.
4. It gives penalty or punishment for persons who do not follow certain standards and rules.
5. It prepares and amends laws, and enforces them to control natural products, thus provide safe and effective medicine.

More than 80% of world population still depends on natural products for their primary health care needs directly or indirectly. Natural products may contain processed or semi processed drugs from plant, animal or mineral origin. There are number of factors that can cause variation in chemical constituents and therapeutic effects. Drugs may contain plant parts or material in crude or processed state as active ingredient along with some excipients. Effectiveness of natural products can vary due to several reasons like growing conditions such as soil, fertilizers, climate, insect control, harvesting procedure, curing procedure, handling conditions like processing, packing, storage and shelf life. Unfortunately, the number of patients experiencing negative health consequences caused by the use of herbal or natural medicines has also been increasing now-a-days. Poor quality of medicines, including raw medicinal materials is one of the major causes of reported adverse reactions. On this background, regulatory requirements for natural products are becoming more important day by day.

11.2 REGULATORY ISSUES RELATED TO NATURAL PRODUCTS

- Most of people have common assumption that natural products are safe and without side effect. In reality, natural products can also have serious side effects and toxicity.

- All natural products come from diverse background and have intrinsic variability in chemical constituents and therapeutic effects also.
- Lack of standardization parameters, absence of marker compound create problem for quality control of natural product.
- Most of the time, in case of traditional medicine, there is no documentary evidence about not only safety but efficacy also.
- Even there is no harmonization between regulatory bodies which regulate natural products. Natural products are not uniformly regulated in different countries and rules have many variation and ambiguity.

11.3 REGULATIONS IN INDIA

From thousands of years, India has rich tradition of medicinal systems including Ayurveda, Siddha etc. Mughal and British rule influenced India culturally and socially in many ways. Mughal invasion introduced Unani system in India. British introduced there reductionist approach now called as Allopathy or Modern Medicinal system. These all systems along with Homoeopathy co-existed and also flourished and influence each other to form Indian system of medicine. After independence, revival of Indian System of medicine was started again. As India become assignee to WTO and TRIPS, these regulations were again modified to fit with global regulations. In 2014, Indian Government made separate Department of AYUSH to foster these traditional systems. So, the original British laws were changed from time to time to better regulation of natural products.

Table 11.1: Laws Regulate Medicines in India

Sr. No.	Law	Year
1.	Drug and Cosmetic Act	1940
2.	Drug and Magic Remedies Act	1954
3.	Central Council of Homoeopathy Act	1973
4.	Central Council of Indian Medicine Act	1973
5.	Medicinal and Toiletries Preparation Act	1995

In 1940, during British India, after recommendation from Chopra committee original 'drug bill' was converted into 'Drug Act 1940'. Rules were drafted in 1945 and came into force from 1947. Original drug act was later modified by addition of cosmetics in 1962 and became 'Drug and Cosmatic Act'. In 1982, Ayurveda, Siddha and Unani means ASU drugs were included into Drug and Cosmetics Act. ASU formularies and textbooks were added for confirmation of these drugs at this point.

Manufacture of ASU drugs:

According to Drug and Cosmetic Act 1940, Govermnet of India and subsequent amendments there are different regulations for manufacture of ASU drugs:

PART XVII-

Rule 161: Labelling, packing and limit of alcohol in ASU drugs

Rule 161 A: Exemption in labeling and packing, provisions for export of ASU drugs

Rule 161 B: Shelf life or expiry of ASU drugs

PART XVIII

Rule 162: Duties of Inspectors specially authorised to inspect the manufacture of ASU drugs

Rule 162 A: Qualifications of the State Drug Licensing Authority for Licensing of ASU drugs

Rule 163: Procedure for dispatch of sample to Government Analyst and its receipt by the Government Analyst and provision of Pharmacopoeial Laboratory for testing of ASU drugs

Rule 163 A to G: Different regarding functions of Pharmacopoeial Laboratory, testing, sampling, recording of results, fees, signatures etc. for testing of ASU drugs

Rule 164: Method of test or analysis to be employed in relation to Ayurvedic (including Siddha) or Unani drugs

Rule 165: Qualifications of Government Analyst

Rule 166: Duties of Government Analyst

Rule 167: Qualifications of Inspector

PART XIX

Rule 168: STANDARDS OF AYURVEDIC, SIDDHA AND UNANI DRUGS

Rule 169: Permitted Excipients

1) ASU DTAB (Ayurvedic, Siddha and Unani Drugs Technical Advisory Board)

ASU DTAB was formed According to section 33C, Chapter IV of Drug and Cosmatic Act 1940. According to Drug and Cosmatic Act 1940, Chapter IV A have provisions relating to Ayurvedic, Siddha and Unani Drugs for formation of Board. According to section 33 B, these provisions will be applicable only to Ayurvedic, Siddha and Unani drugs.

Function of ASU DTAB:

To advise central as well as state government on technical matters related to this subject.

Composition:

In ASU DTAB, first four members are *ex officio* members and remaining members are nominated by Central Government for period of three years and also can be re-nominated. ASU DTAB shall consist following members:

Table 11.2: Constitution of ASU/DTAB

Sr. No.	Member	Appointment nature: *ex officio* / nominated by central Government	Total number of members	Tenure
1.	The Director General of Health Services	*ex officio*	1	--
2.	The Drug controller of India	*ex officio*	1	--
3.	The principal officer dealing with Indian System of Medicine in Ministry of Healh	*ex officio*	1	--
4.	The Director of Central Drug Laboratory, Calcutta	*ex officio*	1	---
5.	Person holding the appointment of Government Analyst under section 33F, to be nominated by the Central Government	Central Government	1	3 years
6.	Pharmacognocist	Central Government	1	3 years
7.	Phyochemist	Central Government	1	3 years
8.	Two from amongst the members of the Ayurvedic Pharmacopoeia Committee, one from amongst the members of the Unani Pharmacopoeia Committee and one from amongst the members of the Siddha Pharmacopoeia Committee	Central Government	4	3 years
9.	Teacher in *Dravyaguna* and *Bhaishajya Kalpana*, to be nominated by the Central Government	Central Government	1	3 years
10.	Teacher in ILM-UL-ADVIA and TAKLIS-WA-DAWA-SAZI	Central Government	1	3 years
11.	Teacher in *Gunapadam*, to be nominated by the Central Government	Central Government	1	3 years
12.	Persons, one each to represent the Ayurvedic, Siddha and Unani drug industry.	Central Government	3	3 years
13.	Persons, one each from among the practitioners of Ayurvedic, Siddha, and Unani Tibb system of medicine	Central Government	3	3 years

Working:

- All nominated members will be working for three years and will be eligible for re-nomination from Central Government.
- The Central Government shall appoint a member of the Board as its Chairman for smooth functioning.
- This board with previous approval of government makes bye-laws for working of ASU DTAB. This can be done by fixing a quorum and regulation of own procedure and code of conduct.
- The functions of the Board can be exercised not withstanding any vacancy.
- The central government will appoint a secretary of the board that will provide the board clerical or other staff as necessary.

2) ASU DCC (Ayurvedic, Siddha and Unani Drug Consultative Committee):

Formation:

Ayurvedic, Siddha and Unani Drug Consultative committee was formed according to Drug and Cosmetics Act 1940, Chapter IV, Section 33D.

Composition:

- There will be two persons nominated by the Central Government as representatives of that Government.
- Not more than one representative of each state nominated by the respective State Government. State Government can appoint maximum one representative.

Function:

The Ayurvedic, Siddha and Unani Drugs Consultative Committee shall meet when required and guide Central Government. This committee can regulate its own procedure on matters related to ASU Drugs.

11.4 REGULATION OF MANUFACTURE OF ASU DRUGS - SCHEDULE Z OF DRUGS AND COSMETICS ACT FOR ASU DRUGS

Regulation and Manufacturing of ASU Drugs:

The drug and cosmetic Act 1940 was introduced in 1940 as national policy for alternative and traditional medicine. In year 1969, Ayurveda, Siddha and Unani drugs were added as separate chapter by Act 13 of 1964 in the act. Later in 2008, guidelines for evaluation and analysis under ISM (Indian System of Medicine) were included in Drug and Cosmetic Rule 1945. In 2014, separate ministry on AYUSH is formed. AYUSH opt for governance, education, regulation, development and growth of ISM. AYUSH has control over many subordinate offices; several autonomous bodies (research councils, professional council, pharmacopoeia laboratories, national institutes, academy and hospitals). It works for the good health and to outreach the healthcare to our people. It provides safe, efficacious, and affordable medicines.

Table 11.3: Different provisions related to ASU drugs according to the Drugs and Cosmetics Act, 1940 Chapter IVA

No.	Section	Purpose
1	33B	Application of Chapter IVA.
2	33C	Ayurvedic, Siddha and Unani Drugs Technical Advisory Board.
3	33D	The Ayurvedic, Siddha and Unani Drugs Consultative Committee.
4	33E	Misbranded drugs.
4.1	33EE	Adulterated drugs.
4.1.1	33EEA	Spurious drugs
4.1.2	33EEB	Regulation of manufacture for sale of ASU drugs.
4.1.3	33EEC	Prohibition of manufacture and sale of certain ASU drugs.
4.1.4	33EED	Power of Central Government to prohibit manufacture etc., of Ayurvedic, Siddha or Unani drugs in public interest.
5	33F	Government Analysts.
6	33G	Inspectors
7	33H	Application of provisions of sections 22, 23, 24 and 25.
8	33I	Penalty for manufacture, sale etc., of ASU drugs in contravention of act
9	33J	Penalty for subsequent offences
10	33K	Confiscation
11	33L	Application of provisions to Government departments
12	33M	Cognizance of offences
13	33N	Power of Central Government to make rules.
14	33O	Power to amend first schedule

Common Points:

Controlling and maintaining of quality, safety and efficacy of ASU drugs is herculean task. Formulation of standard for ensuring safety and quality of polyherbal/herbal and mineral drugs involve many steps. This is done by different approaches:

Preparations of Guidelines and Standards:

- For ASU drugs, manufacturing license, Good Manufacturing Practices (GMP) and adherence to standards of drugs as prescribed in the pharmacopoeia and formularies are mandatory. Authoritative, classical textbook with formula is most important step in case of ASU drugs. This is to ensure ASU drugs will have good quality, safety and efficacy.

- Pharmacopoeias and formularies contain detail information about the biological source, synonyms, description, properties, TLC fingerprinting, important formulations, therapeutic indication, and details related to identity, purity, strength. Pharmacopoeial committees set standards for quality, purity and strength of drugs and approve drug formularies. This is most important step to avoid confusion related to ASU drugs.

Governing Bodies:

- Statutory bodies like Ayurveda, Siddha, Unani Technical Advisory Board (ASU DTAB) and Ayurveda, Siddha, Unani Drugs Consultative Committee (ASU DCC) are formed under the Drugs and Cosmetics Act to advise Government. These bodies give advice to state and central Government on technical matters and for securing uniformity throughout the country and also help in the administration of the acts, provisions and rules.
- ASU DTAB and ASU DCC are also help to attain the uniformity in the administration, implementation of Drugs & Cosmetics Act, 1940 Chapter IV (related to ASU drugs) throughout India.
- The Drugs & Magic Remedies Act, 1954, is useful for regulation of objectionable advertisements & publicity relating to certain drugs and magic remedies.
- This law is important for ASU drugs as most drugs are from traditional background.

Regulating Bodies:

- To maintain the quality and to facilitate drug standardization & testing of ASU drugs, Pharmacopoeial Laboratory of Indian Medicine (PLIM) was started in 1970 and the Homoeopathic Pharmacopoeial Laboratory (HPL) was started in 1975 for checking quality of respective medicines.
- There is provision of testing laboratories according to Drug and Cosmetic act 1940. In addition to reputed laboratories, other labs are also involved in preparation of pharmacopoeial standards and monographs and Standard Operating Procedures (SOPs) for ASU drugs.
- Separate Pharmacopoeial Committees have been formed for ASU drugs. Monograph preparation is one of the important things for ASU drugs. So far, 326 monographs of Ayurveda drugs in 4 volumes, 45 of Unani drugs, 916 of Homeopathic drugs have been published.
- Remaining drugs are also going to be included in monographs on ASU drugs in coming years. Formularies of Ayurveda, Siddha and Unani containing 636, 248 and 745 multi-ingredient classical formulations respectively have been published to facilitate manufacture of drugs with uniform composition and manufacturing procedures and better quality.

- Role of central laboratories like Pharmacopoeial Laboratories, Central Council for Research in Ayurveda and Siddha (CCRAS) laboratories, laboratories of Central Council for Research in Unani Medicine (CCRUM), Council for Scientific & Industrial Research (CSIR) laboratories are importrnt. At the same time, there are several other laboratories of private sector playing important role.

Responsibility of Licensing Authority under Drug and Cosmetic Act for ASU Drugs:

1. To ensure that manufacturing facilities have all the required approved certificates and clearances for manufacturing.
2. The manufacturing facility should comply with the GMP norms.
3. To check whether the documents submitted with license application are complete and the conditions laid down in Rule 158-B are fulfilled to grant or renew the license.
4. To ensure that the contents on the label of medicines are correct and in accordance with labelling provisions.
5. To ensure quality check of adequate number of ASU & H drug samples taken from manufacturing sites and market.
6. To monitor advertisements of ASU & H drugs appearing in print and electronic media for misleading claims.
7. To make the lists of licensed manufacturers and products and upload in the website.
8. To take regulatory action against defaulters acting in contravention of the provisions of Drugs & Cosmetics Act and Drugs & Magic Remedies Act and rules thereunder.

Quality control and standardization of ASU drugs is done by traditional as well as modern approach. Quality has to be checked for both raw and finished products. Many methods from organoleptic, microscopic, physical, chemical fingerprinting, biological assaying is available for checking quality. Testing of heavy metals, pesticides and microbial load have been developed for quality control and standardization of ASU drugs. Several chromatographic fingerprint profiles are also included in Ayurvedic Pharmacopoeia. Identification and estimation of active therapeutic ingredients and marker compounds with reference to which drugs of Ayurveda, Siddha and Unani can be standardized are under development. Chapter IV of Drug and cosmetic act explain the details about misbranded, adulterated and spurious drug related to ASU.

As per the Regulation of manufacture for sale or distribution of ASU drugs, no person is allowed to sale or distributes the substandard drugs. Central Government has the power to prohibit the manufacture, sale or distribution of ASU drug which may fail the prescribed norms.

Regulation of Manufacture of ASU Drug:

ASU drug is considered as misbranded when:

- If drug is coloured, coated, powered or polished that damage is concealed, or if it is made to appear of better or greater therapeutic value then that drug can be considered as misbranded drug.
- Also, if drug is not labelled properly or if its label or container or anything accompanying the drug have any statement, design or device which makes any false or misleding claim then this durg is considered as misbranded drug.

ASU drug is considered as adulterated drug when:

- If drug contain any filthy, putrid, decomposed substance.
- If drug is prepared, stored, packed in bad condition, injurious to health.
- If container is exposed to harmful substances.
- If contain other than permitted colours.
- If contain harmful or toxic substance, injurious to health.
- If mixed with any other substance so that quality is decreased.

According to this law, spurious drug is the one:

- If it is sold, or offered or exhibited for sale, under a name of another drug; or
- If it is an copy or imitation of, or is a substitute for, another drug or resembles another drug in a manner which can deceive,
- If the drug have similar label or container with another drug, unless it is plainly and conspicuously marked so as to reveal its true character and its lack of identity with such other drug; or
- If the label or container have the name of an individual or company claiming to be the manufacturer of the drug, which individual or company is bogus or does not exist; or
- If it has been substituted, replaced with by any other drug or substance partly or completely; or
- If it purports to be the product of a manufacturer of whom it is not truly a product.

According to section 33EEB, any person cannot manufacture any ASU drug for sale or for distribution except in accordance with such standards, if any, as may be prescribed in relation to that drug. This clearly indicates, while manufacturing of ASU drugs all regulatory provisions must be followed.

Government can prevent sale, manufacture or distribution of any ASU drug;

- If any misbranded, adulterated or spurious drug is used.
- If labeled ingredients and actual ingredients in medicine are not matching.

Penalty for manufacture, sale of ASU drugs:

Any Person himself or by any other person on his behalf:

- Manufactures for sale or for distribution of ASU drugs found to be adulterated under section 33EE, or without a valid licence under section 33EEC, shall be punishable with imprisonment for a term which may extend to one year and with fine which shall not be less than two thousand rupees.
- Manufactures for sale or for distribution of ASU drugs found to be spurious under section 33EEA, will have punishment of imprisonment for a term which shall not be less than one year but which may extend to three years and with fine which shall not be less than five thousand rupees.
- Contravenes of any other provisions of Chapter IV or any rule made under this chapter, shall be punishable with imprisonment for a term which may extend to three months and with fine which shall not be less than five hundred rupees.

QUESTIONS

1. Explain need for regulation of herbal drugs.
2. Explain in detail herbal drug regulatoins in India.
3. Describe in detail functions and composition of ASU DTAB.
4. Write a note on ASU DCC.
5. Explain schedule Z of drugs and Cosmetic Act for ASU drugs.
6. Write responsibility of licensing authority under Drug and Cosmetic Act for ASU durgs.
7. Write in detail regulation of manufacture of ASU drugs.

❖❖❖

UNIT-V

Chapter...12

GENERAL INTRODUCTION TO HERBAL INDUSTRY

Objectives

- To learn about present scope and future prospects of herbal drug industry.
- To know about plant based industries and institutions in India.

12.1 HERBAL DRUG INDUSTRY: PRESENT SCOPE AND FUTURE PERSPECTIVES

Global Scenario:

Herbal drugs are gaining importance in recent years, because of the increasing demand for natural medicines. According to the World Health Organization (WHO) report around 70% to 80% of people worldwide rely on herbal sources for their primary healthcare treatment. Affordability and accessibility are two main factors behind popularization of herbal drugs. According to global herbal drug market over the forecast for the period during 2017-2023, market is expected to reach $ 111 billion by the end of 2023; this market is projected to growing at a CAGR of ~ 7.2 %. According to the American Botanical Council, it was reported that the sale of herbal supplements was increased by 7.7% in the United States in 2016.

USA is driving force for Indian pharmaceutical industry; this has affected Indian pharmaceutical industry in positive way. Important reason for massive boom in Indian herbal drug industry is the law passed in the United States by Bill Clinton government in 1994. 'Dietary Supplements and Health Education Act' also known as DSHEA have changed entire Indian herbal drug export scenario by opening US market. Taking natural advantage of this law, many small scale companies started to export herbal drugs as nutraceuticals or dietary supplements. USFDA's rules regarding New Chemical entity (NCE) were not applicable to herbal drugs, so launching of herbal drugs in USA became much easier. Herbal extracts, isolated phytochemicals, enriched fractions, sport nutrition, health drinks, supplements, processing, packing and other many various types of industries witnessed steep growth following implementation of these rules.

Current Status in India:

Pharmaceutical industry in India is one of the fastest growing sectors for last few decades. According to the Department of Pharmaceuticals, Ministry of Chemicals and Fertilizers, domestic pharmaceutical market turnover in 2018 was US$ 18.12 billion and exports revenue was US$ 17.28 billion. In the same year 2018, Indian Ayurvedic industry was about 4.4 billion US$. This clearly indicates importance of herbal drug industry in terms of revenue. More than 60 % of people are using directly or indirectly natural products for their primary healthcare needs. Actually in developing countries like India more number of people depends on herbal drugs.

Herbal medicines are produced by several thousand companies in India, but most of them are quite small. This includes numerous small units that make their own small extraction set up or processing unit. The entire Ayurvedic product market in India is more than one billion US dollars. The industry was dominated by very few major companies for many decades. In recent years, few small companies have showed growth so that there are 30 companies today doing a million dollars or more business per year to meet the growing demand for Ayurvedic medicine. As importance of herbal drugs is increasing, many multinational big pharmaceutical exporters are also reviving their strategy in favour of herbals. The products category called as 'fast moving consumer goods' or FMCG companies are also entering in herbal business. Most of bigger Ayurvedic companies produce food, nutraceuticals, soaps, shampoos and other essential things rather than actual medicine. While few produce only classical Ayurveda and others having traditional herbal ingredients in the composition of toiletries. According to National Medicinal Plant Board fact sheet, India is world's one of the 17th mega biodiversity countries. India is estimated to have more than 7000 known plant species used as medicinal plants out of 17000-18000 total flowering plant species. For the year of 2014-15, apart from export, only domestic demand of medicinal plants estimated was 1,95,000 MT and actual consumption of herbal raw drug was 5,12,000 MT. In the same year, the export demand of medicinal plants estimated about 1,34,500 MT with export value of 3211 Crore. There are 1178 species used in trade of herbal drugs, of which 242 species have trade value in excess of 100 MT/year. India has high mountains, long sea shore and deserted landscape making it unique source of wide variety of plant material. In addition to this, India has more than 5000 years old unique traditional system of herbal medicines called Ayurveda, still in practice. Also co-existence of other systems like Unani, Shiddha and Homoeopathy resulted in flourishment of herbal drug industry. According to Mckinsey report, number of doctors in India in 2020 will be 9,40,000 from 6,70,000 as that of in 2005.

The Indian government and non-government organizations have been collecting statistics on the Ayurvedic system in India. Following data about the manpower and institution shows importance of Ayurveda in India. Total numbers of registered Ayurvedic medical practitioners are 366,812 and number of dispensaries 22,100. While total number of manufacturing Ayurvedic medicine units are around 8,400. The four key suppliers in Ayurveda are Dabur, Baidyanath, Himalaya and Zandu, which together have about 85% of India's domestic market. This clearly shows that there are many very small manufacturing units in herbal industry.

India has about 500,000 medical doctors. Out of these 60% of registered physicians are from non-allopathic systems of medicine. Some states of India like Kerala have good presence of Ayurvedic medicine. Moreover many Ayurvedic practitioners in small villages are also not registered. There are about 400,000 Ayurvedic practitioners and over 170,000 homeopathic physicians.

India has about 500,000 medicinal doctors (similar to the number in the U.S., but serving nearly 4 times as many peoples. Reliance on Ayurvedic Medicine is heavy in certain regions of India, such as Kerala in Southwest. Many Ayurvedic practioniners in small villages are also not registered.

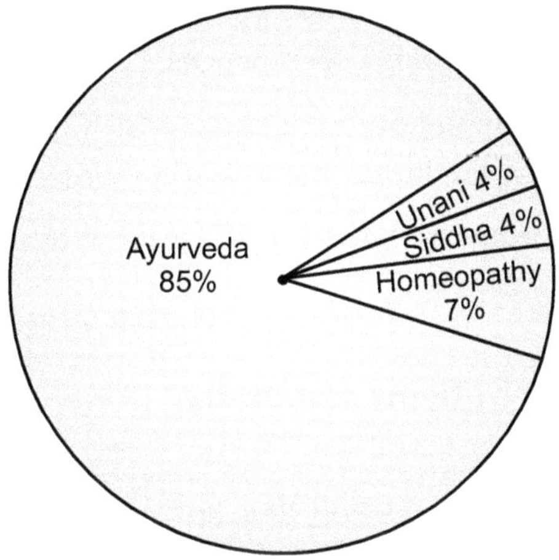

Fig. 12.1: Proportion of manufacturing units of different systems

(Source: Department of Ayush, Government of India**)**

Major part of India's export almost 64% comes from raw materials and extracts. Finished herbal products have only 36 % of the total exports of India. In 2008, the total quantity of exported medicinal plants including plant extracts was around 57880 MT. The number one export herbal drug from India by means of volume is Psyllium constituting 35.6 % of total exports of medicinal plants and second one is Senna (18.9%). The total value of plant crude drugs exported (excluding extracts) was ₹ 354.8 crores corresponding to a quantity of 56,500 MT.

According to Directorate General of Commercial Intelligence and Statistics, Government of India, the annual export of India's herbal sector added to 807 crores. This includes exports worth 354.80 crores relating to plant crude drugs, 161 crores relating to plant extracts and 291 crores to drugs of AUS. While the import amounted to 37,483 MT (173 Crores) and Gum Arabic is number one importuned drug by quantity (12,731 MT; 34 %).

Major Problems for Indian Herbal Industry:

Availability of authentic raw material is one of the important challenges for herbal drug industry. Every small company wants to enter in US or foreign market as these are most lucrative markets. On this background, companies may face some problems such as:

- Presence of differing regulatory requirements and the limited market in foreign countries are the major hindrances for exporting.
- Standardization and quality control of raw materials and herbal formulations emerged as the major challenge for Indian herbal drug manufacturing firms as availability of marker compound is becoming difficult.
- Non-availability of sufficient regulatory guidelines to control herbal drugs. In case, available guidelines are not implemented properly good manufacturing practices, good agricultural and collection practices.
- Poor implementation of Drugs and Cosmetics Act, 1940 is considered as major hindrance for the Indian herbal drug industry.
- Some important herbal drug industries in India:

Table 12.1: Herbal Drug Industries in India

Sr. No.	Name of industry	Year of establishment	Location
1.	Baidyanath Ayurveidic Bhavan Ltd.	1917	Kolkata
2.	Dabur India Ltd.	1884	Ghaziabad
3.	Zandu	1910	Mumbai
4.	Charak Pharma Pvt. Ltd.	1946	Mumbai
5.	Hamdard Laboratories	1906	Delhi
6.	Patanjali Ayurved	2006	Haridwar
7.	Shri Shri Ayurved	2003	Bangalore
8.	Shri Dhutpapeshwar Ltd	1872	Mumbai
9.	Sandu Pharmaceuticals Ltd	1899	Mumbai
10.	Himalaya Drug Company	1930	Bangalore
11.	Vicco Laboratories	1952	Mumbai
12.	Aarya Vaidya Shala	1902	Kottakal, Kerala

Patenting of Herbal Drugs in India:

The following study analyzes the patenting aspects of herbal drugs in India for the last decade.

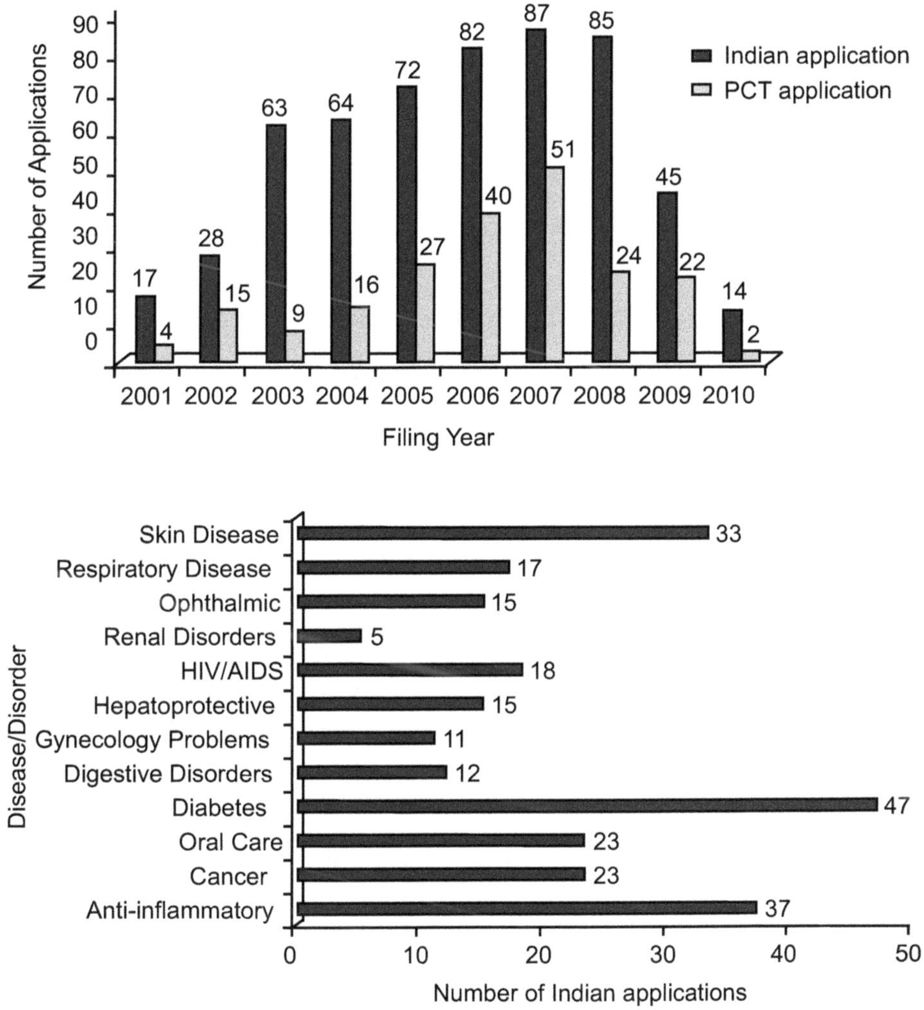

Fig. 12.2: Patent analysis

(**Source:** Niharika Sahoo et. al. Herbal drug patenting in India: IP potential, Journal of Ethanopharmacology, Elsevier)

Last two decades have witnessed increased awareness related to intellectual property rights about herbal drugs. This has resulted in a gradual increase in patent by Indian institutions. At the same time, Indian individual inventors have maximum applications and grants.

- Among research organizations, CSIR, Hindustan Unilever, Avesthagen, Piramal Life Science, Sahajanand Biotech and Indus Biotech are major companies which have the maximum patents granted in India, US and EU respectively.

- These patents are mostly related with diabetes, cancer, cardiovascular diseases, asthama, arthritis and inflammatory disorders. Herbal formulations development for treatment of AIDS, hepatitis, skin disorders and gastrointestinal disorders is new promising area.
- Most of these patent claims are related with novel multi-herb compositions with synergistic action. Indian research organizations are more active than companies in filing for patents.
- From government organizations, CSIR has maximum number of patent applications not only in India but also in abroad. Research organizations and herbal companies have many patents related with isolation and standardization of chemical constituents and new compositions for therapeutic use.
- Pharmaceutical companies like Ranbaxy, Lupin and Panacea Biotech are also having different patents on herbal drugs.

Future Perspectives:

As more number of people wants herbal drugs in the modern framework or formulation, in coming years this field is going to witness steep growth.

- Proper help from government especially from AYUSH is helping to gain awareness about herbal drugs.
- As mentioned earlier, major profit share come from export business therefore more emphasis is needed to increase export of herbal drugs. Promotion of TCM (Traditional Chinese Medicines) by government of China is main reason behind successful capture of foreign market by traditional Chinese medicines. Similar pattern can also be applied for Indian herbal drugs.
- Development of monograph, reference marker compounds, facility for analysis is needed for good quality herbal drugs.
- Financial assistance, provision for knowledge transfer, Good Agricultural and Collection Practices, organic farming are some of the key areas in future.
- Proper implementation of provisions of the Drugs and Cosmetics Act of 1940, development of elaborate guidelines on quality control aspects, and development of marker-based standards are needed to produce safe and effective herbal medicines can boost herbal drug industry in India.
- In years to come, evidence-based studies are becoming important for establishing the safety and efficacy of herbal products in the domestic and export market.
- In future, strong scientific and technological advancement in the field of herbal drugs is much needed along with regulatory harmonization to enjoy commercial success in other countries.

12.2 A BRIEF ACCOUNT OF PLANT BASED INDUSTRIES AND INSTITUTIONS INVOLVED IN WORK ON MEDICINAL AND AROMATIC PLANTS IN INDIA.

On 9th November 2014, The Ministry of AYUSH was formed for optimal development and propagation of AYUSH systems of health care. Earlier the Department of Indian System of Medicine and Homeopathy (ISM&H) which was created in March 1995 was renamed as Department of Ayurveda, Yoga and Naturopathy, Unani, Siddha and Homoeopathy (AYUSH) in November 2003, with focused attention for development of Education and Research in Ayurveda, Yoga and Naturopathy, Unani, Siddha and Homoeopathy.

In India, there are, two statutory councils like Central Council for Indian Medicine (CCIM) and Central Council for Homoeopathy (CCH); Two laboratories namely Pharmacopoeial Laboratory for Indian Medicine (PLIM), Homoeopathy Pharmacopoeia Laboratory (HPL); Eight national institutes namely National institute of Homoeopathy (NIH), National Institute of Ayurveda (NIA), National Institute of Unani Medicine (NIUM), National Institute of Naturopathy (NIN), National Institute of Siddha (NIS), Institute of Post-Graduate Training and Research in Ayurveda (IPGTRA), Rashtriya Ayurved Vidyapeeth (RAV), Morarji Desai National Institute of Yoga (MDNIY); And more than 450 colleges like Ayurveda (240), Unani (39), Siddha (07), and Homeopathic (185).

Indian pharmaceutical industry is leader in production of low cost generic drugs. Indian pharmaceutical industry is largest in terms of volume of generic medicines produced worldwide. Indian Drug Manufacturers' Association (IDMA) was formed in 1961 to provide support to its members who have provided affordable quality medicines. On this background, plant based industry is budding and has its own advantages and disadvantages.

Research institutes which are currently working on areas related to herbal plants can have different backgrounds. Plant based research is carried out mainly in area like botanical, ethanobotanical, phytochemical, pharmacognostical, pharmacological, preclinical, clinical, formulation and toxicity studies. While strong presence of traditional system of medicine, most of the research based in these institutes revolves around this. Isolation of phytochemicals, checking of biological activity, bioprospecting, characterization by using chromatography, herbal formulation development are some of the important areas.

Role of CSIR:

The most prominent effect of herbal drug research was availability of TKDL (Traditional Knowledge of Digital Library). After the biopiracy case of Indian herbal drugs like Curcuma and Neem, this initiative was taken named as TKDL. In this project, all traditional knowledge in different local languages and texts was documented in electronic form and given to all patent offices throughout world. Because of this, good information base become available for herbal industries also. Apart from this, CSIR labs all over India are involved in research related to herbal drugs and have maximum number of patents in this area.

Role of Indian Council of Medical Research (ICMR):

The Indian Council of Medical Research is one of the oldest and largest research institutes in India which is involved with the formulation, co-ordination and promotion of biomedical research.

- Various research initiatives of ICMR have resulted in validation of traditional treatment of *Kshaarasootra* (medicated Ayurvedic thread) for anal fistula, *Vijayasar* (heart wood of *Pterocarpus marsupium Roxb.*) for diabetes mellitus, encouraging micro- and macro-filaricidal activity of *Shakotak* (stem bark of *Streblusasper Lour.*). In experimental studies an iridoid glycosides fraction isolated from root/rhizomes of *Picrorhiza kurroa* Royle ex Benth. (As Picroliv) for viral hepatitis.
- One of the most important works done by ICMR is development of monograph and quality standards. This includes research works on different Indian medicinal plants. There are thirteen volumes of quality standards which contain 449 Indian medicinal plants and three volumes of 90 phytochemical reference standards; fifteen volumes of review monographs on 4167 medicinal plant species. The development of quality standards and mful for herbal drug industry. Monographs are also helping regulators, pharmacopoeial bodies for good quality herbal drugs or traditional medicine preparations.
- At the same time, ICMR is working on many thrust areas from Indian perspectives like management of liver disorders, lymphatic filariasis, diabetes mellitus, tuberculosis, vector borne diseases, tropical diseases, non-communicable diseases, epidemics, nutrition, clinical trial, cancer.

Some Important Herbal Research Institutes in India:

Role of NMPB in India:

National Medicinal Plant Board of India comes under Ministry of AYUSH, Government of India. This is one of the important institutes doing research in herbal drugs. NMPB's main objective is the development of medicinal plants sector.

- NMPB mainly focuses on cultivation of medicinal plants, to meet increasing demand for medicinal plants through *in-situ* & *ex-situ* conservation and augmenting local medicinal plants and aromatic species of medical significance.
- It works on development of co-ordination between various ministries/ departments/ organizations for implementation of policies / programs on medicinal plants.
- The NMPB also promote research & development related to medicinal plants, trainings, creating awareness and promotional activities like creation of herbal gardens.
- NMPB also support programs like development of Good Agricultural and Collection Practices (GACPs), development of monographs, preparation of standards for quality, safety and efficacy; development of new agro-techniques, mechanism for certification of quality of raw drugs, seeds and planting material. Overall helps to develop herbal research.

Table 12.2: Some Important Research Institutes in India Related to Herbal Drugs

Sr. No.	Name	Type	Location	Website
1.	Central Council for Research in Yoga and Naturopathy (CCRYN)	Research Council	New Delhi	http://ccryn.gov.in/
2.	Central Council for Research in Ayurvedic Sciences (CCRAS)	Research Council	New Delhi	http://www.ccras.nic.in/
3.	Central Council for Research in Unani Medicine (CCRUM)	Research Council	New Delhi	http://ccrum.res.in/
4.	Central Council for Research in Homeopathy (CCRH)	Research Council	New Delhi	https://www.ccrhindia.nic.in/
5.	Central Council for Research in Siddha (CCRS)	Council	New Delhi	http://siddhacouncil.com/
6.	All India Institute of Ayurveda, New Delhi (AIIA)	National Institute	New Delhi	https://aiia.gov.in/
7.	Rashtriya Ayurveda Vidyapeeth (RAV)	National Institute	New Delhi	http://www.ravdelhi.nic.in/
8.	National Institute of Ayurveda, Jaipur (NIA)	National Institute	Jaipur	http://nia.nic.in/
9.	National Institute of Homoeopathy (NIH)	National Institute	Kolkata	http://www.nih.nic.in/
10.	National Institute of Siddha (NIS)	National Institute	Chennai	https://www.nischennai.org/
11.	National Institute of Unani Medicine (NIUM)	National Institute	Bengaluru	http://www.nium.in/
12.	National Institute of Naturopathy (NIN)	National Institute	Pune	http://punenin.org/
13.	Morarji Desai National Institute of Yoga (MDNIY)	National Institute	New Delhi	http://www.yogamdniy.nic.in/
14.	Institute of Post Graduate Teaching & Research in Ayurveda (IPGT&RA)	National Institute	Jamnagar, Gujrat	http://www.ayurveduniversity.edu.in/uniipgtra.php

Contd...

15.	North Eastern Institute of Ayurveda and Homoeopathy (NEIAH)	National Institute	Shillong	http://neiah.nic.in/
16.	North Eastern Institute of Folk Medicine (NEIFM)	National Institute	Pasighat, Arunachal Pradesh	http://neifm.nic.in/
17.	Pharmacopoeia Commission of Indian Medicine & Homoeopathy (PCIM & H)	Commission	Ghaziabad, Uttar Pradesh	http://pcimh.gov.in/

Table 12.3: Herbal Research Institutes/Centres in India

Name	City	Postal Code	E-mail
CCRAS (Central Council for Research in Ayurveda and Siddha)	New Delhi	110001	ccras_dir1@rnic.in
RRL (Regional Research Laboratory)(CSIR)	Jammu-Tawi	180001	qazi_gn@yahoo.com
NBRI (National Botanical Research Institute) (CSIR)	Lucknow	226001	r.tuli@nbri.res.in
Gujarat Ayuneda University	Jamnagar	361008	info@ayurveduniversity.com
Bhavan's SPARC	Mumbai	400049	bhaspa@bom5.vsnl.net.in
National Institute of Ayurveda	Jaipur	302002	nia@ raj.nic.in
ACARTS	Mumbai	400008	clinpharm@hathway.com
Arya Vaidya Shala	Kottakal	676503	mail@aryavaidyasala.com
Interdisciplinary School of Health Sciences	Pune	411007	shs@unipune.ernet.in
Banaras Hindu University	Varanasi	221005	directorims@satyam.net.in
CIMAP (Central Institute for Medicinal and Aromatic Plants)	Lucknow	226015	director@cimap.res.in
ICMR (Indian Coucil for Medical Research)	New Delhi	110029	icmrhqds@sansad.nic.in
National Medicinal Plants Board	New Delhi	110001	ccras_dirl@nic.in
Indian Drug Manufacturers	Mumbai	400018	publications@idmaindia.com

Contd...

Regional Medical Research Centre (ICMR)	Belgaum	590010	oicrmrcblm@yahoo.co.in
PERD Centre (Pharmaceutical Education and Research Development)	Ahmedabad	380054	perd@.perdcentrecom
CCRUM (Central Council for Research in Unani Medicine)	New Delhi	110001	ccrum@del3.vsnl.net.in
NISCOM (National Institute of Science Communication)	New Delhi	110012	niscom@sirnetd.ernet.in
IMPCOPS (Indian Medical Practitoners Co-operative Pharmacy & Stores Ltd.)	Chennai	600041	admin@webhealthcenter.com
IHMMR (Indian Institute of History of Medicine and Medical Research)	New Delhi	110062	root@hamduni.ren.nic.in
Zandu Foundation	Mumbai	400025	zanduho@giasbm01.vsnl.net.in
Pharmexcil	Hyderabad	500038	info@pharmexcil.com
Chemexeil	Mumbai	400039	chemexeil@vsnl.com
CDRI (Central Drug Rcscarcch Institute) (CSIR)	Lucknow	226001	icmrredi@ren.nic.in
IMPLANT Centre (Inter-university Medicinal Plant Laboratory for Analysis, Nurture and Therapeutics)	Rajkot	360005	rrkalariya@sauuni.ernet.in
NIMHANS (National Institute for Mental Health and Neurosciences)	Bangalore	560029	sidda@nimhans.kar.nic.in
Panjab University	Chandigarh	600014	webmen@puchd.ac.in
LM College of Pharmacy	Ahmedabad	380009	mukeshgohel@hotmail.com
NBPGR (National Bureau of Plant Genetic Resources)	New Delhi	110012	root@nbpgr.delhi.nic.in
NPRC (Nicholas Piramal Research Centre)	Mumbai	400013	recruitment@nicholaspiramal.co. in
NCL (National Chemical Laboratory)	Pune	411008	rs.malge@nel.res.in
TBGRI (Tropical Botanical Garden & Research Institute)	Thirtiuantpuram	695562	director_tbgri@rediffmail. com

Contd...

BHU ((Banaras Hindu University)	Varanasi	221005	vc_bhu@sify.com
Podar Hospital	Mumbai	400018	rapamc@rediffmail.com
Botanical Survey of India	Kolkata	700001	envisercal2.vsnl.net.in
FRHLT (Foundation for Revitalisation of Local Health Traditions)	Bangalore	560024	Darshan.shankar@frlht.org.in
IASTAM (International Association for the Study of Traditional Asian Medicine)	Mumbai	400012	iastamindia@vsnl.net
ADMA (Ayurvedic Drug Manufacturing Association)	Mumbai	400012	amam2003@sify.com

(**Source:** Ashok D. B. Vaidya et. al. Current status of herbal drugs in India, Journal of Clinical Biochemistry and Nutrition)

QUESTIONS

1. Write current status and future prospects of herbal drugs industry in India.
2. Which are different problems for Indian herbal industry?
3. Enlist different herbal drug industries in India.
4. Write in detail plant based industreis in India.
5. Write in brief about different herbal research institutes in India.
6. Describe in detail Indian and Global scenario of herbal drug industry.

❖❖❖

Chapter...13

SCHEDULE T- GOOD MANUFACTURING PRACTICES OF INDIAN SYSTEMS OF MEDICINE

Objectives

- To know about schedule T and its components.
- To understand the principles, importance of GMP.
- To understand Good Manufacturing Practice of Indian systems of medicine

13.1 INTRODUCTION

Indian Systems of Medicines:

India has the unique tradition of six recognized Indian systems of medicine mainly Ayurveda, Siddha, Unani and Yoga, Naturopathy and Homoeopathy. The formulations of Indian systems of medicine are made from products obtained from plant, animal, mineral or marine origin. This formulation may contain single or multiple ingredients or combination of different formulations. The formulations may be herbal, herbo-mineral or mixture of two or more natural substances; extracts of medicinal plant (aqueous extract or hydro-alcoholic extract or any other extract).

The poor quality formulations may contain toxic elements or intentionally added toxic elements which are hazardous to consumer health. Medicine cannot exert its desired therapeutic effect if it contains fewer amounts or no active principle. To avoid such conditions, the manufacturer should follow some uniform guidelines to ensure consistent batch to batch quality and to prevent harm to consumers. Good Manufacturing Practices and compliance with pharmacopoeial standards of drugs are mandatory for the manufacturing of licensed products. Since 23rd June 2002 Government of India has made the GMP mandatory for all units to regulate the quality of Ayurvedic, Siddha and Unani drugs (ASU drugs). Schedule T of Drug and Cosmetic Act under rule 155-B of Drugs and Cosmetics Rule, 1945 describes GMPs. From 23rd June, 2000 it is applicable to new A.S.U. manufacturing units. Two years time is given for units registered prior to 23rd June 2000 to comply with the guidelines.

13.2 GOOD MANUFACTURING PRACTICES

13.2.1 Definition

The practices which are essential to conform to the guidelines recommended by agencies that are involved in the authorization and licensing of the manufacture and sale of products such as food and beverages, cosmetics, pharmaceutical products, dietary supplements, and medical devices etc. are termed as Good Manufacturing Practices.

The regulatory framework and for monitoring the quality, safety and efficacy of drugs belonging to Ayurveda, Siddha and Unani (ASU) systems provisions are given under the Drugs and Cosmetics Act, 1940 and Drugs and Cosmetics Rules, 1945. The State Governments appoints Licensing Authorities to supervise the enforcement of legal provisions for the manufacture and sale of ASU drugs. Drugs and Cosmetics Rules, 1945 given under the Drugs and Cosmetics Act, 1940, classify drugs under given schedules. It also provides guidelines for the storage, sale, display and prescription of each schedule. It consists of Schedule T which gives various regulations and requirements for manufacture of Ayurvedic, Siddha and Unani products (ASU).

Under the Drugs and Cosmetics Act, Ayurveda, Siddha, Unani Drugs Technical Advisory Board (ASUDTAB) and Ayurveda, Siddha, Unani Drugs Consultative Committee (ASUDCC) are statutory bodies. Their main function is to advise the Central and State Governments on technical matters and to maintain uniformity throughout the country in the administration of the Act. For strengthening of state pharmacies, Drug Testing Laboratories and Enforcement Mechanism, Department of AYUSH has implemented a Centrally Sponsored Scheme of Quality Control of ASU&H Drugs

13.2.2 Types of ASU Drugs

- **Classical/Shastriye/Traditional:** These formulations contains Ayurvedic, Siddha or Unani drug intended for internal or external use or use in the diagnosis, treatment, mitigation or prevention of disease or disorder in human beings or animals. These are manufactured using the formulae described in the authoritative books specified in the Schedule I of the Act.
- **Patent or Proprietary:** These formulations should contain ingredients or natural substances mentioned in the authoritative books.

13.2.3 Objectives of GMPs

The main objectives of Good Manufacturing Practices for ASU Drugs are to ensure that:

- Raw material should have desired quality, should be authentic and free from contamination.
- Proper standards should be maintained during manufacturing of drugs.
- Proper measures should be implemented to ensure desired quality.
- Manufacturer should sale desired quality of drugs.

- To achieve these objectives every licensee should adopt proper methodology and procedure as prescribed in rules. These methods should be well documented; manuals are prepared which should be ready for inspection. The registered Vaidyas, Siddhas and Hakeems who prepare medicines for their patients and not selling in the market are exempted from the Good Manufacturing Practice (GMP) as per IMCC Act, 1970

13.2.4 Importance of GMP

The conventional pharmaceutical dosage forms are produced from synthetic material using specific techniques to achieve reproducible results. But dosage forms based on traditional systems of medicines like Ayurveda, Homeopathy, Siddha and Unani are produced from herbal ingredients. These herbal drugs are obtained from various geographical and commercial resources so they vary in chemical composition and therapeutic properties. Also there are various factors such as diverse physical, chemical nature, cultivation, collection practices, method of preparation; primary processing and adulteration etc. which can directly influence the quality of ASU (Ayurveda, Siddha and Unani) medicines. Hence, implementation of Good Manufacturing Practices during production of ASU medicines is extremely important to assure quality of medicines.

13.2.5 Basic Principles of GMPs

As per guidelines for Inspection of GMP compliance by ASU drug industry published by Department of AYUSH in 2014, the basic principles of GMPs are as follows:

- All manufacturing processes are clearly defined and controlled. All critical processes are validated to ensure consistency and compliance with specifications.
- Manufacturing processes are controlled; the changes in the process are evaluated as they can impact the quality of the drug.
- Clear and unambiguous language should be used for writing instructions and procedures.
- Proper training should be given to operators to carry out and document procedures.
- Records are made manually or by instruments during manufacture that ensures that manufacturing is carried out as per prescribed procedures and desired quantity and quality of the drug achieved was as expected. Deviations in the procedure are evaluated and well documented.
- All the records of manufacture (including distribution) are retained in a comprehensible and accessible form which describes complete history of a batch to be traced.
- Proper system is maintained to trace the record of any batch of drug from sale or supply.
- Complaints about marketed drugs are considered, the causes of quality defects are investigated, and appropriate measures are taken and to prevent recurrence.

The company can fulfill the GMP requirements by many ways while setting up its quality program and manufacturing process. It is the company's responsibility to determine the most suitable way to maintain effective and efficient quality process.

13.3 COMPONENTS OF GMPS

GMPs are described in two parts:

Part I: General requirements for Good Manufacturing Practices.

Part II: List of machinery, equipment and minimum manufacturing premises recommended to manufacture Ayurvedic, Siddha and Unani medicines.

13.3.1 Part I: Good Manufacturing Practices for ASU Medicines

The manufacturing premises should have sufficient facilities to run the daily routine smoothly. The adequate space should be there for:

- Receiving and storage space for herbal material, packaging material and other raw materials;
- Sufficient area to carry out manufacturing process.
- Separate section to check quality of products.
- Storage space for finished goods.
- Space for office.
- Storage area for rejected goods or drugs.

To start Ayurveda, Sidha and Unani Medicine manufacturing unit, minimum area requirement is 1200 square feet with separate cabins and partitions for each activity. To manufacture unani and ayurvedic medicines in same premises, additional 400 square feet area is required.

13.3.1.1 Infrastrucutre Requirements

1. **Location and Surroundings:** The factory building for production of Ayurveda, Siddha and Unani medicines should be located away from any factory producing disagreeable or obnoxious odour or fumes or excessive soot, dust or smoke. The construction should be such that it should avoid contamination from open sewerage, drain, public lavatory etc.
2. **Buildings:** The hygienic conditions should be maintained and building production area should be free from cobwebs and insects or rodents. Adequate facility for light and ventilation should be provided. The floor and the walls of building should not be damp or have cracks. The premises used for manufacturing, processing, packaging and labeling should comply with the provisions given in the Factory Act. The building should be:
    - Compatibility with all manufacturing operations carried out in the same or adjacent premises.
    - To carry out orderly and logical arrangements of equipment and materials, to avoid the risk of mix-up of different drugs or other components and to avoid the risk of cross-contamination by other drugs or substances and exclusion of any manufacturing or control step adequate working space should be maintained.

- Proper construction and maintainance should be there to prevent entry of insects and rodents. The walls, floors and ceilings should be smooth, free from cracks and easy for cleaning and disinfection. The walls of manufacturing area should be impermeable and clean. The flooring should be smooth and even. It should avoid dust or waste products.
- The processing area should possess proper drainage system. The manufacturing area should have proper and safe sanitary fittings and electrical fixtures.
- Furnace or Bhatti area should have tin roof and proper ventilation and should have provisions to prevent flies and dust.
- In case of fire, appropriate safety measures and proper exits should be there.
- Drying space should have proper flooring, wire-mesh window, glass pans or other material. The separate spaces should be available for drying of raw material, in process medicine or medicines should be dried before packing.

3. **Water Supply:** The adequate provisions should be made to provide pure water in manufacturing area and water for washing the premises.
4. **Waste Disposal:** The waste water and the residues generated from the manufacturing sections and laboratories may be harmful to the workers or public health. It should be disposed off after suitable treatment as per pollution control authorities guidelines to make them harmless.
5. **Cleaning of Containers:** The adequate arrangement should be made for washing, cleaning and drying containers such as glass bottles, vials and jars. The arrangement should be separate from the manufacturing operations.
6. **Storage Area:**
   - Adequate and separate space should be maintained for storage of starting and packaging materials, intermediates bulk and finished products, products in quarantine, released, rejected, returned or recalled, machine and equipment spare parts and change items.
   - Storage area should be properly ventilated and should be moisture free. Appropriate house-keeping and control measures for rodents, pests and vermin should be there in warehousing area and records should be maintained. For material storage proper racks, bins and platforms should be provided.
   - The materials and products should be protected from adverse weather conditions during receiving and dispatch.
   - In same warehouse quarantine area should be separately maintained and should give assurance of segregation. The entry into these areas should be restricted.
   - The separate sampling areas should be there in the warehousing area for active raw materials and excipients. During sampling in any other area, contamination, cross-contamination and mix-up should be avoided.

- Poisonous substances should be safely stored. Adequate fire protection measures should be there and comply with the rules of the concerned civic authority.
- Safe, separate and secure areas should be maintained for printed packaging materials.
- The sampling and dispensing of sterile materials should be performed under aseptic conditions. Within the manufacturing facility specific area should be dedicated for the same.
- To avoid spillage, breakage and leakage of containers regular testing should be done.

7. Raw Materials:

- All raw materials should be stored in the raw materials store. The containers for raw materials storage should be selected based on the experience and properties of the particular raw material. The container should protect the quality of the raw material and prevent it from damage due to dampness, microbiological contamination or rodent and insect infestation etc.
- The raw materials should be stored under controlled environmental conditions; they should be stored in separate cabinets. The care may be taken during designing of containers, cabins or areas in the raw materials store, to handle the following different categories of raw materials:
    - Metallic raw material.
    - Raw material of mineral origin.
    - Raw material from animal origin.
    - Fresh herbs.
    - Dry herbs or parts of plant.
    - Excipients.
    - Volatile oils or perfumes & flavours.
    - Plant concentrates/extracts and exudates/resins.
- Each container in which raw material is stored should be properly labelled. The label should indicate name of the raw material, source of supply and status of raw material such as 'UNDER TEST' or 'APPROVED' or REJECTED'. The labels should clearly mention Batch No. or Lot. Number and the date of receipt of consignment, for easy identification of the particular supply.
- All the raw materials should be sampled, should be used only after approval and testing by the in-house ASU experts (Quality control technical person) or by the Government approved laboratories. The rejected material should be stored in separate areas. Procedure of 'First in first out' should be adopted for raw materials testing. Records of the receipt, testing and approval or rejection and use of raw material should be properly carried out.

- All containers and closures should be adequately cleaned and dried before packing the product. Proper arrangement should be there to store packaging materials such as bottles, jars, capsules etc.
- Finished goods after proper packaging should be stored in finished goods stores marked as "Quarantine". After checking the quality, packing and labeling of finished products by expert, then it should be stored in area marked as 'Approved Finished Goods Stock'. These approved finished goods should be dispatched to market as per demand. The records of distribution should be properly maintain. The finished goods store should have adequate arrangements for Ayurvedic, Siddha and Unani drug which needs special storage conditions.

8. Working Space:

- **Manufacturing area:** For orderly and logical arrangements of equipment and materials, to avoid the risk of mix-up of different drugs or other components and to avoid the risk of cross- contamination by other drugs or substances and for easy and safe working manufacturing area should have adequate working space.
- To avoid accumulation of dust pipe-work, electrical fittings, ventilation openings and similar service lines should be properly designed, fixed and constructed. Colour codes are used for service lines for identification and for the nature of the supply, and direction of the flow should be marked.
- **Ancillary area** should have following facilities:

  Rest and refreshment rooms should be built separatly and away from manufacturing and storage areas.

  Adequate number of facilities such as changing room, clothes storing and washing, toilet should be provided. Male and female toilets should be separate away from production or storage areas. The written instructions should be there for cleaning and disinfection for such areas.

  There should be separate maintenance workshops and away from production areas. If required the spares, changed parts and tools to store in the production area, these should be kept in dedicated rooms or lockers. Tools and spare parts for use in sterile areas should be disinfected before use.
- **Quality control area:** There should be quality control section in premises of manufacturer or made available through government-approved testing laboratory. All the tests should be carried out as per the Ayurveda, Siddha and Unani pharmacopoeial standard. In case of unavailability of pharmacopoeia, tests should be conducted according to the manufacturer's specification or other information available. The quality control section should check the quality of the raw materials, in process materials and finished product before sending it to finished goods store. Preferably the tests are carried out by a separate expert.

The following facilities should be there in quality control section:

- The area for quality control section should be 150 sq feet.
- Quality Control Laboratories should be separate from the production areas. Pharmacognostical, chemical, microbiological analysis are carried out in separate areas. For sensitive and sophisticated instruments well maintained separate instrument room with adequate area should be provided.
- For testing of drugs adequate area should be provided for basic installation and for ancillary purposes. The facilities like airlocks and laminar air flow work station should be provided in the microbiology section if necessary.
- To avoid mix-ups and cross-contamination the laboratories should have adequate space. The sufficient and suitable storage space should be available for storage of test samples, retained samples, reference standards, reagents and records.
- The laboratories are properly designed considering the suitability of construction materials and ventilation. Separate air handling units and other requirements should be provided each area. There should be regular supply of water of appropriate quality for cleaning and testing purposes.
- For correct identification of raw drugs the reference books and reference samples should be maintained.
- Records should be maintained for all processes in manufacturing.
- Controlled samples of finished products of each batch should be preserved till the expiry date of product.
- Adequate storage conditions are supervised and monitored for raw materials; semi-finished products and finished products.
- Record of shelf life establishment and storage requirements for the drugs should be maintained.
- For manufacturing patent proprietary Ayurveda, Siddha and Unani medicines, manufacturers should provide their own specification and control references of formulated drugs.
- A specific method or procedure like "Bhavana", "Mardana" and "Puta" are used to formulate Ayurvedic dosage forms, the record of every process should be maintained.
- The results for identity, purity and strength should comply with standards given in respective pharmacopoeias of Ayurveda, Siddha and Unani systems of medicines published by Government of India.
- All raw materials should be checked for fungal and bacterial contamination.
- The Quality Control section should have:
  (a) Expert in Ayurveda or Siddha or Unani who should have degree qualification recognized under Schedule II of Indian Medicine Central Council Act, 1970.

(b) Chemist, with Bachelor Degree in Science or Pharmacy or Pharmacy (Ayurveda) awarded by a recognized University;

(c) A Botanist (Pharmacognosist) with at least a Bachelor Degree in Science (Medical) or Pharmacy or Pharmacy (Ayurveda) awarded by a recognized University.

- As explained under Section 35(ii) the manufacturing unit should have a quality control section or the quality control provisions will be carried out from a recognized laboratory for Ayurveda, Siddha and Unani drugs; under Rule 160-A of the Drugs and Cosmetics Act. All the records of tests conducted by outside recognized laboratory should be maintained.
- It should have equipments recommended and indicated in Part II-C.

9. Personnel:

- For manufacturing of dosage forms of Ayurveda, Siddha and Unani drugs competent technical staff with prescribed qualifications and practical experience should be appointed.
- The separate head should be appointed for Quality Control Laboratory. The competent full time technical staff should monitor testing of drugs.
- For Quality Assurance and Quality Control operations qualified and experienced personnel should be appointed.
- Technical and Quality Control personnel should strictly follow written duties assigned to them.
- Adequate number of personnel should be employed proportional to the workload.
- The licensee should ensure that all personnel in production area or into Quality Control Laboratories should receive proper training as per duties and responsibility assigned to them. The regular in-service training should be provided.

10. Health, Clothing, Sanitation and Hygiene of Workers:

- Healthy workers free from any contagious diseases should be employed in the factory. They should be free from Tuberculosis, skin and other communicable or contagious diseases.
- All employees should be trained to maintain proper hygiene. Instructions related to this should be displayed in change-rooms and other strategic locations.
- As per nature of work, proper uniform with cloth or synthetic covering for hands, feet and head should be given to employees. The climate should be healthy.
- To maintain personal hygiene, adequate facilities such as clean towels, soap and scrubbing brushes should be provided.
- Separate lavatories for men and women should be there which must be away from the processing rooms. The cloth changing facilities and lockers to keep personal belongings should be provided to workers.
- The starting materials, packaging materials, in-process materials, and drug product which may adversely affect the quality of products should not be handled by a person with apparent illness or open lesions until he recovers from illness.

- Instructions are given to all employees to report about their illness or abnormal health condition to their immediate supervisor so that appropriate action can be initiated.
- Raw materials, intermediate or finished, unpacked products should not be touched with bare hands.
- In production, laboratory, storage and other areas smoking, eating, drinking, chewing or keeping plants, food, drink and personal medicines should be strictly avoided as they might adversely influence the product quality.
- Medical Services: Adequate first aid facilities should be provided. Medical examination of workers at the time of employment and periodical checkup should be done once a year to avoid infections. All the records should be well maintained.

11. Manufacturing Operations and Controls:

- Under the direct personal supervision of approved technical staff all manufacturing operations of Ayurveda, Siddha and Unani medicines should be performed by trained personnel. The name of the product, batch no., batch size and stage of manufacture should be clearly indicated on labels of vessels and containers used in manufacture and storage. Each label should be signed and dated by the authorized technical staff. Products not prepared under aseptic conditions are required to be free from pathogens.

Precautions to be taken to avoid mix-up and cross-contamination are:

- Mix-up and cross-contamination of drug material and drug product with environment dust can be avoided by using proper air-handling system, pressure differential segregation, and status labelling and cleaning.
- The records and Standard Operating Procedures should be maintained properly.
- The materials under-process should be properly labelled to prevent mix-ups during production stages. Also current status of all equipment used for production should be indicated.
- There should be separate packaging lines. Before the closing hour cleaning of left-over of the previous packaging operations, including labels, cartons and caps should be done.
- Work area, packaging lines, printing machines, and other equipment must be clean and free from any products, materials and spillages before packaging operation. Records should be kept.
- Printing details should be correct and checked regularly. Every detail should be authorized in writing.
- Proper conditions of temperature, humidity and cleanliness should be maintained in manufacturing area.
- Authorized persons should ensure that, all the employees should be in proper uniform.
- There should be segregated secured areas for recalled or rejected material and re-processed or recovered material.

12. Sanitation in the Manufacturing Premises:

- Validated cleaning procedure should be carried out in manufacturing area so that to keep it free from waste, dust, debris and other similar material.
- The manufacturing areas should not be used for storage of materials except in-process material.
- Records of routine sanitation programme should be maintained. It should indicate specific areas to be cleaned and cleaning intervals; cleaning procedure, equipment and materials to be used for cleaning; and personnel assigned to and responsible for the cleaning operation.
- There should be adequate working space and storage space to avoid mixing up.
- Production areas should be well maintained.

13. Machinery and Equipments:

- Machinery and Equipments based on type of operation, size and the nature of product to be manufactured, suitable equipment such as manually operated or operated semi-automatically (electrical or team based) or fully automatic machinery should be made available. The machinery is required various operations such as crushing, grinding, powdering, boiling, mashing, burning, roasting, filtering, drying, filling, labelling and packing etc.
- The layout and design of the equipment should be such that it should avoid the risk of errors and easy to clean and maintain, avoid cross-contamination, free from dust or dirt and any adverse effect on the quality of products. Log book should be maintained for each equipment.
- The parts of the production equipment should be non-reactive, additive or adsorptive and should not affect the quality of the product.
- To avoid accidental contamination, non-toxic/edible grade lubricants can be used.
- Defective equipment should be removed or properly labelled.
- The adequate space should be maintained between two machines or rows of machines to ensure easy and smooth working. The list of these machinery and equipments and machinery recommended is indicated in Part II-A of GMPs. Proper standard operational procedures (SOPs) should be maintained for each machine.

14. Documentation and Records:

- Documentation is vital part of the Quality assurance system. It is linked to all aspects of Good Manufacturing Practices (GMP).
- The basic aim of records and documentation is to define the specifications for all materials, method of manufacture and control. It also helps all personnel concerned with manufacture to recognize the information necessary batch release of a drug for sale and to provide an audit trail and investigate the history of any suspected defective batch.
- Documents should be well designed, prepared, reviewed and controlled, as per standard rules.
- Authorized persons should approve, sign the documents and dated.

- Documents should clearly indicate the title, nature and purpose. They should be properly arranged and be easy to check. Reproduced documents should be clear and legible. Documents should be up to date and regularly reviewed. Every entry of a document should be signed and dated.
- All the records should be updated time to time to trace out steps in manufacturing process. Records and Standard Operating Procedures (SOP) should be preserved for at least one year after the expiry date of the finished products.
- The documentation can be carried out by Electronic data processing system. For checking the accuracy of the records a hard copy of Master Formulae and detailed operating procedures relating to the system should be also available. The entry or modification of data in the computer should be made by authorized persons. All the record of changes and deletions should be maintained. Documentation should be 'password' protected. The entry of critical data should be independently checked. Batch records should be protected by a suitable back-up and data should be readily available.

15. Batch Manufacturing Records:

- The batch manufacturing record for each batch should be properly maintained for all ASU drugs by the licensee. The record of list of raw materials, their quantities, tests conducted during the various stages such as taste, colour, physical characteristics, chemical tests and other tests prescribed in the approved books of Ayurveda, Siddha and Unani mentioned in the First Schedule of the Drugs and Cosmetics Act, 1940 (23 of 1940). In-house or pharmacopoeial test on raw material or on in process material and in the finished product should be conducted. All records should be properly signed by Production and Quality Control Personnel. Only approved finished products should be sailed. The records such as date, manpower, machine and equipments used and in process record of various shodhana, bhavana, burning in fire and specific grindings in terms of internal use should be maintained.

16. Master Formula Records:

- The competent technical staff i.e. head of production and quality control should prepare and approve master formula records relating to all manufacturing procedures.
- As per guidelines for Inspection of GMP compliance by ASU drug industry published by Department of AYUSH in 2014, the Master Formula should include:
- Product name with product reference code relating to its specifications.
- Its patent or proprietary name of the product and the generic name, a description of the dosage form, strength, composition of and batch size.
- Name, quantity, and reference number of all the starting materials and any substance that may be deleted during course of processing.
- A statement of the expected final yield with the acceptable limits, and of relevant intermediate yields.

- A statement of the processing location and the principal equipment
- The methods, or reference to the methods, used for cleaning, assembling, calibrating, sterilizing of equipments.
- Stepwise processing instructions.
- Instructions regarding in-process controls with their limits.
- Storage conditions of the products.
- Any special precautions.
- Packing details and specimen labels.

17. Distribution Records:

For each batch of Ayurveda, Siddha and Unani Drugs, records of sale and distribution should be maintained. The record keeping should be carried out till the date of expiry of the batch. But few Ayurvedic, Siddha and Unani medicines like Bhasma, Rasa, Kupi-pakva, Parpati, Sindura, Karpu/Uppu/Puram, Kushta, Asava-Arista etc. do not have expiry date, on the contrary their efficacy increases with the passage of time. Hence, records should be maintained up to 5 years of the exhausting of stock.

18. Packaging Records:

As per AYUSH guidelines authorized packaging instructions should include the following:

- The product name.
- Description of dosage form and composition.
- The pack size, weight or volume.
- Complete list of all packaging material including quantities, sizes, types, with the code or reference number.
- Reproduction of the relevant printed packaging materials and specimens.
- Special precautions.
- Description of the packaging operation.
- Details of in-process controls.
- Significant or unusual discrepancy in the numbers.

19. Record of Market Complaints:

Records of complaint related to marked products should be maintained in separate register by Manufacturers. Along with these complaints, records of investigations, corrective action initiated to prevent recurrence of such market complaints should be maintained. Once in six months the manufacturer should furnish these records to the Licensing Authority. Register should be made available for inspection during any inspection of the premises.

The manufacturer should maintain, the reports of any adverse reaction Ayurvedic, Siddha and Unani in a separate register. Adverse reactions are due to any defect in the product, or are already reported in the literature or are new observations. The investigations are made to confirm it.

20. Quality Assurance System:

Along with modern analytical techniques various quality assurance systems should be required for the control of starting materials, storage and processing. It should ensure the following:

- All ASU products are designed and developed as per specifications of Good Manufacturing Practices, Good Laboratory Practice and Good Clinical Practices Guidelines etc.
  There are adequate arrangements for manufacture, supply, and use of the correct starting and packaging materials.
- Adequate quality control methods are followed for raw materials, intermediate products, and bulk products and other in-process controls, calibrations, and validations etc.
- All the finished ASU formulations are evaluated in accordance with procedures given in official books or respective formularies and pharmacopoeias.
- All ASU products are released for sale only after certification by authorized person and it ensures that each production batch has been produced and controlled in accordance with the requirements of the label claim and other provisions relevant to production, control and release.

21. Quality Control System:

- Quality control systems are responsible for sampling, specifications, testing, documentation, release procedures which ensure desired quality of drug.
- There should be separate quality control laboratory with qualified and experienced staff.
- There should be separate areas for pharmacognostical, chemical, Microbiological testing and export of Ayurveda, Siddha and Unani systems.
- Adequate area storage conditions should be provided for reference samples.
- For sampling, inspecting, and testing of raw materials, intermediate, bulk finished products and packing materials and, monitoring environment conditions, Standard operating procedures should be available.
- For all materials, products, reagents water, solvents, reagents and solvents specifications should be authorized and dated. It should includ test of identity, content, purity and quality.
- Batch of the product should be released for sale or supply after certification of authorised person(s) that it is as per the standards laid down.
- At least twice the quantity of the drug required to conduct all the tests is retained for reference/retained samples from each batch. The retained products are stored for period of three months after the date of expiry of Ayurveda, Siddha and Unani drugs.
- Finished product records should be assessed based on factors such as production conditions, the results of in-process testing, the manufacturing (including packaging) documentation, compliance with the specification, and an examination of the

finished products. It should be signed by in-charge of production and countersigned by the authorized quality control personnel before sale of finished product.

- Quality control personnel should have access to production areas to carry out sampling and investigation.
- Investigation of product complaints should be kept by in-charge of Quality Assurance and records are maintained.
- Periodical calibration of instrument and validation of procedures should be routinely carried out before actual testing of drugs.
- Quality Control Department should approve and maintain each specification for raw materials, intermediates, final products, and packing materials. Periodic revisions of the specifications should be conducted.
- Ayurveda, Siddha and Unani Pharmacopoeia, reference standards, working standards, other reference materials and technical books, as required, should be available in the Quality Control Laboratory.
- Ayurveda, Siddha and Unani products should be tested for stability ensure and assign their shelf life.
- Stability data are always required to support the shelf-life for the finished product which should be provided by quality control department. Chromatographic fingerprinting should be carried out to confirm its stability and to ensure quality of drugs. Assay, and physical and sensory or other appropriate tests may be carried out to know the stability of drugs with known active ingredient. The tests like moisture content, microbial contamination and general dosage form control tests can be conducted to know the stability of drugs. The stability of preservatives and stabilizers should be checked time to time. Samples for stability studies should be stored in the containers intended for marketing. Normally, the first three commercial production batches should be evaluated for stability testing to confirm expiry date. The testing frequency depends on the characteristics of products and should be determined on a case-to-case study. The protocol used for stability study should be documented.

22. Standard Operating Procedures (SOPS):

As per guidelines Standard operating procedures should be maintained for the following:

(i) Receipt of Material:

Standard Operating Procedures and records for the receipts of raw, primary and printed packaging material are maintained in written format. The records should include;

- Material name and quantity of the containers.
- The date of arrival.
- Name of the manufacturer and/or supplier.
- The batch number or reference number.
- The total quantity, number of containers and quantity in each container.
- The control reference number given after receipt.
- Any other relevant information.

For the internal labelling, quarantine and storage of starting raw materials, packaging materials and other materials written standard operating procedures should be prepared.

SOPs should be prepared for each instrument and equipment and these should be placed near to the related instrument and equipment.

(ii) SOPs for Sampling:

The written Standard Operating Procedures are prepared for sampling, which include the person(s) authorized to take the samples.

The sampling instructions should give information about the method of sampling and the sampling plan, the equipment to be used, any precautions to avoid contamination of the material or any deterioration, the quantity of samples, instructions for any required sub-division or pooling of the samples, type of sample container, and any specific precautions taken during sampling of poisonous material.

(iii) Batch Numbering:

The details of the batch (lot) numbering should be included in Standard Operating Procedures so that each batch of intermediate, bulk or finished Ayurveda, Siddha and Unani products can be identified with a specific batch number.

The processing stage and respective packaging stage should have same Batch numbering Standard Operating to avoid confusion.

Immediate records of batch numbers should be maintained using logbook or by electronic data processing system. The record should contain date of allocation, product identity and size of batch.

(iv) Testing:

There should be written procedures for testing materials and products which should include details of the methods and equipment and the tests performed.

(v) Records of Analysis:

The records of analysis should include the following data.

- Material name or product and the dosage form.
- Batch number.
- Specifications and testing procedures references.
- Observations and calculations and limits of tests conducted.
- Dates of testing.
- Initials of the persons who performed the testing.
- Initials of the persons who verified the testing and the detailed calculations.
- A statement of release or rejection.
- Signature and date of the designated responsible person.

The written standard operating procedures and action taken reports should be prepared for:

- Equipment used and its validation.
- Analytical apparatus used and its calibration.
- Maintenance, cleaning and sanitation methods.
- Personnel matters including qualification, training, clothing, hygiene.
- Measures taken for environmental monitoring.
- Pest control measures.
- Complaints received.
- Any recalls made.
- Any returns received.

23. Validation and Process Validation:

The validation being an essential part of Good Manufacturing Practices should be conducted as per specific protocols for processing, testing and cleaning procedures. It should include.

A written summary report of recorded results and conclusions:

Processes and procedures should be established on the basis of validation study and periodically revalidated to achieve the intended results. Critical processes should be validated, prospectively or retrospectively.

In case of new master formula or method of preparation, steps should be taken to demonstrate its suitability for routine processing and should yield a product of consistent quality.

Any significant changes in the manufacturing process should be validated.

24. Site Master Files:

Site Master File is a concise document which contains information about specific and factual Good Manufacturing Practices about the production and/or control of ASU manufacturing prepared by the licensee. As per GMP given in Schedule T components of site master files are:

(i) General Information:

- Brief information of the firm.
- Drugs manufacturing activities as permitted by the State licensing authority (AYUSH).
- Any other manufacturing activities.
- Types of all categories of ASU products with flowcharts mentioning procedures and process flow.
- Number of employees working in firm.
- Any external scientific, analytical or other technical assistance.
- Short description of the Quality Management system;
- ASU products details registered with foreign countries.

(ii) Personnel:

- Organizational chart showing the arrangement for quality assurance, production and quality control.
- Qualification, experience and responsibilities of key personnel.
- Outline for arrangements for basic and in-service training and record keeping.
- Health requirements for personnel engaged in production.
- Personnel hygiene requirements, including clothing.

(iii) Premises: It should include:

- Simple plan of manufacturing unit.
- Nature of construction and fixtures / fittings.
- Brief description of ventilation systems. Details of critical areas and classification of the rooms.
- Special areas for the handling of the poisonous materials.
- Brief description of water systems (schematic drawing of systems), including sanitation.
- Description of planned preventive maintenance programs for premises and of the recording system.

(iv) Equipment:

- Summary usage of major equipment.
- Description of planned preventive maintenance programs for equipment and of the recording systems.
- Qualification, including the recording systems and arrangements for computerized systems validation.

(v) Sanitation:

- Written specifications and procedures for cleaning manufacturing areas and equipment should be included.

(vi) Documentation: It should include documentation related to description of arrangements for the preparation, revision and distribution, manufacture; quality control.

(vii) Production: It should include brief description of production in the form of flow sheets and charts, arrangement details for the handling of starting materials, packaging materials, bulk and finished products, including sampling, quarantine, release and storage; description of arrangements for the handling of rejected materials and products; brief description of general policy for process validation.

(viii) Quality control: It includes description of the quality control system and its activities procedures for the release of the finished ASU products.

(ix) Loan license manufacture and licensee: The procedure conducted for compliance of Good Manufacturing Practices by the loan licensee should be assessed.

(x) Distribution, complaints and product recall: It should include records of arrangements made for recording systems for distribution and arrangements for the handling of complaints and product recalls.

(xi) Self-Inspection: It should include description of any outside, independent and experienced external expert who was involved in evaluating the manufacturer's compliance with Good Manufacturing Practices.

(xii) Export of drugs: It should contains details of ASU products exported to different countries; or any complaints and product recalls.

13.3.2 Part-II

Part A: List of Recommended Machinery, Equipment and Minimum Manufacturing Premises Required for the Manufacture of Various Categories of Ayurvedic, Siddha System of Medicines as per Schedule T of Drugs and Cosmetics Rules 1945

Table 13.1

Sr. No.	Category of Medicine	Minimum Manufacturing space required	Machinery/Equipment Recommended
1200 sq. ft. covered area with separate cabins or partitions for each activity. If Unani medicines are manufactured in same premises an additional area of 400 sq./ft will be required.			
1.	Anjana/Pisti	100 sq. ft.	Mechanised or motorized Kharal, End Runner/Ball-Mill, and Sieves/Shifter.
2.	Churna / Nasya Manjan / Lepa Kwath Churna	200 sq. ft.	Grinder / Disintegrator / Pulveriser / Powder mixer / Sieves / Shifter.
3.	Pills / Vati / GutikaMatrica and tablets	100 sq. ft.	Ball mills, Mass mixer/Powder mixer, Granulator, drier, tablet compressing machine, pill / vati cutting machine, stainless steel trays / container for storage and sugar coating, polishing pan in case of sugar coated tablets, mechanized chatoo, (for mixing of guggulu) where required.
4.	Kupipakva / Ksara / Parpati / Lavana Bhasma Satva / Sindura Kapu / Uppa / Param / Qushta / Jawhar	150 sq. ft.	Bhatti, Karahi / Stainless steel vessels/Patila flask, Multani matti / Plaster of Paris, Copper rod, Earthen container, Gaj put bhatti, Muffle furnace (electrically operated) End/Edge Runner, Exhaust fan, Wooden, S.S. Spatula.

5.	Kajal	100 sq. ft.	Earthen lamps for collection of Kajal, Tripple roller mill, End runner, Sieves, S.S. Patila, Filling, packing and manufacturing room should be provided with Exhaust fan & Ultra violet lamps.
6.	Capsules	100 sq. ft.	Air Conditioner, De-humidifier, Hygrometer, Thermometer, Capsule filling machine and balance.
7.	Ointment/Marham Pasai	100 sq. ft.	Tube filling machine, Crimping machnie / Ointment mixer, End runner / Mill (Where required), S.S. storage container, S. S. patila.
8.	Pak/Avaleh / KhandModak/Lakayam	100 sq. ft.	Bhatti section fitted with exhaust fan and should be fly proof, Iron kadahi/ S.S. patila and S.S. storage container.
9.	Panak Syrup / PravahiKwath Manapaku	150 sq. ft.	Tinctum press, exhaust fan fitted and should be flyproof, Bhatti section, Bottle washing machine, Filter press / Gravity filter liquid filling machine, P.P. capping machine
10.	Asava/Aristha	200 sq. ft.	Same as mentioned above. Fermentation tanks containers and distillation plant where necessary, Filter press.
11.	Sura	100 sq. ft.	Same as mentioned above plus distillation plant and transfer pump.
12.	Ark/ Tinir	100 sq. ft.	Maceration tank, Distillation plant, Liquid filling tank with tap/Gravity Filter/Filter press, Visual Inspection box.
13.	Tail / Ghrit /Ney	100 sq. ft.	Bhatti, Kadahi/S.S. patila, S.S. storage containers, Filtration equipment, filling tank with tap/Liquid filling machine.

Contd...

14.	Asch yotan / Netra Malham Panir / Karnbindu / Nasabindu	100 sq. ft.	Hot air oven electrically heated with thermostatic control, kettle gas or electrically heated with suitable mixing arrangement collation mill or ointment mill, tube filling equipment.
15.	Each manufacturing unit will have a separate area for bhatti, furnace, boilers, puta, etc. This will have proper ventilation, removal of smoke, prevention of flies, insects, dust etc. The furnace section could have a tin roof.	200 sq. ft.	

(**Source:** Revised Draft GMP ASU drugs published by AYUSH)

B: List of Machinery, Equipment and Minimum Manufacturing Premises Required for the Manufacture of Various Categories of Unani System of Medicines as per Schedule T

Table 13.2

Sr. No.	Category of Medicine	Minimum Manufacturing space required	Machinery/Equipment Recommended
1200 sq. ft. covered area with separate cabins or partitions for each activity. If Ayurveda/Siddha, Medicines are also manufactured in same premises an additional area of 400 sq./ft. will be required.			
1.	ItrifalTiryaq/ Majoon/Laooq Jawarish Khamiras	100 sq. ft.	Grinder/Pulveriser, sieves, powder mixer (if required), S.S. Patilas, Bhatti and other accessories, Plant mixer for Khamiras.
2.	Araq	100 sq. ft.	Distillation plant (garembic) S.S. storage tank, boiling vessel, gravity filter, bottle filling machine, bottle washing machine, bottle drier.

Contd...

3.	Habb (Pills) and Tablets	100 sq. ft.	Ball mills, Mass mixer / Powder mixer, Granulator, drier, tablet compressing machine, pill / vati cutting machine, stainless steel, trays / container for storage and sugar coating, polishing pan in case of sugar coated tablets, mechanized chatoo, (for mixing of guggulu) where required.
4.	Sufoof (Powder)	200 sq. ft.	Grinder/Pulveriser, Sieves, Trays, Scoops, Powder mixer (where required),
5.	Raugha n (Oils) (Crushing and Boiling)	100 sq. ft.	Oil expeller, S.S. patilas, Oil filter bottle, Filling machine, Bottle drier, Bhatti.
6.	Shiyaf, Surma, Kajal	100 sq. ft.	End runner, Mixing S.S. vessel.
7.	Marham, Zimad (ointment)	100 sq. ft.	Kharal, Bhatti, End runner, Grinder , Pulviser, Tripple roller mill (if needed)
8.	Qurs (Tab)	100 sq. ft.	Grinder /Pulveriser, Sieves, Powder mixer (where needed), Granulator, Drier, Tablet compressing machine, Die punches trays, O.T. apparatus, Balance with weights, Scoops, Sugar coating pan, Polishing pan, Heater
9.	Kushta	100 sq. ft.	Bhatti, Kharal, SilBatta, Earthern pots.
10.	Murabba	100 sq. ft.	Aluminium vessels 50-100 kgs capacity Gendna, Bhatti.
11.	Capsule	100 sq. ft.	Pulveriser, Powder mixer (where needed), Capsule filling machine, Air conditioner, Dehumidifier, Balance with weights, Storage-containers, Glass.
12.	Sharbat & Jushanda	100 sq. ft.	Tinctum press, Exhaust fan fitted, Bhatti section, Bottle washing machine, Filter press, Gravity filter, Liquid filling tank with tap/liquid filling machine, Hot air oven electrically heated with thermostatic control, Kettle.

Contd...

13.	Qutoor-e-Chashm and Marham (Eye drops, Eye ointment)	100 sq. ft.	Hot air oven electrically heated with thermostatic control, kettle.
14.	Each manufacturing unit will have a separate area for Bhatti, furnaces, boilers, putta etc. This will have proper ventilation, removal of smoke, prevention of flies, insects, dust etc	200 sq. ft.	

(**Source:** Revised Draft GMP ASU drugs published by AYUSH)

Part C: As per schedule T of Drugs and Cosmetics Rules 1945 list of Equipment Recommended For In House Quality Control Section.

1. List of equipments required for Pharmacognosy section:

- Analytical balance of 220 gram capacity with sensitivity of 0.0001 gram
- Binocular research microscope
- Dissection and surgical Instruments
- Electric mantles
- Aluminium slide trays
- Essential glassware and other materials including reagents required
- Hot air oven
- Hot plate
- Micro-slide cabinet
- Micrometers - stage, ocular, linear and net ruled types
- Mixer Grinder
- Prism and mirror type camera lucida
- Refrigerator
- Sledge microtome
- Sieves
- Stereo zoom microscope
- Top-Pan balances of 1 kilogram capacity with sensitivity of 1.0 gram
- Water baths

2. **List of equipments required for chemistry section:**
   - Abbe refractometer
   - Alcohol determination apparatus
   - Analytical balance of 220 gram capacity with sensitivity of 0.0001 gram
   - Boiling point determination apparatus
   - Bulk density apparatus
   - Centrifuge machine
   - Clevenger apparatus for volatile oil determination
   - Essential glassware and other materials including reagents required
   - Conductivity meter
   - Refractometer
   - Polarimeter
   - Viscometer
   - Tablet disintegration apparatus
   - Moisture meter
   - Muffle furnace
   - Electronic balance
   - Magnetic stirrer
   - Hot Air oven
   - Refrigerator
   - Glass/Steel distillation apparatus
   - LPG Gas cylinders with burners
   - Water bath (Temperature controlled)
   - Heating mantles/ Hot plates
   - UV- Visible Spectrophotometer
   - TLC Apparatus with all accessories (Manual)
   - Paper chromatography apparatus with accessories
   - Sieve size 10 to120 with sieve shaker
   - Dehumidifier
   - pH meter
   - Limit test apparatus
3. **List of equipments required for Microbiology section:**
   - Autoclave
   - BOD incubator
   - Colony counter
   - Essential glassware and other materials including reagents required
   - High power microscope

- Hot air oven
- Laminar air flow
- Plain incubator
- Refrigerator
- Serological water bath
- Autoclave
- Colony counter

(**Source:** Revised draft GMP of Ayurveda, Siddha and Unani Drugs published by Ayush)

Part D: Specific Requirements for Manufacturing of Rasaushadhies or Rasamaraunthukul and Kushtajat (herb-mineral-metallic compound) of Ayurveda, Siddha and Unani Medicines as per schedule T of Drugs and Cosmetics Rules 1945

This section provides general and minimum technical requirements for quality assurance and control in manufacturing rasaushadhies or rasamaraunthukuland kushtajat. It includes guidelines for ASU formulations such as Bhasmas, satwa (of Metals and Minerals origin) Drutiparpam, karpu and kushta etc. An expert team including Rasashastra experts nominated by the Department of AYUSH, should inspect manufacturing unit before issue of Good Manufacturing Practices certificate for Rasaushadhies.

1. Manufacturing Process Areas:

For the Manufacturing of Bhasma and Kupipakawa and Rasaaushadhi preparations specific areas should be provided, which should be completely segregated from the production areas used for preparations of plants and animals by product based formulations. The details of areas required are as follows:

- Bhatti or Heating Devise Section for Bhasma and Rasaaushadhi: 100 sq. feet area with proper ventilation, exhaust and chimney is required for heating work. Tin shed can be used.
- 10 sq. feet are necessary for grinding, drying and processing section for Bhasma and Rasaaushadhi. Drying can be carried out in space covered with glass or other transparent material which allow entry of sunrays. The drying can be done in oven with a specific temperature.
- Rasaushadhis related store require 100 sq. ft. with specific size and dimensions suitable to the batch size and as per the conditions of Drugs and Cosmetics Act mentioned under Schedule I official books.

Heating materials such as coal, fire woods, cow dung cakes and other heating devices e.g. electrical heating, oil or gas fired furnace can be used. Properly baked and clean earthen pots of other crucibles and glass containers or appropriate design can be employed. The manufacturing areas should be designed to avoid accumulation of toxic fumes like SO_2, arsenic and mercury vapour etc. Proper ventilation and air exhaust flow mechanism should be there to prevent accumulation of fumes and vapours. Properly designed chimneys or ducts fitted with exhaust systems can be designed. The cleaning of equipment with suitable cleaning reagent is necessary to avoid heavy metal contamination and cross contamination.

Records of temperature should be maintained during the entire Bhasmikaran process, while employing different methods like classical puta, furnace using oil, gas or electricity. The pyrometer and pyrograph can be used to measure temperature. Only authorized personal can access these areas.

2. Quality Control:

[I] For In Process Quality Control following registers should be maintained for ready reference:

(a) Shodhan Register should include:

- Serial number
- Batch no. and size
- Date, time and duration
- Name of the raw-material with quality reference and quantity
- Quantity of shodhana dravya
- Book reference followed
- Methodology

(b) Bhavana and Putta Register should include:

- Serial Number
- Batch no. and Size
- Date, time and duration of process
- Material name and Quantity of starting materials
- Nirvapya dravya quantity
- Bhavana dravya quantity
- Date and Time of starting and completion of Bhavana or Mardana process and duration.
- Type and Number of Puttas
- Time and Date of completion of Puttas
- Colour and texture of the products or standards
- In-process tests followed (Bhasma Pariksha and any other tests)
- Temperature required record of attainment of that temperature.

(c) Grinding Records Register should include: (Finished Products/Intermediate Procedure)

- Serial number
- Batch no. and Size
- Date, time and duration
- Material Name and Quantity

- Equipment used (SS/granite)
- Duration of grinding
- Repeat the grinding if required (number of repetition)

(d) Packing details should include:

- Name of Rasaushadhi
- Type of Dosage Form (e.g. Powder, Pill tablet etc.)
- Quantity of Rasaushadhis in each unit.

[II] Product Quality Control

The starting material - metals and minerals used should be of pharmacopoeial standards to assure desired quality of Rasaushadhi. There should be specific in-house standards to assure uniform quality of products. Various quality control tests such as colour, taste, Varitaratwa, Rekhapurnatwa, Laghutva, Nirudhumatwa, Dntagree, kachakacha, Niruttha, Apunarbhava and Nischandratwa etc. are carried out as per official pharmacopoeia or schedule books. The Particle size of products can be calculated using particle size analyser, physio-chemical properties should be checked with proper analytical instruments. The disintegration time of pills-vati and tablets should also be recorded by disintegration apparatus.

3. Product Recalls:

The name, address of the manufacturing unit or email or telephone number for reporting of any adverse drug reaction by physicians or patients should be indicated in Literature inserted inside the products package. The product should be recalled from market if Adverse Drug Reaction is reported.

Standard operating procedures (SOP) should be followed for storage of recalled Rasaushadhies in a secure segregated area, with specific requirements.

4. Medical Examination of the Employees:

Employees should be medically examined periodically at least once a year for any adverse effect of the drug manufacturing process. The necessary investigations are carried out to check effects on vital organs. During Good Manufacturing Practices inspections, the reports of this examination should be made available.

5. Self-Inspection:

The release of Rasaushadhis should be under the control of atrained person. Also personnel dealing with the production and quality assurance of Rasaushadhis should have undergone specific training. He should have degree in Ayurveda / Siddha / Unani medicine or B. Pharma degree holder.

6. Dosage form of Rasaushadhis:

The dosage forms of Rasaushadhis are prepared using suitable permissible fillers or binding agents mentioned under the Ayurvedic Pharmacopoeia of India or Indian Pharmacopoeia and updated from time to time. The label of medicine should indicate ingredients used along with fillers. The crystalline product may be grinded before packing. The dosage forms should be packed in such way that they are ready for use by the consumer. Grinding and weighting of individual dose of potentially poisonous products should be avoided to reduce chances of adverse drug reaction. The label of hospital bulk pack should clearly indicate 'Hopital Pack'.

7. Area specification/requirement for an applicant companies only to have GMP of Rasaushadhies or Rasamaraunthukul and Kushtajat (Herbo-mineral-metallic compounds) of Ayurveda, Siddha and Unani Medicines:

Table 13.3

Sr. No.	Category of Medicine/ Manufacturing area	Minimum Manufacturing space required (1500 sq. ft.)	Machinery equipment recommended
1.	Pisti/ Grinding area for Bhasma, Phisti, Kushtajat.	100 sq. ft.	Kharal/mechanized/motorized, End runner/Ball-Mill Sieves/Shifter
2.	Powdering area for raw drugs used in Rasaushadhies (Herbo-metallic formulations)	200 sq. ft.	Grinder/Disintegrator/Pulveriser/ Powder mixer/Sieves/Shifter
3.	Pills/Vati/Gutika Matrica and Tablets/Habb making area.	100 sq. ft.	Ball mill, Mass mixer/Powder mixer, Granulator drier, Tablet compressing machine, Pill/vati cutting machine, Stainless steel trays/container for storage and storage and sugar coating, Polishing pan in case of sugar coated tablets, Mechanized chattoo (for mixing of guggulu) where required.
4.	Kupipakva / Ksara / Parpati / LavanaBhasmaSatva / SinduraKarpu / UppuParam / Qushta / Jawhar	150 sq. ft.	Bhatti, Karahi/Stainless steel vessels/Patila flask, Multani matti, Palster of Paris, Copper rod, Earthen container, Gaj Put Bhatti, Muffle furnace (electrically operated) End/ Edge runner, Exhaust fan, Wooden, S.S. sapatula.

Contd...

5.	Receiving and storing raw material	200 sq. ft.	
6.	Quality control section	150 sq. ft.	
7.	Quarantine/Observation	50 sq. ft.	
8.	Finished goods store	150 sq. ft.	
9.	Rejected good store	50 sq. ft.	
10.	Bhatti-Putta area	200 sq. ft.	
11.	Area for water and washing etc.	50 sq. ft.	
12.	Office	100 sq. ft.	
	Total	**1500 sq. ft.**	

(**Source:** Revised Draft GMP ASU drugs published by AYUSH)

QUESTIONS

1. What are ASU drugs?
2. What are GMPs? State its objectives and significance.
3. Write an elaborative note on Good manufacturing practices followed for ASU drugs.
4. Describe different components of GMPs.
5. Discuss in detail about Infrastructural requirements, working space, storage area, machinery and equipments, health and hygiene, documentation and records as per GMPs.
6. How to maintain SOP as per GMP guidelines of ASU drugs?
7. Give specific requirements for manufacturing of rasaushadhies or Rasamaraunthukul and Kushtajat (herb-mineral-metallic compound) of ASU medicines.
8. What is site master file?

❖❖❖

INDEX

❖❖❖

REFERENCES

- Wagner L, Ramos B *et al.* Selecting medicinal plants for development of phytomedicine and use in primary health care, Bioactive Compounds in Phytomedicine, Prof. Iraj Rasooli (Ed.), 2012 In Tech, Available at: http://www.intechopen.com/books/bioactive-compounds-in-phytomedicine/selecting medicinal-plants-for-development-of-phytomedicine-and-use-in-primary-health-care
- Directive 2004/24/Ec of the European Parliament and of the Council; Official Journal of the European Union, L136-85-L136-90, 2004.
- Mahanom H J, Azizah A, Dzulkifly M. Effect of different drying methods on concentrations of several phytochemicals in herbal preparation of 8 medicinal plants leaves. Malays J Nutr. 1999; 5(1):47-54.
- Abascal K, Ganora L, Yarnell E. The effect of freeze-drying and its implications for botanical medicine: a review. Phytother Res. 2005; 19(8):655-60.
- Namjoyan F, Hejazi H, Ramezani Z. Evaluation of drying process on the composition of black pepper ethanolic extract by High Performance Liquid Chromatography with diode array detector Jundishapur. J Nat Pharm Prod. 2012; 7(4): 163–167.
- Molins R. A. Food irradiation: principles and applications, 2001. John Wiley & Sons, Inc.
- D. Rigby, D. Caceres. Organic farming and the sustainability of agricultural systems, Agricultural Systems 2001; 68 (1): 21-40.
- WHO guidelines on good agricultural and collection practices (GACP) for medicinal plants, World Health Organization Geneva 2003. Available at: https://apps.who.int/medicinedocs/en/d/Js4928e/
- Hanem Pathy Khater. Prospects of botanical pesticides in insect pest management, Pharmacologia 2012; 3(12): 641-656.
- Dar SA, Khan ZH, Khan AA *et al.* Biopesticides–Its prospects and limitations: an overview, Perspectives in animal ecology and reproduction 2011; 296-314.
- Rizvi PQ, Ahmad SK, Choudhury RA *et al.* Biopesticides in ecologically-based integrated pest management, Integrated Pest Management, Principles and practice 2012; CABI International, UK, 133-161.
- Tripathi AK, Upadhyay S, Bhuiyan M *et al.* A review on prospects of essential oils as biopesticides in insect-pest management, Journal of Pharmacognosy and Phytotherapy 2009; 1(5): 52-63.
- Saha D, Paul S, S. Hosen M Z, Emran T B *et al.* (2012) Role of Ayurvedic formulation in digestion, International Research Journal of Pharmacy and Pharmacology, 2012;2(8): 187-192.
- Ayurvedic formulary of India, Ministry of AYUSH, Government of India. Available at: http://ayush.gov.in/sites/default/files/AFI-Part-I%20for%20website%2004-01-2018.pdf
- Kokate CK, Purohit AP, Ghokhale SB. (2012) Pharmacognosy, 47th edition, Nirali Prakashan 2012
- Evans WC. Trease and Evans Pharmacognosy, 14th edition, W.B. Sounders 2012.
- Heinrich M, Barnes J, Gibbons S *et al.* Fundamentals of pharmacognosy and phytotherapy, 1st edition Chruchill Livingstone 2004.
- Rai M, Carpinella MC. Naturally occurring bioactive compounds, Advances in phytommedicine series 1st edition 2006; 3, Elsevier.
- Agarwal S.S., Paridhavi M. Herbal drug technology, 2nd edition, University press 2012
- Biren Shah, A. K. Seth. Textbook of pharmacognosy and Phytochemistry, 2nd edition, Elsevier. 2014
- Narayanan P. Intellectual property law, 3rd edition, Eastern Law house. 2005.

- Khan R A, Elhassan G O, Qureshi K A. Nutraceuticals: In the treatment & prevention of diseases –an overview. The Pharma Innovation Journal 2014; 3(10): 47-50
- Singh J, Sinha S. classification, regulatory acts and applications of nutraceuticals for health. IJPBS 2012; 2(1) 177-187.
- Bhowmik D, Gopinath H, Pragati Kumar B *et al.* Nutraceutical–A Bright Scope and Opportunity of Indian Healthcare Market; The Pharma Innovation 2013; 1 (11): 29-41.
- Shinde N, Bangar B, Deshmukh S, Kumbhar P. Nutraceuticals: A Review on current status; Research J. Pharm. and Tech 2014; 7(1): 110-113.
- Report on 'Indian Nutraceuticals Industry Current Scenario & Future Trends' by The Associated Chambers of Commerce and Industry of India, 2017.
- Chintale A G,Kadam V S, Sakhare R S *et al.* Role of nutraceuticals in various diseases: A comprehensive Review. International Journal of Research in Pharmacy and Chemistry; 2013; 3(2):290-99.
- Report Published for the Ministry of Food Processing Industries (MoFPI) by Ernst & Young LLP (EY) and Confederation of Indian Industry (CII), on Health Supplements and Nutraceuticals Emerging High Growth Sector in India, 2017.
- Presentation available on https://www.slideshare.net/ArtiRThakkar/nutraceuticals-march-april-2018-93319066)
- Das L, Bhaumik E, Raychaudhuri U *et al.* Role of nutraceuticals in human health, J Food Sci Technol. 2012; 49(2): 173–183.
- Kumar H, Rajpoot A K. Nutraceuticals: Today's Need For Health Care; European Journal of Pharmaceutical And Medical Research, 2018;5(4):255-262
- Sharma R, Kaur A *et al.* Role of nutraceuticals in health care: A review; International Journal of Green Pharmacy (Suppl) 2017; 11 (3);385-394.
- Boik J. Natural Compounds in Cancer Therapy Promising non toxic antitumor agents from plants and other natural sources, 1st edition, Oregon Medical Press, Minnesota USA.
- Ranzato E, Martinotti S *et al.* Role of neutraceuticals in cancer Therapy. Journal of food research 2014;3 (4): 18-25
- Tripathi Y B., Tripathi P, Arjmandi B H., Nutraceuticals and Cancer Management, Frontiers in Bioscience 2005; 10: 1607-1618.
- Chikwere P, Functional foods and nutraceuticals, wonders in cancer risks - a review, WSN 2017;64: 18-33
- Choudhary M, Tomer V. review on Cardioprotective Effect of Nutraceuticals: The Emerging Evidences, Proc Indian Natn Sci Acad Spl. Issue Part B 2013; 79 (4): 985-996
- Kumar A, Zandi P. Plant Nutraceuticals for Cardiovascular Diseases with Special Emphasis to the Medicinal Herb Fenugreek (TrigonellaFoenum-Graecum L.), Editors: S. K. Basu & G. Agoramoorthy 2014; 4 (3): 189
- Nikhra V. Review Article on Nutraceuticals for Improving Cardiovascular Health and Prognosis in Cardiovascular Disease. J Nutri Diet Probiotics 2018; 1(2): 180009.
- Eman M. Alissa, Ferns G A. Review Article on Functional Foods and Nutraceuticals in the Primary Prevention of Cardiovascular Diseases. Journal of Nutrition and Metabolism 2012: 1-16.
- Nimesh S, Ashwlayan VD. Nutraceuticals in the management of diabetes mellitus. Pharm Pharmacol Int J. 2018; 6(2):114–120.
- Dav G, Santilli F, Patrono C. review Nutraceuticals in Diabetes and Metabolic Syndrome; Cardiovascular Therapeutics 2010; 28: 216-226.
- Derosa G, Limas C P, Macías P C *et al.* Dietary and nutraceutical approach to type 2 diabetes. Arch Med Sci 2014; 10(2): 336-344.

- Kaur G, Mukundan S, Wani V *et al.* Review: Nutraceuticals in the Management and Prevention of Metabolic Syndrome. Austin J Pharmacol Ther 2015; 3(1): 1063.
- Singh A, Reddy K R C. Review on Importance of Nutraceuticals in the Management of Diabetes Mellitus. International Journal of Pharmaceutical & Biological Archives 2015; 6(4): 1-8.
- Kochhar A Pathak N. Nutraceutical Based Approach to Combat Diabetes Mellitus. Curre Res Diabetes & Obes J. 2018; 8(2): 555739.
- Duggan C, Gannon J, Walker W A. Protective nutrients and functional foods for the gastrointestinal tract, The American Journal of Clinical Nutrition2002; 75(5):789-808.
- Mijan M A, Lim BO. Diets, functional foods, and nutraceuticals as alternative therapies for inflammatory bowel disease: Present status and future trends; World J Gastroenterol 2018; 24(25): 2673-2685.
- Larussa T, Imeneo M, Luzza F. Potential role of nutraceutical compounds in inflammatory bowel disease;World J Gastroenterol; 2017; 23(14): 2483-2492.
- Bora K, Sharma A. Phytochemical and pharmacological potential of Medicago sativa: A review Journal Pharmaceutical Biology, 2011; 49(2): 211-220.
- Singh R, Chahal K, Cichorium intybus L: A review on phytochemistry and pharmacology, International Journal of Chemical Studies 2018; 6(3): 1272-1280.
- Ali Esmail Al-Snafi, Medical importance of Cichorium intybus, A review, IOSR Journal Of Pharmacy, 2016; 6 (3): 41-56.
- Ashraf K, Sultan S, Shah S A. Phychemistry, phytochemical, pharmacological and molecular Study of *Zingiber Officinale* Roscoe: A Review; Int J Pharm Pharm Sci 2017; 9(11): 8-16.
- Kumar G, Karthik L, Bhaskara Rao K V. A Review on Pharmacological and Phytochemical Properties of Zingiber officinale Roscoe (Zingiberaceae). Journal of Pharmacy Research 2011;4(9):2963-2966
- Dhanik J, Arya N, Vivekanand. A Review on Zingiber officinale. Journal of Pharmacognosy and Phytochemistry 2017; 6(3): 174-184
- Toppo FA, Akhand R, Pathak A K. Pharmacological Actions and Potential Uses of Trigonella Foenum-Graecum: A Review; Asian Journal of Pharmaceutical and Clinical Research 2009;2 (4): 29-38
- Gupta S, Gupta P, Patsariya S; Phytochemical and Pharmacological review on Fenugreek (Trigonella foenum-graecum); Current Research in Pharmaceutical Sciences 2012; 01: 11-13
- Chaudhary S, Shah Chaudhary P, Chikara S K *et al.* Review on Fenugreek (Trigonella foenum-graecum L.) and its Important Secondary Metabolite Diosgenin; Not Bot Horti Agrobo 2018; 46(1):22-31.
- Yadav R, kaushik R. A Study Of Phytochemical Constituents and Pharmacological Actions of Trigonella Foenum-Graecum: A Review. International Journal of Pharmacy and Technology 2011; 3(2):1022-1028
- Banu D, Tabassum H, Ahmad A *et al.* The medicinal significance of bioactive compound of Trigonella foenum-graecum LA review. Int.J.Res. Ayurveda.pharm 2016;7(4):84-91
- Tyagi S, Patel C J, Dadarwal P *et al.* Importance (*Allium Sativum*): An exhaustive Review; Journal of Drug Discovery and Therapeutics2013;1(4):23-27
- Alam M K, Hoq M O, Uddin M S. Medicinal plant *Allium sativum* A Review; Journal of Medicinal Plants Studies 2016; 4(6): 72-79
- Liyanage D A M, Arawwawala, Horadugoda G.S.P. Hewageegana. Health benefits and traditional uses of honey: A review; Journal of Apitherapy; 2017; 2(1):9-14.
- Saranraj P, Sivasakthi S, Feliciano G D. Pharmacology of Honey: A Review; Advances in Biological Research 2016;10 (4): 271-289.
- Ahmad RS, Hussain MB, Saeed F *et al.* Phytochemistry, metabolism, and ethnomedical scenario of honey: A concurrent review; International Journal of Food Properties 2017; 20(1): 254-269

- Hasan M. R, Md. Islam N, Islam M R. Phytochemistry, pharmacological activities and traditional uses of Emblica officinalis: A review; International Current Pharmaceutical Journal, 2016; 5(2): 14-21.
- Patel SS, Goyal R K. Emblica officinalis Geart A Comprehensive Review on Phytochemistry, Pharmacology and Ethnomedicinal Uses; Research Journal of Medicinal Plants; 2012; 6 (1): 6-16.
- Leung KW, Wong AS. Pharmacology of ginsenosides: a literature review; Chin Med 2010; 5; 20: 1-7
- Lakshmi T, Roy A Geetha RV.Panax Ginseng A Universal Panacea In The Herbal Medicine With Diverse Pharmacological Spectrum,A Review; Asian Journal of Pharmaceutical and Clinical Research 2011; 4(1): 14-18
- Kim K H, Dahae L, Lee HL *et al.* Beneficial effects of Panax ginseng for the treatment and prevention of neurodegenerative diseases: past findings and future directions; J Ginseng Res. 2018; 42(3): 239–247.
- Jain R, Kachhwaha S, Kothari SL. Phytochemistry, pharmacology, and biotechnology of Withania somnifera and Withania coagulans: A review; Journal of Medicinal Plants Research 2012; 6(41): 5388-5399
- Qamar U, Samiulla, Singh LVK, Jamil SS. Phytochemical and Pharmacological Profile of Withania somnifera Dunal: A Review Journal of Applied Pharmaceutical Science 2012; 02 (01): 170-175
- Saiyed A, Jahan N, Majeedi S F *et al.* Medicinal properties, phytochemistry and pharmacology of Withania somnifera: an important drug of Unani Medicine Journal of Scientific and Innovative Research 2016; 5(4): 156-160
- Farag MR, Alagawany M, El-Hack MEA, *et al.* Review Article Nutritional and Healthical Aspects of Spirulina (Arthrospira) for Poultry, Animals and Human; International Journal of Pharmacology 2015;12;36-51
- Nuhu AA, Review Article Spirulina (Arthrospira): An Important Source of Nutritional and Medicinal Compounds; Journal of Marine Biology;2013:1-8, www.slideshare.com
- Shukla AK, Bigoniya P. Herbal, Drug and Food Interaction. International
- Journal of Traditional and Complementary Medicine 2016; 1(2): 0024- 0032.
- Mukherjee P K. Quality Control of Herbal Drugs: An Approach to Evaluation of Botanicals, published by Business Horizons, New Delhi 2002.
- Amoolya S, Shibina K A, Hameed J. Pharmacological Review on the all Cure Plant - Gingko biloba. Int. J. Pharm. Sci. Rev. Res 2017; 43(1): 243-247.
- Damanhouri ZA, Ahmad A. A Review on Therapeutic Potential of *Piper nigrum* L. (Black Pepper): The King of Spices. Med Aromat Plants 2014;3: 161.
- Joshi D R, Shrestha A C, Adhikari N. International Journal of Pharmaceutical Sciences and Research 2018; 9(10): 4089-4101.
- Pasi A. Herb-drug interaction: an overview. International journal of Pharmaceutical sciences and research 2013; 8**:** 3770-3774
- http://shodhganga.inflibnet.ac.in, https://www.webmd.com
- Bijauliya RK, Alok S, Kumar M *et al.* A Comprehensive Review on Herbal Cosmetics. International Journal of Pharmaceutical Sciences and Research 2017;8(12):4930-4949
- Kumar S, Swarankar V, Sharma S, Baldi A; Herbal Cosmetics: Used for Skin and Hair. Inventi Rapid: Cosmeceuticals,2012; (4): 1-7.
- Davinder K, Gajendra R, Om P *et al.* Herbal cosmetics: An overview; International Journal of Advanced Scientific Research 2016;1(4): 36-41
- Talal A, Feda M N. Review Article Plants Used in Cosmetics. Phytother. Res 2003; 17: 987–1000.
- Pullar J M, Carr AC, Vissers MCM. The Roles of Vitamin C in Skin Health, Nutrients. 2017; 9(8): 866.

- Anitha D, Reddy K Y, Venkatesh P *et al.* A review - herbal sunscreen agents on skin protection. European Journal of Pharmaceutical And Medical Research 2016;3(11): 308-313
- Korac R R, Khambholja KM. Potential of herbs in skin protection from ultraviolet radiation. Pharmacogn Rev 2011; 5(10): 164–173.
- Gupta A, Malviya R, Singh T, Sharma P. Indian Medicinal Plants Used in Hair Care Cosmetics: A Short Review. Phcog.J. 2010; 2(10):362-64.
- Shahi Z, Mehrizi M K, Hadizadeh M. A Review of the Natural Resources Used to Hair Color and Hair Care Products. J. Pharm. Sci. & Res. 2017; 9(7): 1026-1030.
- Anushri M, Yashoda R, Puranik MP. Review on Herbs: A Good Alternatives to Current Treatments for Oral Health Problems. International Journal of Advanced Health Sciences 2015; 1(12): 26-32.
- Digra R, Rao NC, Gupta N *et al.* Review on Ayurvedic herbs in dentistry: learn how to manage oral health and tooth decay with these modest herbs? Journal of orofacial research 2014;4(1):41-45.
- Buggapati L. Herbs in Dentistry; International Journal of Pharmaceutical Science Invention 2016; 5(6): 7-12.
- Bhushan SK, Chauhan G, Nagpal D *et al.* Review on Treatment of Periodontal Disease – A Herbal Approach. Int. J. Pharm. Sci. Rev. Res. 2015; 33(2): 126-136
- Ahmed J, Shenoy N, Binnal A *et al.* Herbal oral care: an old concept or a new model? International Journal of Research in Medical Sciences 2014; 2 (3) : 818-821
- Charantimath S, Oswal R. Herbal Therapy in Dentistry: A Review Innovative Journal of Medical And Health Science 2011; 1: 1 – 4.
- Ikoni JO, Elijah IN, Jennifer DA. Advances in Natural Polymers as Pharmaceutical Excipients Pharm Anal Acta 2012; 3: 146.
- Verma P, Gupta S, Kushwah A *et al.* Remarkable Contribution of Natural Excipients in Finished Pharmaceutical Products (FPPs). Int. J. Pharm. Sci. Rev. Res. 2018; 52(1): 7-14.
- Alam MT, Parvez N, SharmaP. FDA-Approved Natural Polymers for Fast Dissolving Tablets. Journal of Pharmaceutics 2014; 1-6
- Singh VK, Chaudhary AK. Ayurvedic Natural Excipients: An Advance Option For Modern Medicaments. International Journal of Pharmaceutical Sciences And Research 2016; 7(12): 4743-4755
- Chavhan SA, Shinde SA, Sapkal SB *et al.* Herbal Excipients in Novel Drug Delivery Systems. Int J Pharmacognosy 2017; 4(7): 208-16.
- Singh P, Tarique M, Arshiya S *et al.* A review on Herbal Excipients and their pharmaceutical applications. Scholars Academic Journal of Pharmacy 2016; 5(3): 53-57
- Hand book of pharmaceutical excipients, 6th Ed, Edited by-Raymond Crowe Paul J Sheskey and Marian E Quinn, Publisher-Pharmaceutical Press.
- Karmakar K. Application of Natural Gum as a binder in Modern Drug Delivery. J Anal Pharm Res 2016; 3(4): 00061
- Kokate C. K., Gokhale S.B., Purohit A.P. Textbook of Pharmacognosy2008, Nirali Prakashan, Pune.
- Doris K, Kwabena K. Dosage Forms of Herbal Medicinal Products and Their Stability Considerations-An Overview. Journal of Critical Reviews 2017; 4 (4): 1-8.
- SwainP, Nayak D P. Design, Development & Evaluation of a Poly herbal Syrup from some herbs used as Energy booster. International Journal of Ayurvedic Medicine 2013: 4(4): 374-378.
- Brahmbhatt T, Shah B, PatelU *et al.* Development and Evaluation of Various Oral Herbal Formulations for Anti-Asthmatic Plant Extract. IJPRBS 2012; 1 (3): 317-327.
- Kaushik A, Chauhan V, Sudha. Formulation and Evaluation of Herbal Cough Syrup. European Journal of Pharmaceutical and Medical Research 2016; 3(5): 517-522.

- Joseph A. Kare P, Nikam PH *et al.* Phytosome: A Novel Revolution in Herbal Drugs;International Journal of Research In Pharmacy and Chemistry 2012; 2(2): 299-310.
- Sharma P, Verma S, Misri P. Global Need for Novel Herbal Drug Formulations; International Journal of Pharmacognosy and Phytochemical Research 2016; 8(9): 1535-1544
- Mishra D, Panda G, Kumar P *et al.* Novel Drug Delivery System for Herbal Formulation In Cancer Treatment. World Journal of Pharmaceutical Research 2017; 6(15):341-353.
- Sarangi M K, Padhi S. Novel herbal drug delivery system: An overview; Arch Med Health Sci 2018; 6: 171-9
- WHO guidelines on good herbal processing practices for herbal medicines; WHO technical report series 1010; 2018.
- World Health Organization guidelines, Available at: http://apps.who.int/ medicinedocs/index/assoc/s14878e/s14878e.pdf
- WHO Expert Committee on specifications for pharmaceutical preparations. Thirty-fourth report. Geneva, World Health Organization, 1996:178–184 (WHO Technical Report Series, No. 863).
- Guideline on stability testing: stability of existing active substances and related finished products (CPMP/QWP/122/02, rev 1 corr).
- Kruse S O et. al. Stability testing of herbal medicinal products, Innovations in Pharmaceutical Technology 2010; 33: 64-68.
- Guideline on Quality of Herbal Medicinal Products/ Traditional Herbal Medicinal Products (CPMP/QWP/2819/00, rev 1).
- World Health Organization guidelines, Available at: http://apps.who.int/medicinedocs/pdf/s5516e/s5516e.pdf
- World Health Organization guidelines, Available at: https://apps.who.int/medicinedocs/en/d/Jh1813e/3.3.3.html
- Source: http://www.ipindia.nic.in/history-of-indian-patent-system.htm
- Thomas Efferth *et al.* Biopiracy of natural products and good bioprospecting practice, Phytomedicine 2016; 23(2): 166-173.
- http://www.ecapproject.org/fileadmin/ecapII/pdf/en/information/thailand/patent_act_2522.pdf
- Traditional Knowledge Digital Library, Government of India. Available at: http://www.tkdl.res.in
- Intellectual property India, Government of India. Available at: http://ipindia.nic.in
- http://www.who.int/medicines/areas/policy/doha_declaration/en/index.html
- Sahai S. India's plant variety protection and farmers right act 2001; Special section: Transgenic crops. Current Science 2003; 84(3): 407-412.
- http://www.patentlawportal.com/information/patentbasics/what-is-patent-law.html
- http://www.patentlawportal.com/information/patentbasics/what-types-of-patents-are-available.html
- Kumar A. Towards patentability of essentially biological processes, Journal of Intellectual Property Rights 2008; (13): 129-138.
- http://www.patentoffice.nic.in/ipr/gi/Girule~1.PDF
- E. Isaac *et al.* Bioprospecting or biopiracy? Intellectual property and traditional knowledge in biotechnology innovation. The Journal of World Intellectual Property (2005), 7, 35-52.
- Delgado G C. Biopiracy: Intellectual property as the basis for biotechnological development: the case of Mexico International Journal of Politics, Culture and Society 2002; 16 (2):299.
- http://www.scidev.net/en/agriculture-and-environment/biodiversity/opinions/holes-in-indian-laws-promote- biopiracy.html 1 SciDev.Net

- Navdanya Cultivating Diversity. Research Foundation for Science, Technology and Natural Resource Policy 1993, Delhi, India.
- AchimLerch (1998) Property Rights and Biodiversity, European Journal of Law and Economics 6, 285-304.
- Robinson D. Confronting biopiracy challenges, cases and international debates 1st ed, London, 2010; eBook ISBN 9781849774710.
- Thomas E *et al.* Biopiracy of natural products and good bio prospecting practice, Phytomedicine 2016; 23(2): 166-173.
- Genevieve Bourdy *et al.* Quassia "biopiracy" case and the Nagoya Protocol: A researcher's perspective Journal of Ethanopharmacology 2017; 206: 290-297.
- World Health Organization guidelines, Available at: http://apps.who.int/ medicinedocs/en/d/Jwhozip57e/ 4.5.html
- Okan A *et al.* Traditional Medicine and Intellectual Property Right., J. Fac. Pharm, Ankara. 2007; 36 (2): 135-151.
- Craig D. Biological Resources, Intellectual Property Rights and International Human Rights: Impacts on Indigenous and Local Communities. In: Peter W., Onwuekwe C.B. (eds) Accessing and Sharing the Benefits of the Genomics Revolution. The International Library of Environmental, Agricultural and Food Ethics, 2007; 11. Springer, Dordrecht.
- Phadtare S, Shinde V, Mahadik K. Regulatory issues and natural product, Pharmatutor-ART 2008-1697.
- Shinde V M, Shinde K V, Potdar M, Mahadik K R. Application of quality control principles to herbal drugs, International Journal of Phytomedicine 2009; 1: 4-8.
- Shinde V M, Shinde K V. Issues related to pharmacognosy, Pharmacognosy Reviews 2008; 2(3):1-5.
- Drug and Cosmetic Act 1940, Available at: https://cdsco.gov.in/opencms/ opencms/en/Acts-Rules/
- Sahoo N, Manchikanti P, Dey S H. Herbal drug patenting in India: IP potential. Journal of Ethnopharmacology, 2011; 137(1): 289-297.
- Sahoo N, Manchikanti P. Herbal Drug Regulation and Commercialization: An Indian Industry Perspective. The Journal of Alternative and Complementary Medicine 2013; 19 (12): 957-963.
- Tandon N, Yadav SS. Contributions of Indian Council of Medical Research (ICMR) in the area of Medicinal plants/Traditional medicine. Journal of Ethnopharmacology 2017; 197; 39-45.
- Vaidya A D B, Thomas P A, Devasagayam. Current status of herbal drug in India: an overview. Journal of Clinical Biochemistry and Nutrition 2007; 41: 1-11.
- Drug and Cosmetic Act 1940, Available at: https://cdsco.gov.in/opencms/opencms/ en/Acts-Rules/
- World Intellectual Property Organization, Available at: https://www.wipo.int/portal /en/index.html
- Arushi K, Arora R. Good Manufacturing Practices: A pathway towards quality ASU medicines. Int J Ayu Pharm Chem 2015; 2 (1): 2-15.
- Revised Draft Gmp of Ayurveda, Siddha And Unani Drugs published by AYUSH 2014. Available on http://ayush.gov.in
- The drugs and cosmetics act and rules published by government of India ministry of health and family welfare. Available on https://upload.indiacode.nic.in, https://pharmafranchisehelp.com
- http://www.slideshare.net/priynkagoswami/herbal excipients.

❖❖❖

SECOND YEAR B. PHARM (SEMESTER-IV) PCI

- **Pharmaceutical Organic Chemistry - III:** Dr. K.G. Bothra.
- **Pharmacognosy and Phytochemistry - I:** S.B. Gokhale, Dr. C.K. Kokate, Dr. A.U. Tatiya, Dr. M.G. Kalaskar.
- **Medicinal Chemistry - I:** Dr. K.G. Bothara.
- **Medicinal Chemistry - I:** Dr. Sanjay G. Walode, Dr. Rakesh Somani, Dr. Chandan R.S.
- **Physical Pharmaceutics - II:** Dr. Ashok A. Hajare.
- **Pharmacology - I:** Dr. Sachin V. Tembhurne, Dr. Rao V.S. Vadlamudi.
- **Pharmacology - I:** Dr. K.G. Bothra, K.K. Bothara.
- **Pharmacology - I:** Dr. C.M. Jangume, Shivakumar S. Ladde, R.D. Wadulkar, Dr. Nitin B. Ghiware.
- **Pharmaceutical Organic Chemistry - III:** Dr. Abhishek Tiwari, Dr. Neeaj Upmanyu, Anup Kumar Chakrabarty.
- **Pharmacognosy & Phytochemistry - I:** Dr. Padmini Shukla, Dr. Shashi Alok, Dr. Prabodh Shukla.
- **Medicinal Chemistry - I:** Dr. Prashant Gahtori, Dr. Abhishek Tiwari, Dr. Archana Gahtori.
- **Pharmacology - I:** Dr. Mahesh Prasad, Dr. Rupesh Gautam, Dr. Kalpesh Gaur, Dr. Mandeep Arora.
- **Pharmaceutical Organic Chemistry - III Simplified:** Dr. K.S. Jain, Dr. P.B. Miniyar.
- **Pharmacognosy and Phytochemistry - I:** Dr. Kuntal Das.
- **Medicinal Chemistry - I:** Dr. Chandrashekhar Narajji, Vibha Chandan Patil.
- **Physical Pharmaceutics - II:** Akshay Shashikant Patil, Dr. Md. Rageeb Md. Usman, Dr. Shashikant D. Barhate, Basawarai Bendegumbli.
- **Pharmacology - I:** Dr. S.B. Bhise, M.S. Bhise, Sowmya B.A.
- **A Practical Book of Pharmacognosy and Phytochemistry - I:** S.B. Gokhale, M.G. Kalaskar, Yogesh Kulkarni.
- **Experimental Medicinal Chemistry - I:** Dr. Rakesh Somani, Dr. Sanjay G. Walode.
- **A Practical Book of Physical Pharmaceutics - II:** Dr. Ashok A. Hajare.
- **A Practical Book of Pharmacognosy & Phytochemistry - I:** Dr. Versha Tiwari, Dr. Shamim Ahmad.
- **A Practical Book of Medicinal Chemistry (Combined Book Sem. IV & VI):** Dr. Abhishek Tiwari, Dr. Rajeev Kumar.
- **A Practical Book of Pharmacology - I:** Dr. Mandeep Kumar Arora.
- **A Practical Books of Physical Pharmaceutics - II (Combined book Sem. III & IV):** Sudip Das, Dr. Shubhrajit Mantry, Ravi Shankar.
- **Experimental Pharmacology - I:** Ghanshyam Panigrahi, Arjun Patra.
- **A Practical Book of Physical Pharmaceutics - II:** Tanvir Y. Shaikh, Dr. Md. Rageeb Md. Usman, Dr. Bharat V.Jain, Basawaraj Bendegumble.

www.ingramcontent.com/pod-product-compliance
Ingram Content Group UK Ltd.
Pitfield, Milton Keynes, MK11 3LW, UK
UKHW051318160826
14477UKWH00027B/688

9 789389 686371